"A landmark event, which will change the course of obstetric care by giving parents the information they need to make the decisions that are best for their own families. Comprehensive, highly readable, sensitive. . .should be read by everyone who cares about someone."

—Marian Tompson
Director, Alternative Birth Crisis Coalition,
American Academy of Medicine

"Clearly the most important book on childbirth available today, Silent Knife *should be read by everyone connected with childbirth, consumers* and *professionals. No other book on the market today offers the complete help to cesarean prevention, including VBAC information and support. . .one of those few books that has the power to change a person's life. In the tradition of* Childbirth without Fear *by Grantley Dick-Read and* Immaculate Deception *by Suzanne Arms, Silent Knife will, I predict, spearhead a dramatic change in American obstetrical practices."*

e *Clegg,*
vareness

"This powerful, thoroug̲   ̲nt step in helping all mothers ̲   ̲.....̲..̲ ̲...̲. ̲to ̲lose ̲confidence in their doctors—a necessary prelude to conquering the doctor-produced epidemic of Cesarean sections."

—Robert S. Mendelsohn, M.D.
Author, Confessions of a Medical Heretic

"Silent Knife *marks the end of an era when a previous Cesarean mandates a woman's submission to surgical intrusion in her future childbearing. It is a book to heal the hearts and minds of women who have suffered alienation in childbirth, and it will bring traditional medicine towards renaissance."*

—Gayle Peterson,
Author, Birthing Normally

"A well-documented and easily read compendium of knowledge about cesarean sections [that will] help women to maintain the sanctity of their bodies and prevent their violation by surgical procedures. Silent Knife is empowering and contains the information which patronizing doctors never expected their patients to have."

—Michelle Harrison, M.D.
Author, A Woman in Residence

"SILENT KNIFE, powerful knife. . .cesarean section is becoming so commonplace, so accepted, that many of us have chosen to be silent, like the surgical knife itself. Silent Knife seeks to restore to all birthing couples the gifts of faith, of belief, of awareness—and it succeeds magnificently."

—Catherine Bemis Romeo

"A powerful and long-needed resource. . .Required reading for all childbirth educators and professionals."

—Donna R. Heath,
Chair, ICEA Cesarean Birth Committee

"Reading Silent Knife is an emotional and spiritual experience from which the reader can grow. The authors plant the seeds of insight and inspiration. The reader must bring them to harvest."
—Beth Shearer & Norma Shulman,
Directors, C/SEC, Inc.

"I am thoroughly impressed with the encyclopedic scholarship of Silent Knife. It will be a valuable resource for many years."
—Lynn Moen,
President, Birth & Life Bookstore

(Reviews continued on back cover)

Silent Knife

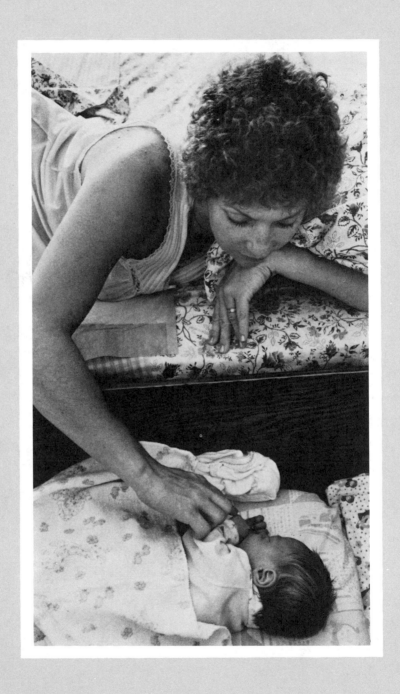

Nancy Wainer Cohen and Lois J. Estner

Silent Knife

CESAREAN PREVENTION AND VAGINAL BIRTH AFTER CESAREAN (VBAC)

Bergin & Garvey Publishers, Inc.
Massachusetts

Library of Congress Cataloging in Publication Data

Cohen, Nancy Wainer.
   Silent knife.

   Bibliography: p.
   Includes index.
   1. Cesarean section.   2. Childbirth.   3. Cesarean section—United States.   1. Estner, Lois
J.   II. Title.
[DNLM: 1. Delivery—Methods.   2. Cesarean section.
WQ 430   C678s]
RG761.C64   1983   618.2   82-24276
ISBN 0-89789-026-4
ISBN 0-89789-027-2 (pbk.)

Published in 1983 by Bergin & Garvey Publishers, Inc.
670 Amherst Road
South Hadley, Mass. 01075

0123456789   056   987654321

Printed in the United States of America

This book is dedicated to our husbands

Paul D. Cohen

And it is here, after months of writing—after hours where the words would not cease, where they would flow from my heart to my hand and then spill from the ink in the pen—that they stop. For there are no words that exist anywhere, nor are there any words that have ever existed, that can even begin to express what your never-ending love, patience, and devotion to me, the children, and my work have meant. I made it through the rain, dear husband, and kept my point of view, but you kept my world protected, and there isn't any way to tell you how much I honor you, respect you, and love you. . .

Martin I. Estner

This marks another milestone for us, the end of another of those passages through which we have traveled and grown together. It is time now for us to move on; but always when I look back, I will remember how your belief in me, your encouragement and your praise, helped to pave the way for this endeavor. Thank you, my husband, friend, lover, labor assistant extraordinaire. Once again you have helped me see that my reach should indeed exceed my grasp, or what's a heaven for?. . .

and to our children

Eric Michael, Elissa Rachel, and Andrea Jill Cohen,

and

Jordana Suzanne and Hillary Joyce Estner. . .

For the children and the flowers
Are my sisters and my brothers.
Their laughter and their loveliness
Could clear a cloudy day.
Like the music of the mountains
And the colors of the rainbow,
They're a promise of the future
And a blessing for today.

⇝ Contents

vi

Chapter 10 • Paternal Perspectives   211

Chapter 11 • Labor Support   223

♣ Foreword

In the current flood of childbirth literature, which ranges from popular magazine articles to whole books, there has been a dearth regarding cesarean prevention and vaginal birth after cesarean. A recently conducted personal survey of some of Boston's well-stocked bookstores revealed a few general books offering an overview of natural childbirth and two books dealing with cesarean birth. None of the books alerted the reader to the perils of cesarean section or ways in which routine medical practices increase the likelihood of cesarean section. As to the VBAC alternative, one book reviewed the situation in approximately three pages, a second devoted a paragraph, and a third about six pages to this subject. No other recognition of this alternative, let alone a book, was available.

Nancy Wainer Cohen and Lois J. Estner have recognized and filled this void with *Silent Knife* and its informative, well-written, and clearly presented material. The authors approach childbirth from various aspects: sociological, emotional, physical, and medical. *Silent Knife* provides a critique of this country's growing reliance on cesarean section, presents methods and strategies to prevent unnecessary cesareans, and will serve as an essential guide to pregnant couples and to health-care professionals.

Over the years I have been condemned both by women who had a cesarean section they considered unnecessary and by women who believed, contrary to my opinion, that they should have had a cesarean. I have never indulged in other than "medically in-dicated" cesareans. However, I have shared the same fears as other obstetricians. Every doctor wants his pregnant patients to have perfect babies. This goal, coupled with the maxims taught in medical school and reinforced during internship and residency, leads to the perpetuation of cesareans and repeat cesareans.

My experience in obstetrics has led me to reject, for the most part, the usual battery of restrictive precautions. The women with whom I work are upright and ambulatory during labor, with no hindrances to having their babies naturally. In addition to their high personal commitment, these laboring women receive good emotional support and ample time to accomplish their work. Within these parameters, we have achieved a very high rate of natural births and over a 70 percent rate of vaginal births after cesareans. In the past few years I have worked with approximately a hundred VBAC women. As I gain experience in this area, I become progressively more convinced that VBAC is low risk and that there are undeniable benefits to vaginal birth over and above repeat cesarean section.

The 1980 Task Force Report of the National Institutes of Health has reinforced the message of popular editorials and contributions from leading obstetricians with its warning about the United States' ever-rising cesarean rate. One primary factor contributing to the burgeoning statistics is that old adage, "Once a cesarean, always a cesarean." Now, however, the documented cases in this country have proven that the risk of vaginal birth after cesarean to both mother and fetus is very low and that the risk of complications imposed by a repeat cesarean are greater than those of VBAC. It is doubtful that the NIH or the American College of Obstetricians and Gynecologists would yet have given their attention to VBAC were it not for such consumer organizations as C/SEC and NAPSAC. With the combined efforts of these concerned groups, it is to be hoped that the cesarean rate will decrease and that VBAC will become the norm, as it is in almost every other country in the world.

After reading *Silent Knife*, I asked myself how any of us obstetricians could allow ourselves the (in)security of performing so many cesareans and repeat cesareans. More and more frequently today, we doctors are being asked to stop hiding behind our scientific tools and to practice our art. This book will help us to do just that.

Leo Sorger, M.D.

⮳ *Preface*

Welcome to our book! It is because we believe that the health and well-being of both mother and child are the most important considerations of any birth experience that we have written *Silent Knife*.

If you didn't have a cesarean, then you almost did, or one or more of your friends did, or you are afraid you might. Perhaps your "natural" childbirth was chemically induced and/or "managed," or resulted in a forceps delivery. You have read about the "cesarean problem" or the "cesarean dilemma" or even the "cesarean epidemic." You have heard the fatalists predict that cesarean section, the ultimate unnatural birth, may soon be the norm, and that some day in the near future, vaginal birth may be the exception. Perhaps you have resigned yourself to "cesarean *birth*," to the "family-centered cesarean birth experience," to the idea that "having a cesarean is having a baby." You have read the army of books that march across the shelves of our country proclaiming and defending the silent knife. We have read them and we have heard it all, too; but we are not resigned.

Before we share with you our knowledge and ideas about cesarean prevention and vaginal birth after cesarean, each of us would like to share a bit of herself. Perhaps then you will be able to appreciate the synergy of our combined efforts.

From C/SEC to VBAC: Nancy's Story

In 1972 our first child was born by cesarean section after an eight-hour, chemically induced labor. Even as I lay on the operating table, I was convinced that this cesarean was unnecessary and that it could have been prevented. Although I was delighted with our beautiful, healthy, 7-pound son, I felt disappointed, cheated, confused, angry, and intensely sad. My empty arms *ached* for my baby (who had been immediately whisked away to the nursery). My *heart* ached for him, too, and for my husband, who had been banished to the waiting room.

Comments from relatives and friends, such as, "What difference does it make how he was born?"; "Aren't you lucky, you won't have to go through labor ever again!"; and "Cesarean babies are so pretty," were well intentioned, but only added to my confusion, my emotional pain, and my deepening sorrow. To think that I might never experience giving birth to my children! To think that my babies would be separated from me and denied their rightful entry into this world. . .

I wrote to my childbirth instructors and asked if there were other women who had anticipated a normal, if not natural, birth, and who had feelings similar to mine as a result of an unexpected cesarean section. My letter was printed in their childbirth newsletter. Although the newsletter was a local one, I began receiving responses minutes after it was sent out—from all other the country! The responses never stopped. I was inundated with letters, phone calls, and even visits to my home—from women who had had cesareans and who had been very upset by the experience.

One of the first women to call was Jini Fairley. Jini and I decided to form an organization. We cofounded "C/SEC, Inc."—"Cesareans/Support, Education, and Concern." It was an organization whose time had come. The concept of prepared childbirth had taken root and was raising couples' expectations about their births. At the same time, however, a dramatic rise in the incidence of cesareans was occurring. This resulted in many couples having operative deliveries that were the antithesis of the happy, awake, and aware deliveries they had planned. Separated from each other, unable to be active participants in their infant's birth, they had no place to turn for information or support until C/SEC's formation in early 1973.

Women wrote to us to share their feelings of being abnormal, of being victimized ("It felt as if I was being raped. I couldn't do anything but wait until it was over"). We learned of anesthetics that didn't take, allergic reactions to medications, babies who were cut during the surgery, and women who were permanently paralyzed as a result of the procedure.

As the months wore on and the volume of mail increased, we were stunned to realize that thousands of women were having their babies surgically, and equally stunned to recognize that their experiences continued to range from *unpleasant* to *horrifying*.

Nine women who wrote to us wanted to help in any way they could. We met, and with ten babies who ranged in age from three weeks to three years—who ate our notes, spilled juice on our research, and sang "Old MacDonald" as we tried to work—we decided we were going to do something. We were going to make a difference.

We did do something. We did somethingS. We talked to doctors, hospital staffs, consumers, newspapers. We got fathers involved in cesarean births and made certain that newborns would be judged on their own merit, not routinely separated from their parents just because they were cesarean infants. C/SEC started cesarean support groups, produced materials, and developed a family-centered slide-tape presentation for use in childbirth classes. We talked about consumer rights and about humanizing the cesarean birth experience, and we did research about medications, anesthetics, and psychological issues. We gave support and caring to frightened, disoriented cesarean couples, and we committed ourselves to making cesarean births joyous, meaningful, family-centered births. C/SEC raised the level of consciousness about cesareans. Its existence prompted further literature, research, and discussion on the subject, which until then had been totally neglected by the public. It was an example of a consumer movement whose loyal and vocal following influenced and effected change nationwide.

In 1974, Paul and I had our second child. Elissa was born, not by cesarean, at a hospital in Boston. We were armed with a great deal of determination, but little support for choosing a vaginal birth after a cesarean. We were obviously very happy to have a healthy baby, excited to have given birth nonsurgically, and relieved not to have been separated from each other as we had been for the cesarean. However, I was still left with feelings of frustration, abandonment, anger, and sadness. Because what we were doing was considered revolutionary—in fact, insane!—there was a great deal of tension at the birth and lots of medical and technical interference (which we felt helpless to refuse).

For the second time, my healthy newborn baby was separated from me, as a "routine hospital policy" (or perhaps as a punishment, this time, for challenging traditional medical authority?). Our beautiful daughter Elissa's birth wasn't a cesarean section, but a cold, unsupported, and unfortunately *typical* United States obstetrical delivery.

In 1977 I left C/SEC to devote my time solely to the issues of cesarean prevention, VBAC, and positive birthing. I felt it a sad commentary on our times that women in the United States have been conditioned to fear labor and birth, and even sadder that so many were choosing a cesarean (or submitting to one) because they felt it was the lesser of two undesirable alternatives.

Paul and I were delighted when, in 1978, I became pregnant again (I had had a miscarriage earlier that year). In May 1979 our third child was born—at home. This decision was not made nonchalantly; it was the culmination of seven-and-a-half years of planning, reading, researching, and soul-searching. Our hard work and intense spiritual questioning brought us to a decision that was 100 percent right, *for us.*

Since Paul and I had made an unpopular decision when we decided to have Elissa vaginally, we were used to the questions and accusations. At that time we had been told that having a baby vaginally after a previous cesarean was outrageous, irresponsible, unthinkable!—how could we consider such an incredible risk? However, some of the same doctors who refused to talk to us then are now promoting VBAC as a much safer alternative than repeat cesarean. Had we not been so determined before, had we not stuck to our unpopular decision, our second child would have been another unnecessary surgical insult.

After Andrea's birth at home, people asked us, "Weren't you frightened?" Our response was an unequivocal NO! We weren't scared! On the contrary, once we have made the decision to stay at home, we felt an overwhelming sense of *peace.* We had competent medical back-up if we needed it and extremely competent midwives who agreed to be with us. Based on our last two birth experiences, it would have taken far more courage and faith for us to go back into a hospital to give birth.

With much time and effort and consideration to every little detail that could affect the birth and the health of our newborn, our dream for a birth as birth *should* be came true. We are still filled with a tremendous sense of joy, pride, exhilaration, gratitude, and awe. Our children were present (something that would have been denied us all at the hospital, since "the facility is not yet prepared or equipped to handle such a situation"—although six months later sibling visitation was instituted as a result of consumer pressure), and they held Andrea before she was minutes old. It was a beautiful, fulfilling family experience. For me, it was a healing experience, too. It feels, I feel, *complete.*

Eric, Elissa, and Andrea will soon be eleven, nine, and four. We are infinitely grateful for our three beautiful children and know that each of their births was a gift to us that will live in our hearts for the rest of our lives.

After Andrea's birth, I continued writing, teaching, lecturing, and counseling. I helped to found the National Cesarean Prevention Movement and joined the staff of Offspring, a childbirth training and counseling center and model for positive birthing. In 1980, Lois and Marty Estner took my childbirth classes. After their daughter Hillary was born, Lois called and said, "Nancy, there has to be a book about VBAC and cesarean prevention!" "I know," I told her. "I've thought about that for months. But I need someone's help!" . . .

Lois's Story

The birth of our first child in 1976 was a joyous and exhilarating event. My husband Marty was with me throughout, I was awake and aware, and our perfect new daughter was happily nursing soon after her birth. Rooming in began almost immediately and prepared us for a very smooth transition from hospital to home a few days later. The weeks and months that followed were filled with the wonder and joy of Jordana. I have come to think of them as "the winter of my content." Jordana's birth, by the way, was a cesarean section.

Although I did not know it at the time, Nancy Cohen and C/SEC had laid much of the groundwork for the family-centered management of my cesarean. Because of the hospital's enlightened maternity care for cesarean mothers, I was able to return home relatively free of the trauma, disappointment, and depression that so often accompany a surprise cesarean. Marty and I rejoiced in the arrival of our lovely daughter and never felt the least bit cheated of the natural childbirth for which we had so diligently prepared. The delivery had been the means to an end; and if the means were less than perfect, well, the end more than justified them.

As I left the hospital, I was given literature from C/SEC and literature from La Leche League to take home with me. C/SEC was of no interest to me—after all, I had no problems with my cesarean—and so it was through LLL, at a leaders' meeting several years later, that I met Nancy Cohen for the first time.

When Nancy learned that Jordana's birth had been by cesarean, she asked if I had thought about VBAC for my next birth. Next birth? But I wasn't even pregnant! Well, never too soon to start thinking about it.

I disagreed. For me, it was too soon. I was having trouble conceiving and felt very superstitious about making birth plans. Also, remember, I had no regrets or complaints about my cesarean and no fear of another one. Me a candidate for VBAC? No way! Marty and I were cautious people, conservative, a bit old-fashioned. No risk-taking for us!

I did become pregnant, and something strange and subtle began to happen to me. I found myself wistfully looking back to the days of our Lamaze classes and our innocent anticipation of Jordana's birth. The thought of a scheduled cesarean delivery for my next baby began to leave me cold and uncomfortable. I would miss the excitement of not knowing when and how labor would begin, and my child would be deprived of his destined birthday. Even more important, I began to hear frightening stories of scheduled repeat cesareans where babies delivered too early demonstrated all the life-threatening problems of prematurity.

The idea of going into labor became more and more appealing. I began to read everything relevant that I could find and to talk with anyone who might know something. What began to emerge was a pretty good suspicion that I did not in fact have to have another cesarean. The more I learned, the more I came to realize that there was far more risk involved in submitting myself to major abdominal surgery than there was in attempting a vaginal delivery. A repeat cesarean for me would be nothing more than elective surgery. I became sure that I did not need it. Now to convince Marty and my doctor.

Marty proved to be the harder of the two to convince. He initially regarded my idea as something akin to suicide and infanticide. I was volunteering to become a maternal mortality statistic, and it was most inconsiderate of me not only to deprive him of his lifelong mate, but also to leave him with a four-year-old and perhaps a newborn to raise. I buried Marty's mound of fears under a mountain of facts about surgical risks and the safety of VBAC. I finished with a reminder that Jordana had never been away from me for a whole week, that the adjustments would be much easier for her if I could be home from the hospital in a few days.

In the end, what convinced Marty of the sensibility of VBAC was simply his faith in me. I had never been one for rash decision-making, and he would just have to go with the trust he had always put in me. We decided together to take Nancy's course and find out what more we needed to know. The next session would begin in a few weeks.

Meanwhile, my first prenatal doctor's appointment yielded a surprise. Not only did my doctor agree to a VBAC, he suggested it! It was unlikely that I would have another breech baby, and so there would be no reason for a repeat cesarean. I was grateful and relieved until I began to reflect upon the management of my 26-hour first labor: the I.V., the artificially ruptured membranes, the Pitocin, the fetal monitor, the epidural, and, finally, the almost inevitable cesarean. In my heart I knew that I was not going to have a vaginal birth with this doctor. He was too impatient, too interventionist, to allow labor to take its own course; and labor intervention is what causes most unnecessary cesareans. By the time Marty and I began Nancy's classes, we had found a new doctor who believed in helping his patients give birth rather than delivering their babies. By the time we finished our VBAC course, Marty was as confident and enthusiastic as I was about our decisions.

After all our months of research, decision-making, and planning, it was Hillary who ultimately defined the terms of her birth. She arrived two weeks early, before a repeat cesarean would even have been scheduled. She chose a day when our labor assistant was away on vacation and our carefully chosen doctor would not be at the hospital. She came so fast that we arrived at the hospital barely in time for her birth. There was no time for intervention, no time even for me to change out of my sundress. Later we wondered how there would ever have been time for a cesarean.

There, in the presence of our darling new daughter, was the confirmation of all that we had known: that a repeat cesarean for us would have been utter craziness. More than that, BIGGER than that: here was our very own empirical evidence that ROUTINE REPEAT CESAREANS ARE AN OUTRAGE.

And so it was not in cesarean section but in vaginal birth that my own anger and energy for this book were conceived. And so it was that Nancy and I met for the second time. . .

The Book

The seeds of our book took root on a Sunday afternoon in February 1981; although it was too early for spring planting, we noticed a promise of warmth in the air. Together we began the first of the countless brainstorming sessions from which *Silent Knife* was to grow.

The task seemed enormous, overwhelming. How to satisfy the desperate needs of the women who were begging us for information that would help them avoid a cesarean, and at the same time appeal to the women who had no idea of the risks and dangers involved in this procedure? How to reach the women who accepted what they saw as their cesarean fate? How to attract those who turned away and said, "It won't be me," when their childbirth educators told them that over 25 percent of the women in each class usually ended up with a cesarean? A book that was to be in any way influential in bringing the cesarean epidemic under control would have to be powerful enough to feed those who hungered for it, but not so strong that it would scare away the timid. It would have to be engaging enough to keep an audience interested, professional enough to be respected by members of the medical community.

We had received more than forty thousand letters from pregnant women and new mothers, and we had developed some idea of the breadth, depth, and urgency of the need for our book.

We wanted all women to come away from our book knowing how much we cared about them and their babies. We wanted to find a way to help them understand how important it was for them to assume responsibility and take control of their births. We wanted our book to give them the information and the confidence to start challenging the medical mythology that has been victimizing them for years.

We wanted so much! We wondered if we could possibly accomplish what we set out to do or if we had set unrealistic goals. We wondered if we should narrow our focus, limit our research, survey our audience, soften our tone—or radicalize it. We pondered over how we could best serve those who picked up our book, knowing how incredibly varied their impressions, experiences, and needs would be. We still haven't found the answers to these concerns; we only know that we have given all that we have to give, and that, above all, this was for us a labor of love.

One striking concern was the vast quantity of information that was buried in professional journals and obstetrical texts and therefore unknown to most laypeople. We knew the book needed to be well researched and thoroughly documented and yet eminently readable. Since we did not want our footnotes to be a major interruption into the text, we decided to first alphabetize and then number our references by chapter. This seemed the least intrusive of the methods we considered, and the one that allowed the sources of our information to be most readily available.

It is fall now. Two planting seasons have passed and our seedlings have their own life. They have basked in the sun and absorbed the rain; they have grown into broad and sturdy trees. It is time for the products of our labor to greet the breezes and weather the forces, in the hope that they will someday bear fruit.

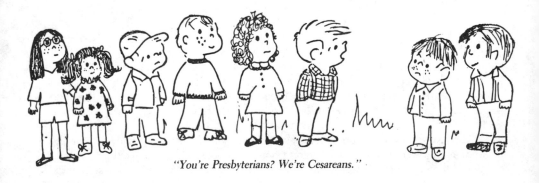

"You're Presbyterians? We're Cesareans."

໑► Acknowledgments

Here's to the friends who come together
To share the search to know
To you I say hello forever
*Love does not end, but it grows.**

In most other cultures, as a woman labors and gives birth, she is surrounded by people who love her and support her. As we labored with *Silent Knife*, countless numbers of people supported us, guided us, and loved us. Their enthusiasm, wisdom, and confidence gave life to our dream and powered our efforts. In particular, we would like to thank the following:

Barbara Adams, Pat Barki, Gail Sforza Brewer, Patty Brumbaugh, Barbara Brown-Hill, Elaine Burke, David Chapin, Betty Clarke, Bernard and Sylvia Cohen, Anne Cornetta, Cathy and Raysh Daub, Gail Epstein, Jini Fairley, Rebecca Feld, Ina May Gaskin, Lu and Rich Gabriel, Debra Gelles, Doris Haire, Michelle Harrison, Jay and Marjie Hathaway, Donna Heath, Ralph Johnson, Joyce Kisner, Janet Leigh, Kay Matthews, Fredelle Maynard, Lewis Mehl, Sue Miller, Marilyn Moran, Judy Norsigian, Peggy O'Hara-McMahon, Jami Osborne, Andy Osborne, Claudia Panuthos, Gayle Peterson, Jim Staton, Lynn Richards, John Romeo, Beth Shearer, Norma Shulman, Annette Simmons, Leo and Kay Sorger, David and Lee Stewart, Norma Swenson, Anne Marie Sullivan, JoAnn Sykes, Lindsa Vallee, Lauri Wolff, Diony Young, and Esther and Tom Zorn.

And to Ethel Wainer, Merton Wainer, and Cathy Romeo, our deepest thanks, for without their unshakable faith, infinite patience, continual assistance, and unconditional love, there would be no book.

In addition to those listed here, we are grateful to all the people who helped us in so many ways. We are grateful to all the women who "aimed above the clouds, rose above the crowds, and started their own 'parades'."† We are grateful to all the little babies who, in spite of doubting obstetricians, anxious staffs, narrow passageways, and many other obstacles, continued to remember the blueprints and followed them to be born. We are also grateful to all the previously sectioned uteri that contracted powerfully and never caused any one of the VBAC women with whom we have worked any cause for concern. And finally, we, Nancy and Lois, thank each other; for as we worked together, our love and respect for each other continued to grow.

Thank you, Jenna Schulman (our editor), for the sensitive and caring way in which you held our manuscript. We admire your skills, your sensitivity, your professionalism, and above all, your sense of humor.

Thank you, Jim Bergin and Judy Garvey, Deborah Huisken, and Jeanne Juster. If ever fate brought a group of individuals together . . .

---

*From "Hello Forever," by Karen Riem.
†From "I Made It through the Rain," by Barry Manilow.

Fools, said I, you do not know:
Silence like a cancer grows.
Here my words that I might teach you,
Take my arms that I might reach you.

—P. Simon
"Sounds of Silence"

1 ᏶ Introduction

Nature has designed a system in which a baby travels through its mother's body in order to be born: from the safety and warmth of her womb to the reassurance and comfort of her arms. It is a process that has worked for eons, one in which each step has a distinct purpose and a specific goal. It is agonizingly detailed, yet very simple. It is extremely precise, yet requires no scientific tools or devices; indeed, outside interferences often confuse the process. The design is beautiful, intricate, unique, delicately balanced, and not easily duplicated. Birth's design was patented years and years ago; the original blueprints are not accessible, nor will they ever be.

When a problem exists in the birth process, whether resulting from external interventions, or inherent in the system as one of its own infrequent mistakes, medical obstetrics can often provide us with procedures to correct it. These procedures are available to assist nature, and we are indebted for their existence. Problems arise, however, when we interfere with Nature's plan, when we egotistically believe that we have a design that surpasses the original, and when we believe that our technology can produce a birth process superior to Nature's own. When we become so confident as to believe that we can reproduce and redesign such a complex event as birth, we are assuming that we can, indeed, play God. Without the original blueprints, we cannot fully comprehend the process, nor can we understand the importance of each step along the way. Each individual birth has its own blueprint, similar, but never identical, to the original plan.

The United States has one of the highest rates of cesarean section births in the world, and the number is increasing daily. In spite of expensive, sophisticated, ultramodern equipment and technology, we still rank fifteenth or sixteenth in fetal and maternal morbidity and mortality. In spite of the fact that "natural"

1

childbirth has become ingrained in our culture, mothers are still being drugged, monitored, shaved, enemaed, starved, needled, "pitted," immobilized, and cut. More and more babies are being drugged, "scalped," injected, pulled out or sucked out with instruments, and restricted from their rightful place: their parents' arms. Indeed, it seems as if women's bodies are losing the ability to give birth without intervention.

When a cesarean is necessary, it is an important, often lifesaving procedure. But far too many cesareans are done unnecessarily, or when they have *become* necessary because of medical interventions, obstetrical interferences, invasive procedures, and attitudes about women, pregnancy, and birth that affect a positive outcome. These factors contribute to the course of labor and delivery and ultimately to the outrageous number of women who are told that they must be cut open in order to have their babies "safely."

In our country, cesareans are glorified. They are referred to as "delivering from above," whereas vaginal birth is referred to as "delivering from below"; and most of us are ignorant concerning the risks and the high number of complications and dangers inherent in the cesarean procedure.

We believe that most of the cesareans that are performed could and should be prevented. We believe that there is an attitude in our country on the part of most health professionals that birth is impossible without tools, tubes, chemicals, drugs, and machines. In our country, we have come to believe that *doctors deliver babies*, not that *women give birth*. This attitude has been adopted and integrated by most people in our culture; it undermines a woman's confidence and influences her choices. Its popularity is responsible for many of the problems that arise. Women come to their births believing that somehow someone else will get their baby out for them, rather than trusting in themselves and their body's ability to open and actively birth their babies.

In our culture, women often come to birth frightened, anxious, malnourished, uninformed, and unsupported. If their labors are not progressing quickly enough, they are given something to hurry things up. If their labors are intense and they are in need of loving guidance and support, they are given drugs to slow things down. They are separated from people in their lives whose presence at their births could do more to calm them than any drug. They are deprived of those who could help them feel relaxed, confident, supported, and able to cope. United States obstetrics surrounds us with men who never have given and never will give birth, and who tell us, "Don't worry. *I* know. *I'll* take care of things."

Physicians in the nineteenth century did a very successful advertising campaign to convince women that birth was an abnormal medical event. Their colleagues in the twentieth century are proving equally successful in convincing us that birth is no longer "just" a medical event, but a surgical event as well. The silence and mystification of the birthing process that has been building through the centuries is ever more frequently punctuated by "knights" who pull out their "swords" to save the "fair maidens," thus turning healthy, normal women into damsels in distress.

We are put into institutions that are otherwise entirely devoted to illness, and "decorated" with the latest "advancements" in obstetrical technology. Doris Haire, past president of the International Childbirth Education Association (ICEA) and author of several articles, including "The Cultural Warping of Childbirth," states, "Of all the 36 countries I have visited to observe maternity facilities, I am absolutely convinced that the United States has to be the most bizarre on earth in its management of obstetrics." Ms. Haire also tells us that the average Dutch health professional would "cringe in fright," looking at our obstetrical practices. We, too, are cringing in fright—and in frustration and sorrow, as well. Because most medical care givers view birth as a medical event, they become active participants (meddlers) in our births, intervening in the natural process and negatively affecting the outcome.

We believe that birth is a natural process that can take place naturally. We believe that every pregnant woman can give birth if she so desires and has the proper information and support. Every woman can find the strength from within to deliver her baby as she integrates feelings of trust and confidence in her body, accepts her particular labor, and appreciates the process of birth. We believe that birth requires teamwork among mother, uterus, and baby, and that all three know instinctively how to work together to complete the process. We believe that many of us start out as low-risk, normal, pregnant women, but are inappropriately labeled and then *become* high-risk as a result of the "system." We believe that iatrogenia (physician-induced damage) contributes to a large proportion of obstetrical complications and emergency situations. We know that postpartum depression is not a normal, unavoidable sequela of birth, but that it is culturally ingrained. We know that the label "high-risk" need not be a lifelong albatross. We believe that birth is a spiritual, emotional, and psychological experience as well as a physiological one. We know that all these experiential aspects must be addressed before we can begin to understand the process and reduce the number of cesareans being performed.

We believe that birth is not a medical circumstance. We believe that birth is a safe passage for both mother and child, and that both are fully equipped for the journey. We know that women are in a vulnerable state during labor and are easily sabotaged in their plans for normal birthing.

We know that many prepared-childbirth classes are ineffective and inadequate. We believe that *cesarean*-childbirth classes are an insult to women. Women and babies need not be subjected to the risks inherent in a major abdominal operation just because it can be a "good experience."

We see a fascination with technology that may someday actually destroy the blueprints for natural birth. We are subjected and exposed to ultrasound, x-rays, electronic monitoring devices, drugs, anesthetics, chemicals, and knives, which in most cases are not beneficial, necessary, or safe. We endure countless vaginal exams, which are invasive and usually unnecessary. We permit our genital areas to be cut, in order, we are told, to accommodate our infants. We are told that it doesn't make a difference if the baby is artificially fed or breastfed or if we room in. We are part of a twentieth-century farce, and, sadly, most of us don't even know it yet.

Can it be that one out of every four or five women in this country needs to be sectioned in order to have her baby safely? Are our bodies no longer able to accommodate our infants? Are cesareans really as safe as we are led to believe? Why are so many babies from seemingly healthy, normal, pregnant women pronounced distressed during labor? Are babies really *unfit* for their journey into the world? And why are so many of these "distressed" babies perfectly healthy when they are born? What of the truly distressed infants—*what is causing their trauma?* Is it truly inherent in "the system," or are we unaware of how our interferences affect our little ones? The answers to these questions are being ignored by far too many, far too often.

Vaginal birth after cesarean is not only safe, but generally safer than its alternative. In spite of the research and evidence and documentation that appear on this subject, most obstetricians in this country continue to perform repeat cesareans simply because a woman has been previously sectioned. There is always an excuse, it seems, why a woman cannot be a candidate for vaginal birth after cesarean (VBAC—pronounced VEE-back) or a vaginal birth in the first place. We know that most women who have had a cesarean are capable of delivering vaginally. This includes women with a diagnosis of cephalo-pelvic disproportion (CPD), prolonged labor (failure to progress, or FTP), or more than one previous cesarean. We have worked with women who have had VBAC breech births, VBAC twins, and many other VBAC "special circumstances."

We know that women who want to birth vaginally after a cesarean are not crazy, selfish, or insane. We know that many cesarean women are bitter and sorrowful. There is great understanding for a man who is unable to get an erection or ejaculate; most people understand that this is a part of his total identity as a male. There is support for feelings of inadequacy, frustration, failure, sadness, and guilt. But there is very little understanding for cesarean women who have feelings of disappointment, sadness, failure, and frustration at not being able to complete the normal womanly physiological process of giving birth. For many women, becoming pregnant and giving birth are integrally and intricately linked with feelings of self-worth and identity. Is it any wonder that so many women in our culture are grieving? To want to give birth in a way that unites us with other women—to all women, to WOMAN—to want to experience each of the cycles of our life, is not insane. It is normal.

We know that most obstetricians believe in the appropriateness/necessity of what they are doing. We are concerned about a system that brings these individuals a set of beliefs that cause them to fear, rather than respect and appreciate, the natural design. We must take a careful look at our obstetrical practices, whether or not that scrutiny upsets or threatens the medical establishment.

We have so much to learn, and we are taking so much time! Meanwhile, more and more women are being needlessly cut. More and more babies are being deprived of their "right of passage." In addition, whole families are becoming the innocent victims of this unnecessary surgery.

Birth is a significant life experience. Its effects are immeasurable and boundless. It needs to be—and can be—a time of peace, exhilaration, joy, and growth that can be treasured for a lifetime.

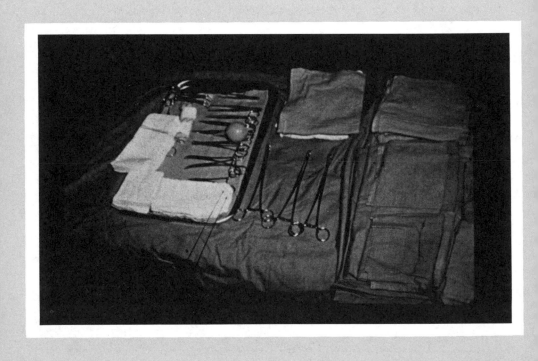

2 ᐧᐁ The Knife Unsheathed: Cesarean Section in the United States

The State of the (Obstetric) Union

The cesarean delivery rate in the United States has reached epidemic proportions. We know that statistics do not make exciting reading, but the facts and figures speak for themselves, and what they have to say is appalling.

The fact is that America has fallen in love with machines, computers, tools, and gadgets. We have not yet entered an era of computerized childbirth, but it is surely not far off. In the meantime, the birthing stage is set with mechanized props that turn a warm, human, natural event into a cold, impersonal performance. We see the cesarean knife as the ultimate symbol of technocratic interference in the process of childbirth.

The "silent knife" is carving a new image of childbirth in our country. Having long ago defined birth as a medical event, America is now on the threshold of accepting it also as a surgical event. As we tolerate one invasive procedure after another in the birthing rooms of our land, we lose our horror of the knife; indeed, we sometimes welcome surgical delivery as the end to a poorly managed labor. Many cesarean mothers describe an initial feeling of relief when the "need" for a cesarean is discovered; surgery provides an escape from the tortures of the hospital labor room.

According to Robbi Pfeuffer's "The Hazards of Hospital Childbirth,"[40] the number of invasive procedures used in hospital deliveries "increases every year."

7

They now include placing the woman flat on her back, restricting her food intake, artificially inducing or stimulating her labor, rupturing her amniotic membranes, routinely using intravenous fluids, analgesia, anesthesia, electronic fetal monitors, episiotomies, and forceps, and routinely separating mothers from their babies. "Routine cesarean section might also be added," Pfeuffer notes, "for in one Boston teaching hospital, one out of every four babies is born by cesarean section."

That figure is outrageous, but, regrettably, it is not atypical. One out of every four babies is born by cesarean section in New York City, too; and the 1979 Massachusetts Health Department statistics listed seven Boston area hospitals with cesarean rates over 25 percent, one with a rate of over 30 percent![22] We have heard rumors of physicians with 80–100 percent cesarean rates. It becomes hard to remember that as recently as 1968, the overall cesarean section rate in the United States was 5 percent,[9] a rate deemed normal by generations of obstetric and nursing textbooks,[11] although a bit high by us. If we (reluctantly) accept a 4 to 5 percent cesarean section rate as "normal," then it is clear that over 80 percent of today's cesareans are an unnecessary surgical intervention! Perhaps we need to take a look at who is doing the intervening.

In "Unnecessary Cesareans: Doctor's Choice, Parent's Dilemma,"[11] Susan G. Doering reminds us that until quite recently, "one could judge a physician by his section rate: the lower it was, the better obstetrician he must be." She recalls Kroener's statement:

> One of the long held principles of obstetrics has been that the cesarean section rate was inversely proportional to the quality of obstetrics practiced. Any physician with a high section rate was evaluated for the quality of his obstetric care and accused of trying to pad his financial remuneration.

As an example of that bygone philosophy, Doering describes the "stress and concern" of a group of Los Angeles physicians who, in 1956, were placed on probationary status by the Joint Committee on Accreditation because their hospital section rate was almost 10 percent. Doering's remark that "things have changed a lot since 1956" is an understatement. Now it almost seems that physicians and hospitals pride themselves on their high cesarean rates, and that high rates are considered synonymous with good obstetric care.

Let us contrast those distressed, concerned Los Angeles physicians with Dr. John Sutherst and Dr. Barbara Case, writing in the April 1975 issue of a British journal, and quoted by Corea: "It may well be that during the next 40 years *the allowing* of a vaginal delivery or attempted vaginal delivery may need to be justified in each particular instance" (our emphasis). When a physician is able to even contemplate such a trend, it becomes apparent that the medical profession is no longer holding itself accountable for its excesses; that, as *Williams*

Obstetrics notes, "in modern obstetric practice, there are virtually no contrain-dications for cesarean section."[41]

This complacent attitude is reflected in the skyrocketing cesarean rate. Between 1970 and 1978, the cesarean birth rate in the United States increased about threefold, from 5.5 percent to 15.2 percent,[33] an almost 200 percent increase. In 1979, officials at the National Institute of Child Health and Human Development (NIH) became concerned about the rising cesarean delivery rate in the nation and decided to hold a consensus development conference on cesarean childbirth. A nineteen-member task force was appointed to gather and analyze data for a preliminary draft report. By the time the conference convened in September 1980, the cesarean section rate in the United States had reached 18 percent, with northeastern states such as New York and Massachusetts running consistently ahead of the national norm.[21] This translates into approximately 14,850 cesareans in Massachusetts and 647,640 cesareans in the country, in 1980 alone.

The regional variation in cesarean rates can be seen on a smaller scale in the rate differences among doctors and hospitals.[55] Diony Young and Charles Mahan, authors of "Unnecessary Cesareans: Ways To Avoid Them," remark that factors such as age, medical training, personal attitudes, habit, location, style of practice, availability of facilities and personnel, financial incentives, and convenience affect the differences among individual physicians. Among individual hospitals, factors such as hospital size and number of beds influence the rate, with more cesareans occurring in the larger hospitals. Additionally, the rate of cesareans is higher in teaching than in nonteaching hospitals. Young and Mahan caution that "an unusually high physician or hospital rate may indicate that the physician or hospital is receiving referrals for complicated pregnancies that require cesarean section." Then again, it may not. More about all this in Chapter 13.

The trend toward rising cesarean rates is "pervasive," according to the NIH conference report, "affecting hospitals and patients in all parts of the country. . . [and] is also evident internationally."[33] But at twice the British rate and approximately four times the Western European average,[22] the United States has by far the highest rates. With 98 percent of cesarean mothers in the United States opting for repeat surgical deliveries in subsequent pregnancies, it is likely that things will get much worse before they get better—unless we, as consumers, begin to exercise our rights and make demands for change. Now.

What has happened to childbirth in America? How have we allowed cesarean section to become an acceptable alternative to vaginal birth? Why did we relinquish our rights as healthy, normal birthing women and join the jonnied ranks of ailing hospital patients? When did we start believing that surgical delivery is safer and better for our babies? These questions and more must be answered before we can even hope to bring the cesarean epidemic under control. Let's start at the beginning.

A Brief History of Cesarean Section

Legend has it that Julius Caesar was born by cesarean section and that the procedure was named after him. It is more likely that the name of the operation comes from the "lex caesaria" of Roman law, which required that abdominal surgery be performed on a dead or dying woman in a late stage of pregnancy to save her baby for the state. It may also come from the Latin "caedre," to cut.

In any case, we know from early mythological references and ancient folklore that surgical delivery has been practiced for centuries. It was first performed to provide a separate burial for the fetus of a dead mother, then to extract a living baby from a dead mother in an effort to save it. Not until the sixteenth century was the surgery performed with the intent to save both mother and baby.

The first cesarean sections in America probably occurred in the late 1700s or early 1800s. The death rate for both cesarean mother and baby was quite high, as uterine suture was not yet practiced, and the importance of sterile techniques had not yet been recognized. In 1882, when Adolf Kehrer and Max Sanger closed the wound of the uterus with silk sutures, the most important advance in cesarean surgery was made.[23]

It wasn't until the late nineteenth century that reports of cesareans became common, and the early 1900s brought the first hospital records of cesarean deliveries. In 1916, when Dr. Craigin originated the phrase, "Once a cesarean, always a cesarean," surgical delivery was still a very conservative procedure done for an absolute contracted pelvis, a recurring condition.[45] By the 1930s, hospital was replacing home as the place to give birth, making surgical delivery a more convenient option[23] and allowing it to become an alternative to high- and mid-forceps on the impacted fetus. With the advent of sterile technique,[54] improved operating methods and anesthesia, and the availability of blood and antibiotics, the risks of cesarean surgery were greatly reduced. Still, the cesarean rate remained fairly stable.

Until the 1960s, hospital birth usually meant delivery under general anesthesia and a lengthy hospital stay, whether delivery was vaginal or abdominal. Then the "back to nature" movement of the '60s made women realize how far from nature hospital childbirth practices had strayed, and the resurgence of the women's movement gave them a strong voice with which to be heard. Maternity care, responding to consumer demand, began to undergo remarkable changes. Childbirth preparation and regional anesthesia allowed women to consciously experience the births of their children, and they insisted that their husbands be made partners in the experience. Maternity care in many of the larger hospitals became family centered, with baby rooming in and siblings coming to visit. By the early 1970s, childbirth environments and practices had begun to be humanized[54] in response to the demands of childbearing families. Each forward step for natural childbirth, however, took the cesarean experience, by contrast, a leap behind. Ironically, it was just at this very time that the cesarean birthrate began to soar.

Factors in the Rising Cesarean Rate

While consumer groups worked to humanize and naturalize the childbirth experience, medical groups were working to eliminate the risks of childbirth to mother and baby. On the surface, it would seem that the two groups would be united in a joint effort, with the potential for phenomenal results. At closer look, however, we see that the new drugs, machines, and procedures espoused by the physicians are often counterproductive and result in more complications than they are intended to prevent. Moreover, the benefits and safety of this "new obstetrics" have yet to be proved.

In "An Evaluation of Cesarean Section in the U.S.," her 1979 report to the Department of Health, Education and Welfare, Dr. Helen Marieskind identifies in order of significance twelve factors that contribute to the burgeoning rate of operative deliveries. Because they will be a recurring topic throughout our book, we would like to present them here in some detail.

1. *Threat of malpractice suits* is the most frequent reason given for the increase. Doctors are concerned about the threat of malpractice suits if a cesarean is not performed and the outcome is a "less than perfect baby." Many physicians feel pressured to practice "defensive medicine" in order to be "covered" if they "produce" a defective infant. They feel that if they have performed a cesarean, they have done everything they can. When questioned, physicians freely agreed off the record that fear of a suit prompted cesareans and that this is commonly discussed among colleagues. Few, however, know of a colleague who has been sued. One obstetrician said that fear of malpractice suits rather than medical criteria is the reason for the rise. Upon examination of data from insurance claims, it is not clear that the threat of malpractice suits for failure to perform a cesarean justifies the rapid increase in cesarean deliveries. However, obstetricians feel "at risk."

2. *The policy of "Once a cesarean, always a cesarean"* has become standard obstetrical practice in the United States. In a 1974 Professional Activities Study, only 0.9 percent of 358 women who had previously had cesareans delivered

vaginally. The subjects were a random sampling from all over the country, with eight cases the most at any one hospital. The repeat cesarean rate in our country is almost 100 percent, and the policy accounts for approximately one-third of the indications for cesarean deliveries in the United States and Canada. Marieskind reports, "In 1976 alone, we could potentially have saved about 95 million dollars had a policy of individual evaluation and subsequent. . .[VBAC] been followed. From all reports, the mothers and babies would have had at least equally as favorable an outcome as from routine repeat cesareans."

3. *Lack of training* makes physicians ill prepared to manage labor. As you will see, we believe that the idea that labor has to be "managed" is responsible for many problems. Many physicians stated that they are not familiar with normal labor but have received extensive training in the use of highly technical equipment. Others commented that the art of obstetrics is no longer being taught, and that residents have little or no experience with vaginal breech deliveries or obstetrical maneuvers such as external version. In most medical centers, anesthesiologists train residents in general, not local, anesthesia. Many physicians complained that regular reviews of deliveries were rarely offered; when they were, only difficult cases were discussed. Patients with similar cases who were successful at vaginal delivery were not discussed. It was also stated that delivery-room nurses' estimates of cesarean sections in particular hospitals were more accurate than the estimates of the chiefs of staff. If that is true, then it is unfortunate that the nurses are not the ones responsible for keeping the records.

4. *Most physicians believe that a cesarean section results in a superior outcome.* "Superior outcome," however, has not been proved. Other factors, such as the availability of neonatal intensive-care units, improved nutrition and prenatal care, and the availability of abortions may be more influential in regard to improvements than acknowledged. In fact, fetal mortality and morbidity rates have shown little change in the decade since the cesarean rate took wings and flew. The United States, with the highest cesarean rate in the world, ranks fifteenth and sixteenth in infant mortality.

In "The Cesarean Epidemic,"[9] Gena Corea states, "there is no evidence whatever that liberal use of the c/section has done ANYTHING TO RAISE THE MENTAL PERFORMANCE OF CHILDREN" (emphasis in original) or to "reduce the incidence of neurological disorders in our population." The belief that birth is a dangerous process for babies is simply unfounded and unsubstantiated. In fact, it is a tried and proven means of entering this world.

Have increased cesarean delivery rates resulted in lower neonatal mortality rates? Dr. Diana Pettiti,[38] a member of the NIH Task Force, used New York City birth certificates from 1968–1969 and 1976–1977 to study the relationship between neonatal mortality and method of delivery. She found that for term deliveries complicated by dystocia or by fetal distress, there were *no significant differences* in neonatal mortality between vaginally delivered and surgically delivered infants. Her conclusion:

> This analysis raises serious questions about the extent to which the rising cesarean delivery rate has had a beneficial effect on pregnancy outcome. . . [and] provides strong evidence for the need to inquire more closely about the risks and benefits of the present high cesarean delivery rate.

"Superior outcome"? Hardly.

Dr. M. G. Kerr* says that it might be "both misleading and dangerous" to attribute improvements in pregnancy outcome to the efforts of physicians. "We may have assumed too lightly that more sophisticated management necessarily brings benefits to women." He concludes, "There is virtually no reliable information to determine the benefits of obstetrical innovations in terms of fetal well being," and points out that even if benefits can be measured, they have to be balanced against the costs—not just hospital costs and doctors' fees, but also "the unwanted side effects of interference in terms of physical trauma, discomfort, emotional and social distress and the detrimental effects this technology may have on the aspects of maternity care." We agree.

5. *The changing indications for cesareans* contribute to the rise. There is increased use of cesarean delivery for cephalo-pelvic disproportion (CPD), failure to progress, and breech presentation. Many doctors commented that a section may be safer than a vaginal breech birth because few doctors had sufficient experience with the latter. Marieskind[23] has questioned whether the seemingly superior outcome of cesareans-for-breech is due to the surgical intervention per se or the fact that cesarean-breech data are being compared with data of vaginal breech deliveries managed by people increasingly unskilled at such deliveries— an extremely important issue. Several physicians stated that no one knows how to do breech vaginals anymore. WHY DON'T THEY LEARN? Dr. Marieskind quoted one physician as follows:

> Section is remarkably safe, but we did have two deaths two years ago, in both of which the operation itself played a role. We have seriously infected patients from time to time. By and large, I think American obstetrics has become so preoccupied with apparatus and with possible fetal injury that the mothers are increasingly being considered solely as vehicles. In many instances, small and uncertain gain for the infant is purchased at the price of a small but grave risk to the mother. I don't think I have to spell out the politics of this for you.

6. *Age, parity, and fertility characteristics* have been cited as contributors to the rise. Older women and women bearing their first babies have increased in the child-bearing population. The declining fertility rate and decrease in average family size have led to the concept of "premium babies." Marieskind states that an analysis of national data does show changing ages, but they are not of significance to justify the increase in cesarean sections. She says that demon-

---

*M.G. Kerr, *Problems and Perspectives in Reproductive Medicine*, University of Edinburgh Inaugural Lecture, no. 61, 1975.

stration of shifts in parity and ages by itself does little toward contributing to an understanding of cesarean incidence.

7. *Economic incentives* are involved: increased earnings for obstetricians—more money for less time, a predictable expenditure of physician time, added length of hospital stay with increased hospital earnings, and greater reimbursement by third-party payment for a cesarean—provide little incentive to support vaginal birth or to adopt a "wait and see" attitude that could culminate in a vaginal delivery. Several physicians stated that they simply "couldn't afford not to do cesareans"[23] because of fear of malpractice suits or because of time constraints involved in attending deliveries and keeping office hours.

Marieskind suggests that a policy of accommodating deliveries to the "working day" also contributes to the cesarean increase.

8. *Technological interventions* appear to contribute to the rise in the cesarean rate. Interventionist procedures have permeated obstetrics. Marieskind reports that while these developments may help some people, they have "side-effects," one of which is increased cesarean sections. (For a further discussion of these "side effects," see Chapter 9.) Marieskind adds:

> There are many who argue that the woman is protected from technology—and therefore the potential of its promoting a cesarean—by the concept of informed consent. Unfortunately, this point of view ignores the practice of many hospitals to *insist* on interventions. It also ignores a very human dilemma; when a woman is pregnant or in labor and is told that "what we'll do will save your baby," she is most unlikely to refuse. . .

9. *Birthweight* is cited as a reason for the rising cesarean birth rate. Bigger babies would contribute to CPD. Marieskind points out that this reason is unsubstantiated because the average birthweight has increased only 2 ounces during the years in which the section rate has doubled. Cesarean section, however, is used as part of an "aggressive approach" to save low-birthweight infants.

10. Management of women with *chronic diseases* like diabetes and heart disease has improved to the degree where these women can now carry a pregnancy to term, and often their medical management includes delivery by cesarean section.

11. *Herpes II* is on the increase in the United States. Infants infected by vaginal herpes as they pass through the cervix can suffer from brain, kidney, or lung damage or can die. To avoid this possibility, the baby is delivered by cesarean. It is generally agreed that if cultures are negative late in pregnancy, if cervical smear shows no shedding, and if there are no lesions present in the vagina during labor, a vaginal delivery is appropriate.*

12. *Miscellaneous other factors* contributing to the cesarean epidemic have been identified. Multiple pregnancy was listed, although opinions differ greatly

---

*Further information about maternal herpes and vaginal birth is available in Chapter 13.

as to appropriate management in multiple gestations. Some physicians advocate cesarean section because the second twin is frequently in a breech or transverse position. Others advocate cesarean only for the second twin.

Several physicians commented that the increase in natural-childbirth classes contributes to an increased cesarean rate. Marieskind reports that a recent study of prepared-childbirth patients showed *no differences in obstetric outcome* between those women who had taken classes and those who had not. Included in miscellaneous factors is the statement by a few physicians that women are really afraid of labor and want a cesarean (sort of like a man fearing intercourse and preferring to be castrated!).

Lastly, Marieskind mentions physician attitude to cesarean section. Cesareans are now regarded as commonplace, she says. This is evidenced by many physicians who predicted that the section rate would climb because they are "just so easy." FOR WHOM, WE ASK? Several physicians asked: "What's so great about delivering from below, anyway?" This, about the miracle of birth, from obstetricians.

Cesareans are done for many reasons. In addition to the legitimate ones, they include power, control, money, fear and prestige. However, we believe that the most important reason is that most physicians totally lack understanding and respect for women and for birth. Repeat cesareans are done for the same reasons, with risk of uterine rupture the *excuse* for this deplorable crime.

The word obstetrician means "to stand before," to stand before a birthing woman in awe and reverence, not before an operating table, knife in hand.

Indications for Cesarean Section

When is a cesarean delivery really necessary? Marieskind divides the indications for cesarean section into two categories: *"absolute indications"* are those that determine that there is no other method by which a healthy, living child can be delivered, while *"relative indications"* are those where the physician determines that a cesarean delivery will offer a better outcome for mother and baby.

Absolute Indications

The absolute indications for a cesarean section are life-threatening and extremely rare. Maternal pelvic contraction is one example. Here the pelvis is clearly incapable of accommodating a mature fetus. Pelvic contraction may have been caused by injury to the pelvis, as in a car accident, or by extreme malnutrition, such as that suffered by American slaves in the early nineteenth century. A normal, reasonably healthy woman rarely has maternal pelvic contraction.

Prolapse of the umbilical cord, where the cord precedes the baby in the birth passage, is another absolute indication for a cesarean, as the pressure of the descending head on the cord can cut off the baby's blood and oxygen supplies. Hemorrhagic conditions also indicate the need for a surgical delivery. These include complete placenta previa, where the entire placenta has implanted over the opening of the cervix, and placenta abruptio, where the placenta separates from the uterine wall before the birth of the baby. Finally, a baby that stubbornly refuses to budge from a transverse presentation must be delivered by cesarean.

"Gray Area" Indications

Between "absolute" and "relative" reasons is a "gray area" of cesarean indications that depend on individual circumstances. In the past, diabetic mothers were almost all delivered by cesarean section to avoid the intrauterine fetal death that frequently occurred if pregnancy went beyond 38 weeks.[33] However, medical advances in the care of the pregnant diabetic are now allowing some diabetic women to carry to term and deliver vaginally. The same is true for women with heart disease. In some cases of placenta previa, if the placenta is only partially covering the cervix, a vaginal delivery is possible. Women with active vaginal herpes have also until recently been delivered by cesarean section, as exposure to the virus during vaginal birth could be lethal to the baby. Now it is known that vaginal birth can be safely achieved, depending on the location of the open herpes lesion. Another fetal indication for cesarean delivery is RH hemolytic disease, where the mother's RH-negative blood and the baby's RH-positive blood are incompatible. This indication is becoming virtually nonexistent, because of new methods of prevention of maternal sensitization. If the fetus is endangered by anemia as a result of RH disease, and the delivery cannot be induced safely and successfully, a cesarean delivery is required.[16] A failed induction to end toxemia of pregnancy may also lead to a cesarean.

However, it is the relative indications for cesarean section that are responsible for the increasing rates. These are the ones that are doctor-determined—and often, we believe, doctor-caused, or "iatrogenic."

Relative Indications

Dystocia   According to the NIH Conference Summary Report, a diagnosis of *dystocia* is responsible for 30 percent of the increased cesarean rates. "Dystocia" is a catch-all term that encompasses two groups of currently accepted indications for cesarean section. The first group includes problems such as cephalopelvic disproportion (CPD) and fetopelvic disproportion, where the baby's head or the whole baby is deemed too large to be accommodated by the mother's pelvis. The second group concerns problems of labor dysfunction, with such names as "failure to progress," "prolonged labor," and "uterine inertia." Of the 130,000 abdominally delivered pregnancies reviewed by the NIH for its study, dystocia was the indication for approximately 43 percent. Additionally, many reports list CPD as the primary cause of cesarean section and the primary indication for one-third to one-half of the operative procedures.[52]

CPD differs from maternal pelvic contraction in that it places the blame for the problem on both the baby and the mother. Because it is common for each successive baby to be a bit larger than its predecessor, many physicians tell a CPD cesarean mother that she will never give birth vaginally. We are happy to report that they are full of beans.

What we want you to remember is that CPD is fast becoming a grab-bag phrase, that it is an easy diagnosis for a physician to make when your baby refuses to simply fall out of you, and that it NEVER contraindicates an attempt at labor or VBAC. Saldana states that "previous fetopelvic disproportion does not rule out the possibility of vaginal delivery";[42] Bartholomew has recommended that patients who were sectioned previously for disproportion should not be denied consideration for vaginal delivery (in Reid and Barton);[25] and Morewood agrees that "a previous cesarean for CPD does not rule out subsequent vaginal delivery."

Ina May Gaskin, author of *Spiritual Midwifery*, tells us that most ladies' pelves are completely adequate in size to give birth to a normal-sized child because of natural selection over millions of years. It is important to remember, she says, that neither the pelvis nor the baby's head is a fixed size. Even if the pelvis is small, a fine natural delivery is still possible, provided the mother is strong and patient, "the rushes strong, and the vibrations good."[13]

In 1946, Heyns reported on the Bantu women in South Africa. He said that these women deliver babies spontaneously, although they have pelves so small that Western women would most assuredly need cesareans to deliver the same size babies. Heyns believes that psychological differences account for stronger uterine contractions, which help the baby be born:

> It is submitted that in the European world there is an unfavorable emotional background which has an inhibitory effect on efficient uterine activity. [When] there is emotional stability supported by unwavering resolution to push through with the task of spontaneous delivery, [any woman can equal] the achievement of the Bantu. Simple dystocia due to contracted bony passages can almost be eliminated by fostering the will in the parturient [that's you!] to deliver herself.*

*O.S. Heyns, "The Superiority of the South African Negro or Bantu as a Parturient," *J. Ob. Gyn. British Empire*, 53 (1946):405.

We need to learn from our sisters in South Africa. They have much to teach us. . .

Another Eastern culture, reported on by Marchand in 1932, believes women are better off dead than unable to bring forth their children by themselves.* They either birth or croak, and they prefer birthing.

A diagnosis of CPD made prior to the onset of labor is particularly suspect. During labor, the muscle fibers stretch, the central portion of the perineum thins, and the connective tissue ligaments of the pelvis soften and relax to give more room;[41] in addition, the flexible bones of the baby's head mold to decrease its circumference.[55] If a squatting position is assumed during pushing, the size of the pelvis may be increased more than a centimeter. A preliminary x-ray in the late stages of pregnancy cannot possibly account for the changes that will occur during labor. What it can do is begin a chain of events that will ultimately lead to a cesarean, for even the slightest mention of CPD is enough to undermine the first-time mother's confidence in her ability to birth. A labor and delivery-room nurse notes:

> The doctor examines the laboring woman and mentions on his way out that he's a bit worried about the pelvic margin. You can see the woman's approach change after that. Her heart goes out of it. Naturally, a few hours later, she's off to surgery.[51]

A woman who has once delivered a baby vaginally is almost never diagnosed as CPD in subsequent deliveries. Marieskind says, "It is possibly significant that while cephalopelvic disproportion can be determined by clinical or x-ray pelvimetry prior to delivery, neither it nor failure to progress can be determined by any quantifiable measure after the birth."[23] CPD is discussed further in other chapters of this book, especially in Chapter 5, in the section entitled "What If My Pelvis Is Too Small?"

"Failure to progress" is the other category of dystocia that by contemporary obstetrical standards necessitates a cesarean. Even as you read these words, thousands of laboring women in hospitals across the land are failing to progress. One of the roots of the problem is Friedman's curve, a graphic definition of "normal" labor patterns based on a study of the labors of a "large number" of women. *Williams Obstetrics* calls the limits set by the Friedman chart "admittedly arbitrary."[41] The NIH Draft Report[33] states:

> Functional definitions of abnormal labor progress, pioneered by Emanuel Friedman, are typically based upon a concept that the slowest progress experienced by a population of laboring gravidas is abnormal. . .the concept that slow progress constitutes abnormal progress permeates current obstetrical thinking, and although less easily documented, may also conceptualize the patient's expectations. Thus,

---

*L. Marchand, "Obstetrics among South African Natives," *South African Med. J.*, 6 (1932):329.

delivery for all patients in *less than 24 hours* has been advocated, as has intervention after *two to four hours* of poor progress in active labor [emphasis added].

"Although less easily documented" than the physician's expectations, the laboring woman's preconceived notions of normal labor do undermine her confidence when progress is slow. "I was found wanting at five centimeters," says the woman in Chase Collins' story "Random Voodoo."[7] Soon after that, she is on her way to a cesarean.

We have so many questions to ask about functional definitions of labor progress. How does one define the "beginning" of labor? (We know women who have experienced mild contractions for days and even weeks!) What is "normal" labor? How does one allow for the notorious slowing down of contractions under epidural anesthesia? What is "poor progress"? Does it generally indicate too-early arrival at the hospital? How is the labor being managed? Is the slowly progressing woman walking and taking nourishment and squatting when she pushes? Is she offered kind words and gentle encouragement when she becomes disheartened? Or is she lying flat on her back, I.V. in place, fetal monitor clattering away, food and drink denied, and all manner of analgesia and anesthesia offered when she shows signs of frustration? Has anyone put a time limit on her labor? We hope not. The idea of an optimum length of labor with its accompanying time constraints horrifies us. We have an image of a blustery physician charging into the labor room, shouting, "Time's up!" (That would be enough to make any uterus stop contracting!) We know that failure to progress is seldom an issue at home births or at midwife-attended births, and we contend that the mere idea of a time limit for delivery can be enough to cause labor dysfunction. In "The Cultural Warping of Childbirth," Doris Haire cites the belief of Dutch obstetricians that "when the labor of a normal woman is unhurried and allowed to progress normally, unexpected emergencies rarely occur."[14] Their belief is shared by the midwives of The Farm in Tennessee, a self-sufficient spiritual and farming community that delivers its own babies. Ina May Gaskin, The Farm's first midwife, cautions:

> The mother's rushes may or may not cause her cervix to dilate at a steady rate. You don't have to have any preconceived notions about what is too long for the first stage. If the mother is replenishing her energy by eating and sleeping, rushes are light, the baby's head is not being tightly squeezed and the membranes are still intact, the first stage can stretch over three or four days and still be perfectly normal.[13]

Few physicians are willing to take such a laissez-faire attitude toward a long labor, and the methods used to speed things along often lead to surgical delivery. We have much more to say about that in our chapter on medical interventions and their consequences.

When we consider that the maternal mortality ratio for dystocia is 41.9 deaths per 100,000 cesarean births as compared with 11.1 deaths per 100,000 vaginal births,[33] the need to evaluate dystocia as an indication for surgical delivery becomes even more compelling. In the meantime, it is important to remember that failure to progress, like CPD, never contraindicates VBAC for future deliveries. Pauerstein found in his VBAC study that "success in giving birth vaginally was not. . . related to the degree of cervical dilation attained in the previous labor or to whether the woman had labored at all."[52]

Prior Cesarean Delivery In fact, success in giving birth vaginally after a cesarean section isn't related to much that occurred in the prior labor. Yet prior cesarean delivery is second only to dystocia as an indication for cesarean section, accounting for almost 30 percent[33] of the increase in the cesarean rate and for over 30 percent[23] of the surgical deliveries performed. In the United States, more than 98 percent[33] of the women who have cesarean sections go on to deliver their next children surgically; in other words, less than 2 percent of cesarean mothers have subsequent children vaginally. The amount of unnecessary surgery performed via elective repeat cesareans is staggering. We are the only country where routine repeat cesarean is a matter of national policy.

When Edwin Craigin made his "Once a cesarean, always a cesarean" presentation to the New York Medical Society in 1916, the cesarean birth rate was less than 1 percent,[33] and the classical incision was in use. This incision extends vertically into the upper segment of the uterus and has a slightly higher potential for instability (1–3 percent) than the lower segment incision (0.5–1.5 percent). The lower segment incision is a low, horizontal "smile" or "bikini" cut that came into use in the 1930s for the purpose of allowing subsequent vaginal delivery. The lower segment incision is used in over 90 percent of current cesarean surgery, yet the idea of VBAC has yet to gain general acceptance with the American medical community.

> Vaginal delivery following cesarean section is neither unique nor experimental. There are several reports in the literature that attest to the feasibility of such a procedure, but the medical profession as a whole seems to exhibit a profound reluctance to accept the fact.[36]

As Douglas remarks, while "most dogmatic medical concepts are noted for their impermanence, Craigin's dogma is self-perpetuating because of fear of legal reprisal."* Fear of malpractice suits, fear of rupture, and fear of the relatively unknown combine to make many physicians reluctant to accept the realities of VBAC.

---

*Douglas, R.G., et al., "Pregnancy and Labor Following Cesarean Section," *American Journal of Obstetrics and Gynecology*, 86 (Aug. 1963), p. 961.

Other physicians, however, are learning to judge each labor on its own merit and not by the records of past deliveries. "The medical literature should encourage medical practitioners to seriously consider allowing a trial of labor," says S. McKay, editor of the ICEA Review; and, indeed, the medical literature is starting to do just that.[52] R. Gordon Douglas reports:

> With all facts entered on the ledger sheet, we have concluded after observing over 3,000 patients who have had a previous cesarean section that vaginal delivery is better for both mother and infant when there is no recurring or new indication for cesarean section. If progress is unsatisfactory or some complication develops during the course of labor, flexibility is maintained and *cesarean section can be resorted to at any time*. I feel that the results so obtained are superior to those obtained by routinely performing an elective repeat cesarean section [emphasis ours].[25]

Those who favor routine repeat cesarean because of its "ease" and "safety" need to be reminded that "all the factors that make cesareans so safe nowadays also serve to make VBAC safe, and more rewarding."[45] We agree with Meehan when he says that "elective repeat cesarean section is meddlesome obstetrics unless there is a recurring indication."[52]

Breech Presentation   One indication for cesarean that is not a recurring indication is *breech presentation*, which occurs in 3–4 percent of all pregnancies. Ina May Gaskin[13] describes three major types of breech presentation. In the complete breech, the thighs and knees are flexed, with the buttocks and feet presenting, and the baby is in a sort of upside-down fetal position. In the

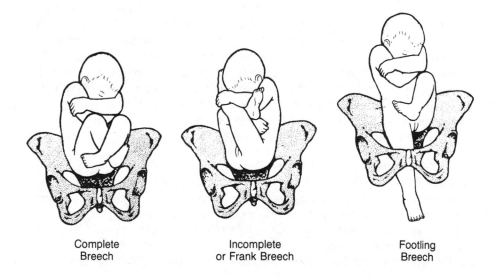

Complete
Breech

Incomplete
or Frank Breech

Footling
Breech

incomplete or frank breech, the baby is in a jack-knifed position, with the buttocks presenting and both feet touching the head. This is the most common breech position and the easiest presentation for a vaginal breech delivery. The footling breech presents one or both feet first and is the least common breech position. Breech presentation is associated with greater risk factors than the vertex (head down) position, yet cesarean delivery for breech babies is a fairly recent trend in American obstetrics. Some blame the increasing use of cesareans for breech on the failure of medical schools to train physicians to perform vaginal breech deliveries. One obstetrician reported:

> *Recently I had two breeches close together, assisted at each delivery by a first- or second-year resident. I discovered that these fellows knew practically nothing about breech delivery. They assumed that every breech was going to be delivered by cesarean section, and when it came to the delivery, they knew nothing about getting the arms out, about delivering the after-coming head, the use of Piper forceps, or any such things. Their first thought was—a breech; we do a cesarean. It seemed to me that there was too much science and not enough art. They knew all about ultrasonic monitoring, scalp sampling, all the ultrasonic things, but nothing about the actual technique and art of delivering a breech.*[23]

Others cite superior infant outcome as the reason for resorting to surgical breech delivery, although this contention is largely unsubstantiated.

In any case, the proportion of breech presentations delivered by cesarean rose from 11.6 percent in 1970 to 60.1 percent in 1978,[33] accounting for another 10–15 percent of the increase in the cesarean rate during those years. Approximately 12 percent of the cesareans performed are done because of breech presentation, and many institutions report that 60–90 percent of their breech presentations are delivered surgically.[23] Some physicians choose to deliver all multiple births by cesarean because often one of the babies is in a breech position. It is important to note here that the dramatic rise in the use of cesarean section for the delivery of breech babies has not been accompanied by measurable improvement in infant outcome. In fact, "there has been no overall decrease in mortality over a 10-year period for the total group of breech presentation."[33] A review of 457 breech deliveries at the Medical Center Hospital in Burlington, Vermont, showed "no significant improvement in death and morbidity rates for breech babies delivered by c/section over those born vaginally."[9]

Fetal Distress So-called fetal distress is responsible for another 10–15 percent of the increase and for 5 percent of the cesareans performed. There is no evidence that the actual incidence of fetal distress has changed; however, the diagnosis of fetal distress has become much more common over the past ten years. Many critics point an accusing finger at the electronic fetal monitor, and we will have much to say about this later (see Chapter 9).

By definition, "fetal distress during labor is a condition resulting from inadequate fetal oxygen supply and carbon dioxide removal."[33] Signs of possible fetal distress are meconium in the amniotic fluid or irregularities of the fetal heart rate. The NIH Draft Report notes, "In some instances infants predicted to be normal may have in fact experienced fetal distress and are depressed at birth. On the other hand, some infants predicted to be distressed appear normal at birth." When fetal distress does in fact occur, it is tragically often the result of interventions in the normal course of labor and birth. Labor stimulants such as pitocin (which is generally accompanied by analgesia to make the exaggerated contractions bearable or used to speed up labor once analgesia has slowed it down) put a great deal of stress on the fetus, as does artificial rupture of the membranes cushioning the baby's head. The common use of the lithotomy (flat on the back) position during labor allows the pressure of the uterus to rest on the inferior vena cava (the main blood vessel bringing blood back to the heart from the lower body) and to cut down the blood supply to the uterus. Lester Hazell[17] warns that there is no way of knowing how many cases of fetal distress are caused by the mother's remaining immobilized on her back because of a fetal monitor or I.V. Any interference in the rhythm and pattern of a woman's labor has the potential for distressing her baby.

More than any other indication for cesarean, fetal distress shows that the emphasis of the medical profession is on the fetus rather than the mother. The view of the baby as a delicate creature endangered by the turbulent forces of birth, a view held by the mother as well as by the physician, paves the way for many labor interventions and problems. In *Birthing Normally*, Gayle Peterson says that when we can see the baby as resilient and ready for the transition to outside the womb, and when we can see labor as a healthy process that stimulates the baby for breathing, then we have achieved the attitude for a healthy delivery.[37] In the meantime, we have to wonder why so many "fetal distress" babies are cut from their mothers' stomachs with Apgar scores of 9 and 10. Fetal distress as an indication for cesarean section is clearly in need of more accurate definition.

Failed Induction   Induction of labor is of two types: medical (use of drugs like pitocin) and surgical (artificial rupture of the membranes). Both types of induction put a great deal of stress on the baby and on the mother, both of whom are unprepared for a violent surge in active labor. The United States Food and Drug Administration has banned the use of oxytocin for elective induction of labor (induction for the convenience of the woman or her physician) because of the potential hazards of prematurity, fetal distress, newborn jaundice, rupture of the uterus, and higher cesarean rate.[53] It is now used primarily as a follow-up to artificial rupture of the membranes, which has a high failure rate and leaves the woman, in the eyes of her physician, highly susceptible to infection. When both surgical and medical induction have failed, a cesarean is performed to protect the woman from infections, which used to threaten within seventy-two hours but which for some reason have recently reduced their delay to only twelve hours. The NIH Summary Report points out the need for a safe and effective method of labor stimulation for those women who should not carry to term because of medical problems such as diabetes and toxemia. For all healthy, normal women, labor induction should be seen as the first step on the road to surgical delivery and, as such, should be heartily avoided.

Prematurity, Low Birthweight Finally, low-birthweight and premature babies are often delivered by cesarean because it is believed that they are unable to tolerate labor. Improved survival rates for these infants may be the result of recent innovations in newborn care rather than of surgical delivery.

The Cesarean Population

Which women are the most likely candidates for cesareans? Statistics show that by today's obstetrical standards, any pregnant woman is likely to fall prey to the knife, but Marieskind's report[23] suggests that women who have the highest incidence of cesarean section are as follows:

1. Women with the least and most education—the 1972 National Natality Survey showed the highest cesarean rate among women who were college graduates.
2. Women with the lowest and highest incomes—that is, women who don't have to pay and women who can afford to.
3. Women of the youngest and oldest ages—women in the under-15 age group are particularly high risk, and there has been a substantial increase in births among this age group. In women over 30, dysfunctional labor and/or malpresentation have been reported to be almost double. One study found that a higher incidence of sedation occurred in older women, that dysfunctional labor could generally be associated with sedation use, and that women 35 years and over were five times more likely to experience cesarean section. "In general, women outside the prime child-bearing years of 20–29 are potentially at higher risk and may have more complications with their pregnancies, thereby making a cesarean delivery more likely."[23]
4. Women with the lowest and highest parity—women who are primiparous (first delivery) or multiparous (six or more deliveries) are more likely to have cesareans. Primiparas generally have a higher rate of CPD, of hemorrhage, of dysfunctional labor, and of pre-eclampsia. According to Marieskind, it seems quite reasonable to expect that the number of complications reported in primiparous women may be in part attributable

to the physician's unfamiliarity with the patient herself and both the physician's and the patient's unfamiliarity with her ability to manage labor and delivery. Older women who are multiparas are more likely to have placental accidents and more likely to have multiple births, which increase the chances of toxemia and hemorrhage.

5. Women with public insurance and women with the most comprehensive private insurance.
6. Women who have no prenatal care and women who have the most prenatal care (perhaps because they are "high risk" to begin with).
7. Women who use general municipal hospitals and women who use exclusive private hospitals.
8. Women with low- or high-birthweight babies.
9. Women with low- or high-gestational-age babies.
10. Women who have lost a baby (and come to this birth with tension and fear).
11. Women with multiple births.
12. Women who are private as opposed to nonprivate patients.
13. Women who have taken childbirth-education classes and expect to be in complete control.
14. White women (a slight difference).
15. Metropolitan women (including high-risk women who have come to the city for better prenatal care).

Still, the most likely candidate for cesarean section is the woman who has already had one, and the uterine scar remains the single greatest indication for cesarean delivery.

For most of this century, the integrity of that scar has been the subject of debate and controversy. When we consider vaginal birth after cesarean, the scar is what makes us hesitate. Our doctors point at it knowingly and sadly shake their heads. It's as if we'd been branded "high risk" down at the O.R. Corral, so that in every obstetric territory they'll know we come from c/section. If we think about straying from the herd, they threaten us with "rupture"—a terrifying idea. "Rupture" is the risk they talk about when they warn us against VBAC. And what are the risks of cesarean section? "Oh, none," they tell us, "it's so safe that there's really no reason not to do it!"

Niles Newton remarks that physicians in the nineteenth century did a very successful advertising campaign to convince women that birth was dangerous. We would add that physicians in the twentieth century have done a very successful advertising campaign to convince women that cesarean section is safe. Right now we'll take "equal time" to give you some very frightening information about cesarean section. Later on in Chapter 5, we will address your fears about uterine instability and show you how sensible VBAC really is.

Risks of Cesarean Section to the Mother

This quotation from N. J. Eastman appeared in an issue of the *I.C.E.A. Review**
that focused specifically on vaginal birth following cesarean section:

> I gather the impression that, except in our own clinic, nothing ever goes wrong
> with a patient who has a cesarean section. Anesthetic mishaps are never mentioned,
> nor does appreciable blood loss or need for transfusion seem to occur (although
> everyone knows that the average blood loss at section is at least 700 cc.). These
> sectioned patients in the literature, however, appear to be immune to pulmonary
> embolism, and the ubiquitous staphylococcus passes them by; as for postoperative
> distention, one gets the impression that this complication is now of historic interest
> only. But in our own experience, the course of cesarean section is not always so
> tranquil, and once or twice a year we are scared to death by some section patient
> who acts up with one or another of these complications. True, we have not lost
> a section case for a good many years, but I wonder sometimes if our luck has not
> about run out. In any event, on the basis of my own experience, I find it difficult
> to believe that cesarean section, even today, is quite as safe as having a haircut,
> statistics to the contrary notwithstanding!

Eastman's skepticism, or at least his admission of it, is unusual. Most physicians would have us believe that a cesarean is a simple little operation, that
it is, indeed, "quite as safe as having a haircut." Not true! "The statement that
cesareans have never been safer for the mother," notes Doering,[7] "simply means
that the surgery is safer now than it was 20 or 50 years ago." Despite all the
wonderful advances in recent medical history that serve to minimize the risks
of cesarean delivery, a cesarean is still major abdominal surgery, with all the
risks inherent in any surgical procedure.

Major Abdominal Childbirth

In order to prevent any further comparisons between a cesarean section and
a haircut, we would like to share with you Dr. Michelle Harrison's description
of the cesarean delivery of a baby. We want to thank Michelle and her publishers
at Random House for allowing us to quote so extensively from her new book,
Woman in Residence.

> In the morning the woman is wheeled on a stretcher to the L&D (Labor and
> Delivery) suite, and then to the delivery room, which doubles as a section room.
> For epidural anesthesia, the woman is placed on the operating table on her left

---

*Vol. 3 (Dec. 1979), no. 3/4.

side. She is told to curl into a fetal-like position to allow a needle to be inserted between the vertebrae of her curved spine. When the needle is withdrawn, leaving a tube in the spine, the woman is placed flat on her back and the table temporarily tilted slightly to lower her head in order to establish a level of anesthesia that is high enough to make the woman's abdomen numb, but won't affect her ability to breathe. There is only a fine margin of both safety and comfort: if the level is too low, she will have pain during the surgery; if it is too high, she will have difficulty breathing and will require mechanical assistance.

The woman's bladder is next catheterized and the tube left in the bladder to keep urine draining. During the surgery the bladder is cut away from the surface of the uterus as there is a greater risk of perforating or cutting into it if it is full.

Preparation of the surgical site consists of scrubbing and draping the abdomen, with only that portion to be cut left exposed. It is similar to any other surgical preparation except for the inhibited discussion if the woman is awake.

I had been wondering why I always got so covered with blood and amniotic fluid during a Caesarean section, while the surgeon would come out so much cleaner. I would be soaked through my gown, my greens and my underwear. It was finally explained to me: "The table is tilted slightly so the blood and fluid run onto the assistant and not onto the surgeon."

As soon as the woman is draped, the anesthesiologist tilts the table to one side and signals for the surgeon to begin. The surgeon takes a scalpel from the nurse and with one strong and definite motion creates a crescent-shaped incision along the woman's pubic hairline. As the skin is cut, the subcutaneous tissue bulges upward as though it had been straining to get through all the time. Within moments this fatty tissue, interconnected by thin transparent fibers, becomes dotted and then covered with blood that oozes out of tiny vessels. With scalpel and forceps—delicate tweezers—the surgeon cuts deeper beneath the subcutaneous tissue, to a thick layer of fibrous tissue that holds the abdominal organs and muscles of the abdominal wall in place. Once reached, this fibrous layer is incised and cut along the lines of the original surface incision while the muscles adhering to this tissue are scraped off and pushed out of the way. The uterus is now visible under the peritoneum, a layer of thin tissue, looking like Saran Wrap, which covers most of the internal organs and which, when inflamed, produces peritonitis. The peritoneum is lifted away from the uterus and an incision is made in it, leaving the uterus and bladder easily accessible. The bladder is peeled away from the uterus, for the baby will be taken out through an incision in the uterus underneath where the bladder usually lies. When a Caesarean is done as an emergency procedure and speed is essential, the bladder is not removed and instead the incision is made much higher in the uterus. This produces weaker scar tissue and greater chance of rupture during a subsequent pregnancy and labor.

The uterus of the pregnant woman is large, smooth and glistening. Shaped like a huge pear, the top and sides are thick and muscular, the lower end thin and flexible. With short careful strokes of a knife, a small incision is made through the thinner segment. Special care is taken not to cut the baby or the membranes surrounding the baby which, if still intact, now bulge through the tiny hole in the uterus. The room becomes silent: the quiet presence of the baby about to be born causes time suddenly to stop.

The obstetrician extends the initial cut either by putting two index fingers into the small incision and ripping the uterus open or by using blunt-ended scissors and cutting in two directions away from the initial incision. If the membranes are still intact, they are now punctured with toothed forceps, and the fluid spills out onto the table. In the normal position, the baby's head is down and under the incision, so the obstetrician places one hand inside the uterus, under the baby's head, and with the other hand exerts pressure on the upper end of the uterus to push the baby through the abdominal incision. The assistant also uses force now to help push the baby out. Once the baby's head is out, the throat is immediately suctioned with a small ear syringe, and then the shoulders and rest of the body are eased out. Held in the air, the baby usually begins to cry. The cord is clamped and the baby handed over to a nurse holding a warmed towel. Sometimes, en route to the nurse, the infant is momentarily held over the woman's head with its genitals facing down into the mother's face, as she is told, "Look, it's a boy/girl!" The assumption is always made that the woman wants most to know and see the sex of her child. For many women, including those delivering vaginally, this is all they see of their babies at the time of delivery.

The rest of the surgery is more difficult for the woman. There is more pain and women often vomit and complain of difficult breathing as we handle their organs and repair the damage. This period may also be more difficult because there is no longer the anticipation of waiting to see the baby born. Sometimes the woman is given sedation for the rest of the surgery.

The placenta separates from or is peeled off the inside of the uterus. Then, since the uterine attachments are all at the lower end, near the cervix, the body of the uterus can be brought out of the abdominal cavity and rested on the outside of the woman's abdomen, thus adding both visibility and room in which to work.

With large circular needles and thick thread a combination of running and individual stitches is used to sew closed the hole in the uterus. A drug called pitocin is added to the woman's IV to help the uterus contract and to decrease the bleeding. Small sutures are used to tie and retie bleeding blood vessels. The "gutters," spaces in the abdominal cavity, are cleared of blood and fluid. The uterus is then placed back in the abdominal cavity. The bladder is sewn back onto the surface of the uterus, and then finally the peritoneum is closed. Now sponges are counted to be sure none have been left inside the abdominal cavity, and then the closure of the abdominal wall begins.

Muscles overlying the peritoneum are pushed back in place, and are sometimes sewn with loose stitches. Fascia, the thick fibrous layer, is the most important one, since it holds all the abdominal organs inside and keeps them from coming through the incision, especially if the woman coughs or sneezes. Therefore this layer is closed with heavy thread and many individual stitches so that, even if a thread breaks, the stitches won't all come out. The subcutaneous tissue, most of which is fat, is closed in loose stitches that mainly close any air spaces which might become sites for infection. Skin, the final layer, is closed with silk or nylon thread or metal staples. The appearance of the final scar is generally considered important, since many people judge whether a surgeon is good or not by the scar's appearance.

A dry bandage is placed over the woman's incision and then taped to her skin. The drapes are removed. A baby has been born.[15]

However, for far too many women and their infants, the trauma is not over.

Maternal Death

In "Complications of Cesarean to Mother and Infant,"[3] Madeleine Shearer summarizes the physiologic costs of cesarean section to the mother. Some of these are pain and depression, gas, infection, hemorrhage, adhesions, injury to adjacent structures, blood transfusion complications, aspiration pneumonia, anesthesia accidents, cardiac arrest, and death.

Death. Although we tend to think of cesarean section as a life-saving rather than a life-threatening procedure, the maternal mortality rate for cesarean patients is not insignificant. Evrard and Gold, in their eleven-year study of maternal death associated with cesarean section in Rhode Island,[12] found that "the risk of death from cesarean section was 26 *times greater* than with vaginal delivery" (emphasis ours). A recently completed analysis of maternal deaths in Georgia showed a mortality ratio of 59.3/100,000 births by cesarean section as compared with 9.7/100,000 vaginal births.[33] A California study showed the risk of maternal death associated with cesarean section to be two to three times greater than that for vaginal delivery.[39] All of these studies took into account the conditions that necessitated the cesarean and only included deaths that were due to the surgery itself.

Maternal mortality statistics are difficult to assess because maternal death is notoriously underreported (or covered up!). The *Ob./Gyn. News* for July 1980 describes a study of cesarean sections performed in Georgia in 1975, where eleven deaths were determined by routine surveillance of death certificates. Upon further investigation, five more cesarean-associated deaths were identified. By obtaining additional information from the medical examiner's reports, the hospital records, the police reports, and the women's physicians and families, researchers attributed nine of the total sixteen deaths to the surgery itself. The reported cause of death in those nine cases was pulmonary embolism, in six women, and complications of anesthesia, in three. In this article, Dr. George L. Rubin stated that earlier studies had underestimated the risks of cesarean sections and that physicians should carefully assess the risks whenever they are considering performing a section.

Maternal death is defined as one related to pregnancy and/or the process of childbirth. An article in the Winter 1981 issue of *NAPSAC News* warns that "the time span of consideration" for maternal death often extends only to the sixth week following a live birth, so that the death of a mother after this time span is not attributed to pregnancy-related causes even when it should be. Additionally, many maternal deaths that occur closer to the time of birth are not recorded as maternal mortalities because the woman with severe complications has been moved from maternity to another wing of the hospital and is no longer considered a maternity patient.

The NAPSAC article cites a study of childbirth-related deaths that found a significant number of maternal deaths to be due to complications of cesarean delivery. Yet the death certificates of many of these women made no mention whatever of the cesarean surgery or even of the fact that they had been recently pregnant. This article suggests that maternal deaths in the United States may be double the rates reported. "Theoretically," it says, "the period of time during which a maternal death could occur would begin with conception and extend through the year following birth."

The NIH Draft Report cites the fact that maternal deaths are underreported in vital records—probably seriously underreported—as one of the major problems in data evaluation. Most of the NIH data on maternal mortality comes from the Professional Activities Study (PAS), an organization that collects data from a large number of hospitals throughout the United States and provides the largest single tabulation of information on cesareans in the country. Of interest to us is the PAS finding[33] that the relative risk of maternal death in a repeat cesarean delivery increased during the eight-year period 1970–1978. (We thought you might like to have that bit of information to offer your doctor when you are discussing VBAC with him!) The NIH Task Force determined that "cesarean delivery carries about four times the risk of maternal mortality of a vaginal delivery" and that "cesarean delivery for previous cesarean carries two times the risk of maternal mortality of all vaginal deliveries."[33] We believe these figures to be conservative.

Maternal Illness and Disability

The NIH Task Force also determined that maternal morbidity (disease) rates are generally five to ten times higher after cesarean delivery than after vaginal delivery:

A cesarean delivery is a major operative procedure and as such is associated with many complications leading to maternal morbidity that are never encountered in a vaginal delivery. Examples of these complications include operative injuries to the urinary tract and bowel, wound abscess, wound dehiscence, evisceration, operative and postoperative hemorrhage, and paralytic ileus. In addition, complications such as pulmonary emboli, venous thrombosis, and anesthesia related morbidity are more common following a major operative procedure. Consequently, maternal morbidity associated with cesarean delivery is substantially higher than the morbidity associated with a vaginal delivery.[33]

"Infections constitute the greatest portion of this morbidity," the NIH Summary Report concluded, and "the most common infections are endometritis, urinary tract infections, and wound infections." But hemorrhage is also not uncommon, with the average blood loss following cesarean section estimated to be about 1000 cc., double the usual blood loss following vaginal birth.[38]

Most of the studies we have read report a 50 percent morbidity rate associated with cesarean section. What this means is that 50 percent of all new mothers delivered by cesarean section have some serious illness such as infection or hemorrhage![11] "Almost half of all cesarean patients had one or more operative complications," Madeleine Shearer found in her study, "including a respectable number of severe complications which compromised future child-bearing or were potentially lethal."[44]

McGaughey et al. add that "maternal morbidity in repeat sections is high."[25] Their study of pregnancy and labor following cesarean section showed that the complications of repeat cesarean section "were of sufficient magnitude in many cases to cause severe, even if limited, disability," and that "the incidence of wound infection and disruption, pneumonia, bladder injury, septicemia, and pelvic thrombophlebitis indicates that the procedure is not benign."

Like maternal mortality, maternal morbidity associated with cesarean section is seriously underreported. Few follow-up studies are done once women leave the hospitals, and physicians do not talk about the postoperative complications they treat—especially not with their pregnant clients. Few women are even remotely aware of the risks to which they subject themselves when they submit to surgical delivery. No one tells them about the risks of infection and hemorrhage. No one tells them about the risk of adhesions that result in intestinal obstruction, or the risk of postoperative urinary-tract symptoms resulting from the adherence of the bladder flap to the uterus. No one talks about possible injuries to the bladder during abdominal delivery. The only risk that is discussed with the cesarean patient, if she is lucky and there is time, is the risk of anesthesia; and while she is made to feel that she has a voice in the decision about which one to use, she generally does not have the option to refuse it altogether. The role of anesthesia is an important consideration when assessing the risks and benefits of cesarean section, for anesthesia is a necessary component in the operative procedure.

Exposure to anesthesia always carries a risk which, Marieskind notes, increases with each successive episode;[23] and, given the current policy of repeat cesarean section, most cesarean mothers will undergo additional surgery for subsequent pregnancies. The possibility of an anesthesia accident is a risk inherent in any surgical procedure, but it has the potential for being doubly tragic in cesarean surgery because there are (at least) two patients involved. Maternal deaths related to anesthesia continue to occur, and most of these are avoidable.[33] But in every case, use of anesthesia can cause serious problems. Appropriate selection and better technique can reduce these risks. Both the physician and the mother have responsibilities in this regard.

> The best that obstetricians can do is to be aware of the knowledge about drug effects on the mother, the labor, and the fetus, and when they are truly indicated, use the minimum amount of the apparently safest medication to achieve the necessary result. Similarly, the mother must also make herself aware of the results which may ensue from medications used during labor, and temper both her demands and her acceptance of such medications with that knowledge.[26]

A knowledge of the types of anesthesia used for cesarean section and their inherent dangers is essential to every pregnant woman.

General anesthesia works quickly and requires less skill to administer than other anesthesia. Its well-known disadvantages are an unconscious mother, the hazard of aspiration of gastric contents into the lungs (a common cause of anesthetic death), and a depressed newborn. In addition, women are generally groggy and depressed themselves for days following the use of general anesthesia. Having missed not only the birth but also the critical bonding period, they often feel alienated from the baby and from the birth experience itself. Mothers who have had general anesthesia have much more difficulty integrating and accepting their cesarean sections.

Because of those disadvantages, most women today who are allowed a choice select regional anesthesia instead. Regional anesthesia is of two types: spinal and epidural. Spinal anesthesia involves the injection of a local anesthetic into the lumbar subarachnoid space. Its disadvantages are its effects on the baby and its possible complications: hypotension (reduced blood flow), total spinal blockade with respiratory paralysis, anxiety and discomfort, spinal headaches, and bladder dysfunction. The incidence of maternal hypotension after spinal anesthesia, estimated to be as high as 80 percent, is a contributory factor to maternal anesthesia-related morbidity.

Lumbar epidural anesthesia also involves the injection of a local anesthetic into an area of the spine, but this time into the epidural space. Often a catheter is inserted so that reinforcement of pain relief may be provided, as larger doses of local anesthetic are required than with the spinal. The disadvantages are the greater amounts of anesthetic required, the effects on the baby, and the possibility of inadvertent spinal anesthesia when the dura is accidentally punctured. As with spinal anesthesia, epidurals also carry the risks of hypotension and convulsions, or even cardiac arrest due to central nervous system stimulation.

An additional concern with epidural anesthesia is the likelihood of "spottiness" in pain relief. Areas called "windows" may be unaffected by the anesthesia, with the result that the women can feel everything that is going on in that particular spot—cutting, pulling, stitching, everything! As you can see, choosing your anesthesia is really deciding which is the least of the evils.

Seldom mentioned in connection with cesareans and drugs is the cesarean mother's increased need for postpartum drugs. It's as if no one wants to talk about how much she is going to hurt. The fact that the surgery is so painful is often a surprise and a difficulty. There is a catch 22: you can take medication and be too groggy and weak to hold the baby, or you can not take it and be in too much pain to care about holding the baby. "My baby and I, we just lay there and cried together," one woman wrote, "he in his bed and I in mine— I couldn't even lean over to pick him up." In "Unnecessary Cesareans: Doctor's Choice, Parent's Dilemma," Susan Doering says,

> Not only are 50 percent of surgically delivered women actually sick postpartum, but virtually 100 percent experience a great deal more pain, weakness, problems moving around, and difficulties caring for their newborns. In my own research, I observed that women who had been delivered by cesarean were significantly more negative about their birth experience, were much more miserable physically, required far more drugs postpartum, experienced more serious and longer-lasting depression, and did not "feel like a mother" . . . till much later than the vaginally delivered women. Many other researchers have reported on the shock, deep disappointment, feelings of failure, and other negative emotions experienced by cesarean mothers postpartum. Surgery is never a pleasant experience, but becoming a mother through major abdominal surgery is particularly difficult. Helpless, dependent newborns cannot wait until their mothers "recover"—they need mothering at once.[11]

When we look upon the cesarean section as major abdominal surgery, we are able to see the risks of a whole range of physiologic complications. When we look upon it as the birth of a baby, we need to examine its potential for psychological trauma and consequent mothering difficulties. The psychological complications can be as debilitating as the physiological ones.

Psychological Complications

Gayle Peterson says, "How a woman gives birth has been found to influence her confidence and ability to mother."[37] The cesarean mother is at a decided disadvantage; she is a mother, yes, but she has not given birth. Having lost control over her childbirth experience, she is likely to feel cheated, disappointed, angry, frustrated, guilty, regretful, helpless, and depressed. In addition, she may experience a sense of failure, distaste for her scar, and envy of those who have given birth vaginally. These are not healthy feelings with which to welcome a newborn, and others will soon grow impatient with her.

Often there is little sympathy for a cesarean mother the first few days after surgery. "C'mon, Sally, let's get going here. You've only had a baby. Let's not pamper ourselves. Hop out of bed!" (Hop? Hop? How about a shuffle?) No one would expect someone who had just had an appendectomy to begin caring for another person within hours after the operation; yet the cesarean mother, having undergone the same kind of major abdominal surgery, is expected to do just that. Or, at the other extreme, she is separated from her baby immediately after delivery and only allowed to see him for a few moments every four hours. ("You must get your rest, dear. We're taking lovely care of him in the nursery!") There is a balance, and it's up to the hospital staff to find it. Those who tend to the cesarean mother postpartum need to remember that the psychological assimilation of the birth process is generally longer for her than it is for the mother who delivers vaginally.[51]

In "The Cesarean Section Patient Is a New Mother, Too," Betsy Bampton and Joan Mancini advise nurses to pay special attention to the cesarean mother's needs as a maternity patient. They emphasize the importance of communicating with her—before the surgery, to prepare her; during the surgery, to reassure her; and after the surgery, to comfort her. They also point out the importance of making sure that the new cesarean mother has access to her baby immediately after the delivery and often thereafter. Providing her with emotional and physical comforts and the opportunity to get to know her baby in a nonthreatening way will give her the time and energy to try to integrate all that she has just gone through.

> The cesarean section patient needs to relive her labor and delivery experience so she can finalize her pregnancy, face the separation from her fetus, and integrate this experience into her life pattern. The experience may be traumatic. She may misunderstand events, forget moments of the experience or her response to it because of fear and apprehension.[4]

On the other hand, the new cesarean mother may feel fine, be delighted with her baby, and take her departure from the hospital without any extraneous emotional baggage. The woman who readily accepts her cesarean experience is not necessarily healthier, just different.

Risks of Cesarean Section to the Infant

When we talk about the risks of cesarean section, it is sometimes easy to forget the smaller, less verbal, and more helpless patient involved. But the risks of surgical delivery to the infant must not be overlooked; they are very real, quite dangerous, and too common. Among those listed by Madeleine Shearer[44] are jaundice, fewer quiet and alert periods after birth, iatrogenic respiratory distress, neonatal drug effects, abnormal or suspect neurological exams, low birthweight, neonatal acidosis due to maternal hypotension, inadvertent infant-to-placenta transfusion, and neonatal death.

We have long known about the danger of anesthesia to the unborn child, and this is the most obvious fetal risk of all surgical deliveries, in first and repeat c/ sections combined. Doris Haire[14] warned us years ago about the role that medication plays in our "staggering incidence of neurological impairment." She cautioned that an infant who showed no signs of respiratory distress and scored well on the Apgar scale could, upon closer investigation, show lingering signs of oxygen deprivation resulting from obstetrical medication administered to the mother. She told us that "we can no longer assume that the apparent recovery of an asphyxiated infant after successful resuscitation is a guarantee that the infant has come through unharmed." Ms. Haire went on to say that a baby with a heartbeat after cardiac massage may appear to be recovered but, in fact, may be "irreversibly brain-damaged."

Our confidence in drug-testing programs should have been weakened by what happened with Thalidomide and DES. Yet many of us continue to assume that science and government protect us and our infants from drug-related tragedies. All pregnant women should be warned that the Food and Drug Administration has no regulations whatever regarding drugs and the child-bearing woman. It does not require that obstetrical drugs be proved safe for the fetus.[9]

It takes only seconds or minutes for anesthesia (or in fact any medication) to cross the placenta and enter the circulatory system of the unborn infant; it takes days and even weeks for the newborn's immature excretory system to rid his body of the effects of these medications. The sluggishness and depression exhibited by the medicated newborn may mask other problems that require immediate attention.[23] At the least, they serve to interfere with the infant's suckling reflexes, thus preventing him from getting the full immunologic advantage of his mother's colostrum and inhibiting the start of the breastfeeding relationship.

In addition to lower Apgar scores and an "alarmingly high incidence of asphyxia,"[52] cesarean newborns exhibit problems such as a greater intracellular water content, wet lung, lower blood volumes, and lower plasma levels.[3] Dr. Mary Ellen Avery, in a study of the effects of cesarean delivery on the fetus, concluded that "morbidity and mortality are greater among infants delivered by cesarean section."[3]

Fetal mortality rates are even more difficult to determine than maternal mortality rates. Some figures show greater mortality rates among vaginally delivered babies, which would tend to support those cesarean advocates who claim better results from surgical delivery. However, R. Gordon Douglas [25] gives us three reasons why their claims are unjustified:

1. When a fetus is known to be dead, a physician will not perform a cesarean. Therefore, intrauterine death becomes part of the vaginal-birth mortality statistics.

2. When a fetus is very small for date, it may be delivered vaginally. Thus, many premature or low-birthweight babies, who are known to be high risk, may be part of the vaginal-birth statistics.

3. A baby known to have severe congenital abnormalities will not be delivered by cesarean and so is likely to join the vaginal-birth mortality statistics.

Douglas concluded that there is "no evidence that vaginal delivery per se is responsible for a higher perinatal mortality than cesarean section. In fact, our data indicated that a number of infants delivered by elective cesarean section were premature and died as a result of pulmonary complications."[25]

For elective repeat cesareans, fetal mortality statistics are available, and they are high.[46] Studies have shown death rates varying from three to seven times higher in babies delivered by scheduled cesarean than in those whose mothers were allowed to start labor.[3] A 1969 study showed that 1 out of 100 mature infants died after elective primary or repeat cesarean with no trial of labor. Benson determined that neonatal mortality was twice as high in infants delivered by repeat cesarean without labor when compared to a vaginally delivered control group.[11] He also found that four times as many cesarean babies had dangerously low five-minute Apgars (0.3 range) and that reasons for favoring vaginal delivery were evident at both the four-month and one-year pediatric neurologic exams.

Petitti reports that a comparison of neonatal mortality rates for 1976–1977 for vaginally delivered infants with those delivered by repeat cesarean showed a higher rate of neonatal mortality in the repeat cesarean group for all birthweights.[23]

These studies support Douglas's contention that "cesarean section should not be done until there is definite evidence of labor."[25]

The villain in elective cesarean delivery (whether it be primary or repeat) is iatrogenic prematurity, or the doctor's miscalculation of the baby's readiness to be born. (This also occurs commonly in inductions.) In addition to low birthweight, the danger of prematurity is an immature respiratory system, which can cause respiratory distress syndrome (RDS) or hyaline membrane disease (HMD). Prematurity is estimated to exist for 5–22 percent of c/section babies as compared with 6–7 percent of babies born vaginally.

Respiratory problems in the premature newborn are caused by a deficiency in alveolar surfactant. Surfactant develops in the lungs at about 36 weeks and helps get oxygen to the body tissues. There is a test to measure its presence and thus the lung maturity of the baby: The pulmonary phospholipids in surfactant are synthesized by the lung and secreted into the amniotic fluid.[23] A sample of fluid can be removed by a procedure called "amniocentesis," which itself carries many associated risks (see Chapter 8). The fluid is analyzed, and the ratio of two of the phospholipids, lecithin and sphingomyelin, is used as the internal standard. This is called the L/S test. Like all the other tests, it measures only one aspect of fetal maturity and has the potential for being inaccurate, but it's better than most educated guesses when a woman must be sectioned without benefit of labor.

Much of the perinatal mortality and morbidity from iatrogenic prematurity is preventable. First of all, the physician should encourage his patients to work toward vaginal birth after cesarean rather than elective repeat section. If VBAC is impossible, he can wait until the woman goes into labor before he delivers her by cesarean. This has the advantage of establishing fetal maturity and stimulating lung action in the fetus (the "thoracic squeeze") by the contracting uterus. It also thins out the uterus and minimizes blood loss. [23]

Second, the physician must be convinced that a simple clinical estimate of fetal age and maturity is not an adequate means of determining optimal birth date. He must learn to routinely perform the available tests for maturity on any woman for whom labor is contraindicated. While the L/S test has the potential for greatly reducing the risk of iatrogenic prematurity, the trial-of-labor test has the potential for pretty much eliminating it altogether. Saldana[42] found that infants delivered following a trial of labor had reached optimal fetal growth and maximum lung capacity.

We have looked at how cesarean section endangers mothers and at how it endangers infants. Now let's look at how cesarean delivery threatens the mother/infant relationship.

Risks of Cesarean Section
to the Mother/Infant Relationship

In "Bonding: How Parents Become Attached to Their Babies," Diony Young states that "a positive childbirth experience appears to create in the mother an increased self-esteem and self-confidence."[53] This, in turn, may foster maternal bonding. On the other hand, Young tells us, "A negative birth experience, where fear and pain predominate, may adversely affect a mother's feelings toward her child." Because a cesarean delivery is so often a negative experience colored by fear and pain, the cesarean mother and child are at a decided disadvantage as they begin their life together. Often the mother is medicated, sluggish, depressed, angry, disappointed, and all those other feelings we've mentioned. The baby is groggy or fussy because of the effects of the anesthesia and other complications. And these two are supposed to be gazing into each other's eyes with everlasting love?! Add to this the hospital procedures that routinely separate cesarean mothers from their newborns, and this couple is off to a very difficult start.

Recently, because of the studies by Marshall Klaus[19] and others, there has been a great surge of interest in the issue of bonding—the early development of the unique attachment between mother (and father) and baby. Research by Klaus and by Salk[43] demonstrated that the first 24 hours postpartum are a crucial period for the development of the normal mother/infant bond. Moreover, it was pointed out that hospital routines, which generally separated babies from their mothers during that postpartum period, served to inhibit rather than encourage the mother's nurturing instincts.

It wasn't long before parent groups, studies in hand, began to bang on the doors of hospital administrators demanding change. And it wasn't long before the hospitals responded to consumer demand and began to institute rooming-in, whereby mother and baby became roommates and touched, stared at each other, got to know each other, smiled at each other, and bonded. Although rooming-in has become pretty much standard fare in hospitals across the country, it is still routinely denied many cesarean mothers. The cesarean newborn is still required by too many hospitals to spend the first 24 hours—bonding time!—in a special-care nursery, in an artificial warmer, alone and apart from the one person who knows his needs best, away from what Doris Haire calls "the most logical of warming devices," his mother's arms.

The immediate results of all this are that the mother is more a hospital patient than a mother, and the baby is lying alone, at the peak of his sucking reflex, not learning how to nurse. Both Klaus and Salk demonstrated that maternal response and nurturing are adversely affected a full one month after birth when the mother and her baby have been thus separated.[14] (It's significant that of all the risks associated with cesarean section, this risk to the mother/infant bond is the one that makes consumer groups the most irate. Forget morbidity and mortality: bonding is the issue around which they rally. "You can take my health, and you can take my life, but you can't take my relationship with my child!" they seem to say.)

What are the long-range effects of early mother/baby separation? Klaus and his associates feel that the "battered child syndrome" may be one.[2] Lynch reported, in a study of child abuse, that bonding failure is related to the mother's pregnancy, her labor, her delivery, and the amount of neonatal separation she endured.[*] Also mentioned in this study was the high incidence of prematurity among abused children. Others question whether the mothers of abused children have a higher cesarean rate than that of the general population. Given the greater likelihood that the cesarean baby will be premature and will be separated from his mother immediately postpartum, the implications for his future warrant further examination.

Despite all of these physiological and psychological maternal and fetal risks,

---

*M. Lynch, "Ill-Health and Child Abuse," *Lancet* (16 Aug. 1975):317.

the force that ultimately turns the cesarean tide may well be the economic cost of cesarean section to the consumer.

Costs of Cesarean Section

The costs of a cesarean vary widely throughout the United States, but they are always greater than the costs of a vaginal delivery. In general, physicians charge about a third more for a surgical delivery, and the hospital stay for both mother and baby is about double. Marieskind[23] warns that sometimes there are additional charges for the use of the operating room, the use of the recovery room, additional supplies, anesthesia, lab work, pharmacy items, I.V. equipment, blood transfusions, oxygen, and x-rays.

All of these expenses also hold true for the cost of a repeat cesarean as compared with a trial of labor and a vaginal delivery. In a study by Shy et al.,[46] the cost difference between an elective repeat cesarean and a VBAC averaged $500 per patient. As we have already mentioned, the Marieskind report estimated that "in 1976 alone, we could potentially have saved about 95 million dollars had a policy of individual evaluation and subsequent vaginal deliveries been followed." Many are starting to look at midwives and homebirth as a way to cut costs and avoid the interventions that lead to cesareans. Mahan, as reported in the *ICEA Review* in 1979, predicts that when the insurance companies and the professional service review organizations start to realize the tremendous cost savings of VBAC, they will exert economic pressure to end the practice of routine repeat cesareans.[52] But until that happens, American babies will continue to be "from their mothers' wombs untimely ripp'd."

Conclusions

In its summary statement, the NIH Task Force concluded that the rising cesarean section rate is "a matter of concern." Its members agreed that the cesarean trend could be stopped and indeed reversed "while continuing to make improvements in maternal and fetal outcomes."

We also conclude that the rising cesarean section rate is a matter of concern. It is a matter of grave concern. The cesarean epidemic must be brought under control. Too many mothers and their babies are being needlessly exposed to avoidable risks, and too many physicians are refusing to admit it. As it becomes increasingly apparent that the medical profession is not going to put constraints upon itself, it becomes more and more obvious that we, the consumers, are going to have to take control.

In the meantime, the silent knife continues to slash its way across the stomach of America, maiming our confidence in our bodies and murdering our hopes and dreams for our children's births. Its quick, stealthy flash cuts through to the core of our being, stripping us of our illusions of control and leaving us wounded and vulnerable.

Hear now the voices of its victims.

3 ❧ *Voices of the Victims*

Letters and calls from cesarean mothers have poured into C/SEC's office and Nancy's home since 1973. To date, they number well over forty thousand. They come from all over the United States and beyond. Most contain pleas for caring, understanding, support, and information.

We invite you to read excerpts from some of these letters. As you will see, the letters speak so eloquently on their own that no commentary is necessary.

LETTERS FROM CESAREAN MOTHERS

Last June, after fifteen hours of hard labor I underwent a cesarean section for which I was totally unprepared. The problems I've had and some I'm still having I'm sure are all stories you've heard so I won't go into detail. Basically it has made me feel less than a total woman. I felt like I had failed. Now I'm sure in my head that the feeling is silly but my heart aches. It's been almost a year and I believe I'm starting to be able to sort out my feelings; however, it has been a long hard year and I feel sure that if I had someone whom I could have gone to and knew they understood because they had been through it too, I might have gotten over this a lot quicker.

—Michele (North Carolina)

I had my first child by cesarean eighteen months ago. It was a long labor and then I developed a wound infection and ran a 103° temperature for four days. My baby, who I waited for for so long to be with, was kept from me for over twenty-four hours . . . . About half of my incision broke open.

I am absolutely determined to try a vaginal delivery the next time. My OB told me all the standard "horror stories," but I'm not convinced. I strongly feel the risk lies in major surgery. He finally said that he would consider it only if I would consent to a cesarean the minute that my labor deviated from the "normal" in the least bit. This idea terrifies me, since it smacks of the typical type of patronizing that obstetricians have always given women to shut them up. I'm terrified that once I'm in the hospital in labor, I will be badgered and bullied into consenting to anything the doctor wants to do. I would dearly love to have a home birth but my doctor is against home births in any case, and laughed at my "foolish notion." Then, he showed me the record of my pelvic measurements that he took when I was entering my ninth month of pregnancy. I am smaller than normal in every way, but when I was measured almost two years ago, he told me that my pelvis was adequate for a vaginal delivery. I don't see why it was okay then and too small now.

I'm so frightened of becoming pregnant again for fear of being manipulated by people who are considering themselves instead of me and my baby and my precious toddler. I desperately need advice and encouragement. Please help me. If you were able to have vaginal deliveries, and one of them a home birth, maybe there's hope for me.

—Jocelyn (New Jersey)

I am a nurse, and one of your classic examples of unnecessary primary cesarean. My physician told me I had CPD. I was young, inexperienced, and uneducated. The fact that I only labored two hours didn't strike me as being an unfair trial of labor until later, unfortunately! My baby was groggy for days from the general anesthesia, sucked poorly, and coupled with the fact a diuretic was ordered unbeknown to me, my breastfeeding was a total failure. All in all, not a pleasantly memorable birth experience.

—May (New Hampshire)

Four years ago my doctor decided it would be best for me and my baby to have a cesarean birth operation. The baby was breech. The baby was fine but they couldn't bring me out of the general anesthesia and I was put on a respirator to survive. I suffered very much. It was a terrible experience.

Now my husband and I are considering having another child, but I am terrified because of my first experience. The doctor says he will give me another cesarean because he believes it is too much of a risk to attempt a vaginal delivery.

—Theresa (New York)

Whale

"Like a beached whale"–
the phrase
keeps bubbling up –
Flopped
gracelessly
upon unyielding sand
and pebbles
I lie
on the hard confines
of
this narrow bed
clothed in
white sheets
pain
and slow ticking time

Later. . .
heaved over
onto
my left side
I complain
tremulously
resenting this disturbance
of my tenuous
hold on the spasm
screaming up my back

Rubber gloves
grope
measuring
assessing
probing your skull
to monitor
your fragile
pounding
heart

(Do anything –
get this child
out)
You don't exist –
my cramping uterus
is numb now
to the sensuous pressure

of your limbs
heels
knees
fists
head
bum
wriggling so long
within
you
are
stone now
muscled and gripped
tight in my belly
The dials flip
and gibber
"You must
get this child out"
Voices squeeze
tight
rubber hands
grope again
inside

Bed races
mazing
through halls
into white lights
flashing off
icy steel

I'm lugged
from bed
to table
a gasping mask
a beached whale
a vein opened
feet cold
your hand please
needled
into a vortex
spinning light
metal on metal
voices
sucked
spiralling
down

(don't rip me
open yet
I'm not gone)
Welcome
oblivion
from the terror
of your birth/your death
plucked from
my belly
beached
on unconscious sands

—*Maggie Fehlberg* (Toronto, poem written 1½ years after her cesarean section)

My labor began "two weeks late" according to the doctor, although it was the day I predicted. Fetal monitors were hooked up and the doctor ruptured my bag of waters. It did not speed up the dilation. Later, I was pushed into the delivery room—stirrups and drapes covering everything. Who the hell can push with legs flying in the air! I was exhausted. My last meal was fifteen hours ago! I was an employee at the hospital, but despite my medical backup I got fouled up. I plan on delivering my next baby vaginally. If my doctor doesn't agree to it I'll simply find someone who will.

—Dianne (Arizona)

I need helpful information on finding the courage and strength to go about finding willing doctors and an understanding hospital. I would prefer a home birth, for I really believe that a hospital is no place to have a baby, and I really believe, too, that the hospital caused the reasons for the cesarean birth of my son in May. I'm not pregnant again, yet, but I would like more children. I don't want more repeats of the nightmare experiences that began my career in motherhood. I don't want my body and my newborn babies "stolen" from me again, for that is how I felt from the first step I took through the hospital doors. I don't know if I could try a home birth next time—the "risks" involved have been thoroughly drilled into my head, but then, no-one can tell me, really, what the risks are, or how great, or are they really that much less in a hospital.

The cesarean support group here hasn't been very helpful—the people I've talked to have left me feeling I should just resign myself to future cesareans, that a vaginal delivery is a nice idea, but not a very likely reality. Not very encouraging. I can't seem to talk to anyone, either, about how I feel, that the cesarean was a horrible accident, that hospitals and their personnel really don't know what labor and childbirth families are all about. The magic lump in my tummy was suddenly a disease that must be cured at all cost and with great speed, and my baby was an incidental by-product, like a tooth handed back after it's been pulled for causing a toothache.

My "tooth" is now five months old, trying desperately to crawl, and has filled my life with company and joy, and I can think of nothing better to do than sit and watch him grow, count his smiles, and return his laughter. When people ask what I'm going to do when he's weaned, expecting me to go back to work I say I'll get pregnant and start all over again. I would like to bring my son's brothers and sisters into the world a little less dramatically. Any help would be greatly appreciated.

—Deborah (Maryland)

The cesarean was more frightening than anything I have experienced. No one would tell me what was happening. I hadn't thought my blindness a significant handicap until then.

—Peg (Michigan)

What I don't know what to do with are my feelings of rage and frustration. Is it possible that these feelings have been with me for six years? It feels like they have! Even as I write I feel my throat closing and tears coming to my eyes. Can you tell me if this is normal, do other women feel this way, too, even after so long?

—Henrietta (New Hampshire)

I'll have to switch hospitals. I found out from nurses here that some women have VBACs but they are "accidents."

—Sandra (New York)

I went into labor two and a half weeks late (the doctor had set my due date two weeks earlier at the beginning of the pregnancy). Anyway, I actually could have been right on time according to my own calculations. When I went to the hospital, they immediately put the fetal monitor on me, in spite of our objections, "only for an hour." It was never removed, and was recording the contractions as hard when they weren't and vice versa. So I know it is (or can be) quite inaccurate. There were so many manual checks for dilation by different nurses, doctors—you name it, and almost always during contractions. I understand this is supposed to be easier for them but does not do much toward the mother-to-be's concentration and relaxation. Before long there was an I.V. of sugar water. Then after six hours and still only dilated to nine, I was told to push although I didn't feel like it. When the head did not come down, I was sent for x-rays to see if there was room. By now I was losing control, being passed around so much. There must have been room, because they decided a forceps delivery was in order. So I was moved from the birthing room to the delivery room. They gave me the shots into the vagina but couldn't reach the baby's head with the forceps so back to the birthing room. I was still being advised to push with each contraction, although I still felt no impulse to "bear down." This included pushing while riding on the table down the halls. As you can see, our "planned natural birth experience," was already quite the opposite. I was beginning to just want "that thing" removed, as if he were only a rock or something.

The doctor told me since there were problems, I needed an emergency c/section, and I was pushed to the operating room (lots of rides through the halls, "jumping" on and off the table for a girl who only wanted a quiet delivery in the birthing room!). My husband was told he must wait in the father's room and I was operated on. I was allowed to see my baby long enough to ask if I could hold him, and to be told "NO." Meanwhile my husband was frantic with worry. After the baby was "born," I asked someone to please go tell my husband. They said, "when they had time" they would. We later discovered he wasn't informed for half an hour or more after the birth. He also had to practically fight a doctor in order to be allowed to see me in the recovery room and only saw our son through the nursery window. There is no reason for the delay, our son was not sick. His first Apgar score was eight, in five minutes was nine. A nurse told me that is good for a c/section baby.

Recovering from a spinal is no picnic as your whole body shakes uncontrollably and it's awful not to be able to wiggle your feet "on command." I realize we could have asserted ourselves more, but it hit us with no warning, and we were scared that something was terribly wrong. My doctor said the reason for the c/section was "swollen tissue." Obviously, pushing when one is not fully dilated could certainly contribute to that.

We have since moved from that city. I do not feel that I ever needed that cesarean, and will certainly do all in my power to avoid another one "just because I already had one." Especially since they took x-rays and must have felt there was plenty of room.

Please forgive me for rambling on so. I must say it felt good to get it out—I am so very bitter. People say, "just be glad you are both healthy, and now you have a son";—I am I am!, and that does make me feel guilty. But I also feel cheated and do not trust doctors since we had really trusted this one. Five of seven couples in our Lamaze class alone had c/sections and I overheard a nurse say she couldn't believe how many were being done lately! Neither can I.

The worst thing is wondering, deep down inside, "what if"—what if I refused to have another c/section and it really was warranted? and on and on. . . .

—Sue (Wisconsin)

Our Heavenly Father must be sad when He looks down upon the things that so many doctors are doing concerning the most sacred of all things—the miracle of birth.

—*Linda* (Virginia)

I am in the position of trying to convince the four OBs in the group to allow me a trial of labor instead of being routinely scheduled for a repeat cesarean. If I go into labor, I have no control over which doctor will be on duty. The first told me I'd lose my baby and need a hysterectomy. He did admit he knew of women who delivered vaginally, but only because they came in fully dilated.

—*Mary* (Pennsylvania)

My baby's face was cut by the doctor when he did the cesarean. They covered her with a blanket—nobody told me.

—*Sarah* (Massachusetts)

Excuse me for saying that our first experience at natural childbirth was not a "wonderful" one. The labor was excruciating but the cesarean was worse.

—*Sharon* (California)

I need information on cesarean sections. My doctor wouldn't listen to me. He insisted my dates were off. I made a total of seven trips to the hospital for tests. I was going nuts. When it was all over, the doctor said I was probably right.

—*Tammy* (Indiana)

I get mad any time I talk about my first birth to anyone. First you cry, then you are mad.

—*Marcy* (Georgia)

I've found a doctor who says he's willing to treat me as a normal pregnancy. He said if anything happened it would probably occur before the onset of labor. However, his standard procedures for delivery are no eating, episiotomy, spinal anesthesia, breaking the water, and a c/section if I'm past my due date. If I need a c/section my husband will not be allowed. I'm thinking of a home birth. This decision brings me peace.

—*Ilene* (New Jersey)

My daughter was born four years ago by cesarean. I was eleven days past my due date when my water broke. When I went to the hospital I was informed for the first time that my child was in the breech position and a cesarean was needed. I was completely taken off guard and very upset, but they asked me what was more important, "a healthy baby" or "a normal birth." I conceded, of course, to the c-section and my daughter was born a perfectly healthy beautiful baby without my ever even experiencing a labor pain. I did, however, develop a staph infection from the hospital and was pretty ill. I was put on antibiotics and continued nursing my baby. One week to the day after going off the antibiotics my daughter became deathly ill—her illness was never diagnosed but she nearly lost her life. Miraculously, she made a complete recovery and has never had any repercussions (unlike her parents, who were never the same after all that).

—*Shirley* (Massachusetts)

Our first child was born by cesarean section in February of 1978. Our second child is due this July and we are in kind of a quandary, trying to decide whether or not to go for a trial of labor.

I have talked with about four or five doctors and they seemed to be split down the middle; half for, half against. The statistics I was given were that approximately 1 percent of women having a trial of labor, rupture . . . and approximately one-third of that 1 percent require a hysterectomy as a result of the rupture. I know that those statistics sound good with only one-third percent of a chance that I'd have a hysterectomy. But as some people have put it, why take the chance at all?

The hospital that we'll be delivering at is the most progressive in the area as far as delivery procedures and maternity care. They have birthing rooms and rooming in, and will use the Leboyer method when they can. For c/sections they give an epidural rather than a spinal and husbands are allowed to be present, and I can have the baby to nurse right away. This is all what I've been told. (Perhaps I should get it in writing.) In other words, they seem to make a c/section as close to a normal delivery as it could possibly be.

However, for some reason, I still feel a strong desire to experience a normal delivery. Perhaps it's an ego trip. I felt like a real failure after my son was born. If that's the reason then I think perhaps it would be stupid to take the risk just for the sake of my ego. But whatever the reason, I really feel the desire to try.

Perhaps you need to know the circumstances of his birth . . . About a week after my due date my bag of waters sprung a leak and sealed up again, this at about five o'clock on Wednesday. But no labor pains came. We waited a few hours and then consulted a homeopath who recommended blue cohosh. After taking the pills every couple of hours I started having light labor pains. They lasted on into the night but never got any stronger. By morning all I had was a temperature. So we went to the hospital. They were real busy when we got there, so we had to wait around for a couple of hours or so. Then they broke my bag of waters, put me on Pitocin, strapped a monitor around my belly, laid me on my back, told me not to roll over and left. My temperature at this point was 100.4°. I was in labor for about four hours and there was no significant change. I think I was only dilated about three or four centimeters. Plus my temperature had gone up to 100.8°. So they gave me a spinal and half an hour later we had a 6 lb. 15 oz. baby boy. They cleaned out all the infection that was in the uterus and my temperature disappeared right away. My son never even had one. There were no further complications. Still we were both isolated—me for three days in post surgical and my baby in the nursery for six days. For the three days before I got to meet our son, my husband would go down to the nursery for several hours every day and rock him and sing to him and take Polaroid pictures and bring them to me. Finally, I got to see him and everything was fine. Now he's two years old and a very nice, even-tempered child, though he's always been clingy, and has only slept through the night about four times in his whole life. How much of that has to do with his birthing I guess we may never know.

I hope you can help us. I think we are just so full of doubts and conflicting feelings that we can't bring ourselves to make any decision. I don't know anyone around here who has had a trial of labor so I have no first-hand accounts to refer to. Everyone seems as doubtful as we are. Perhaps I am just asking for support and encouragement . . . someone to give me twenty great reasons for taking the risks of a trial labor. I really don't relish the idea of a hysterectomy. I am only twenty-six years old and I think we might like to have a third child.

—Bim (Maryland)

I live within a mile of several large maternity hospitals. All day long I hear them cutting.

—Rose (Massachusetts)

Do you know of any long-term studies on mother's reactions to unscheduled cesareans? All the ones I have end when the mother goes home from the hospital. Then the researchers conclude there is minimal negative reaction. This can't be true. All the cesarean mothers I see are frustrated, scared and sad.

—Ella (Texas)

Having a c/section is like running a marathon and being right near the finish line, and getting tripped by someone's foot.

—*Claudia* (Massachusetts)

The doctors and general public in this area have been brain-washed. Is it possible to re-educate the doctors and birth educators?
. . . They all say it is dangerous to allow a trial labor!

—*Beth* (Florida)

My baby was delivered by cesarean because my water broke and they said it was dangerous. My baby was seven and a half pounds and very healthy. I don't want another cesarean if I can find a doctor who will do it. Mine won't. Another cesarean? Thanks, but no thanks.

—*Mary Beth* (Colorado)

*I am your basic "Once a cesarean—*don't want *to always be a cesarean."*

—*Terry* (New Hampshire)

My first baby was a c/section, my second a vaginal, my third a section. My sections were very trying emotionally and physically. I was upset because we had taken Lamaze and had the best possible attitude about birth. My second was an eleven-hour uncomplicated labor. With my third, we thought there would be no problem. They broke my water, but labor didn't occur, so they used Pitocin and after eight hours they did another cesarean. I was very upset.

—*Claire* (U.S. Air Force, stationed in Germany)

The times I try to explain to others the depths of my disappointment and heartache over my c/section, the words just won't come out right. After months of trying to push these feelings aside, I no longer can. I always felt guilty thinking I was just feeling sorry for myself, that I was ungrateful for my healthy child.

—*Robin* (Michigan)

Upon our recent prenatal exam, I was asked the classic question, "When would you like to schedule your next c/section?" I replied, "I wouldn't."

—*Jerolyn* (California)

The father of my child fears for my life. For me—I care less—as a repeat section is as difficult to accept as death.

—*Maryann* (Tennessee)

The situation here is that people are becoming "thankful" for cesareans as a means of "producing" healthy babies. Surely we can apply ourselves to discovering natural birth processes that would provide optimum safety and well-being for mothers and babies. There is a long struggle ahead. They have only just started spreading the "joy" of epidurals.

—*Claudine* (England)

How excited I was to read of your work and research on vaginal delivery after cesarean birth! My little girl is four and a half months now, but I still have much sadness over the fact that our well-planned and very prepared home birth ended up being a cesarean in the hospital. I feel cheated in a way and am still blaming myself and feeling like I did something wrong. She is healthy and happy and I am grateful for that, but it still doesn't erase my disappointment in not being able to have her the "real way."

Of course when I think of ever having a second child, I want very much to have a vaginal birth. But I am confused and scared and reluctant to even think of getting pregnant again. Whatever it was—I want very much to hope and believe that it could be different next time.

—*Crystal* (Massachusetts)

They told me it was necessary to operate. I was very upset, mostly because of the attitude of the doctor. My obstetrician was called out of town due to a family emergency. The doctor who took over was very unfeeling and cold. At least as far as I was concerned. Perhaps because I wasn't his regular patient. I still feel cheated! I had a general anesthetic and didn't get to see my baby right away. When they did bring him to me in the recovery room, I was so groggy and half blind without my glasses, that all I saw was a blur.

I was given the "classical" incision and I also resent that very much. It left an awful scar and messed up my navel. Sometimes I feel a little foolish because I think perhaps I shouldn't have these negative feelings and should just be thankful I'm alive and have a beautiful healthy son. Perhaps the doctor didn't attempt the "bikini" incision because I'm overweight and he assumed I didn't need to worry about it ever showing. I am still left with the impression that because I wasn't his regular patient, he wanted to hurry up and do things in the quickest way possible to get it over with.

I want to have my next baby vaginally and at home, if possible. The last part is my ideal, but I'm not absolutely adamant about it. I want a live, healthy baby and be alive to enjoy it.

But first I have to get pregnant again. I'm having trouble conceiving. It took me a year to become pregnant with my first. In the three years since Kevin was born, I have used absolutely no method of birth control, and have had no luck at all. I'm 34 years old now and want to have more children before I get much older.

—Linda (Illinois)

After nine hours of labor I was told to push, even though I was at nine centimeters. My cervix began to swell. The doctor insisted on Pitocin to increase dilation. Finally he wouldn't wait and insisted on a section. At least we were able to convince them to allow me a local (spinal) which they don't normally do, and to allow my husband into the OR (a first). At first I was so grateful to the doctors—I had a gorgeous healthy eight-pound three-ounce daughter. The past few months we've gained enough distance and we're becoming more and more angry . . . You are at their mercy and they threaten you with birth defects . . . I didn't have any intention of writing so much. It is now obvious to me that I'll have to write the whole story out in detail so I can exorcise the ghost . . .

—Judy (New Jersey)

My doctor insisted on measuring my pelvis with x-rays. When I refused, he exploded into a tirade about dead babies and brain damage.

—Jeanne (New York)

The birth of my daughter was the worst experience of my life and I am not looking forward to having another baby because of it—although I truly would like to be the mother of a second child.

. . . . My doctor warned me I might have to have a cesarean because he thought

I was so small. . . . When I was in early labor my doctor examined me and decided to do a cesarean. He had seen me the day before and could not tell I needed this surgery but now he knew I did. . . . How could he know this? I know small stature does not mean small pelvic structure, though this seemed to be his reasoning. . . . . The things that happened to me were demeaning and awful.

—Michele (Florida)

My first child was an emergency cesarean after failure to dilate past four centimeters. I questioned if my next child had to be another cesarean since my baby had complications due to the surgery, and my doctor said yes, it wasn't worth the risk.

My second child was born by elective cesarean with wet lung—a condition quite common in c/sections, but still very serious. It took four days before he could breathe on his own. Consequently, I am anxious to know if it's possible to have another baby without a cesarean.

—Cam (Minnesota)

Monday I developed a cold sore on my lip and was separated from my baby again. I became a familiar figure with my nose pressed against the glass of the nursery, having to watch my daughter be bottle fed. The next morning I looked at my belly and found it dripping with a clear brownish fluid—my incision draining . . . the resident ordered a fancy device which allowed the dressings to be changed without new adhesive. My belly looked like a Buster Brown shoe, all neatly laced up . . . . Wednesday my abdominal incision began to come apart. It is unnerving to say the least to have your body open up almost literally before your eyes. Another resident examined it and said that I shouldn't worry, that in five years I'd just have a white line about this big (holding his fingers about an inch apart). I wondered where he'd studied bedside manner. I hadn't even held my daughter! I thought I was going crazy.

—Elizabeth (Virginia)

The spinal didn't take but surgery continued regardless. The worst blow was my doctor's pronouncement later that the section probably wasn't necessary.

—Laurie (Tennessee)

I missed even the contractions! I'm so eager to know pushing. Anytime I ask my doctor a question with a little bit of medical knowledge on my part he gets intimidated and ignores me.

—*Elaine* (Massachusetts)

All alone in the "birthing room," Andy and I were both positive that I was going to die. There was no one to tell us what to expect or that our fears were normal or that I should be eating and drinking and walking and squatting and taking a hot shower and being held and loved and reminded that I was there to have a baby. We cried and we waited to die!

. . . At 6:30 the doctor came and checked me and I was three-and-a-half to four centimeters dilated. Not far enough. He ruptured the membranes of the amniotic sac and then told me things would now pick up and in half an hour to an hour we would see our baby. In the meantime, just in case, they were going to get the OR ready for our cesarean. A student nurse was assigned to me against my wishes. It took two tries to get the needle for the spinal in the right place (and I still have a backache in the mornings in that spot). I couldn't feel myself breathe from the anesthesia and because I was partially shaved, painted orange, draped in green, I.V. in one arm, the BP cuff on the other, and strapped down spread-eagle on the table to have my baby. No one could (or would) take one of my hands and let me feel my chest move as I took a breath. Andy, poor thing, was in the OR with me. I say "poor thing" because I think he was sure he was there to watch his wife be sacrificed to some chrome and green god.

—*Jami* (Massachusetts)

My husband was told he could be with me. But they detained him so long signing forms he missed the birth and they told him there was no use in his being there while I was being stitched.

—*Emily* (Washington)

I was never told I had to have a cesarean until I was admitted into the labor room. I wasn't even given a chance to start labor. What was frightening was that my doctor's partner, whom I had never seen before, performed the surgery. Also what was strange was that he had to perform three other cesarean births before mine.

—*Olympia* (New Mexico)

When I arrived at the hospital, in very intense labor, the delivery nurses treated me like a piece of meat, and crudely strapped me up to a fetal monitor. With the doctor confirming the fetal distress, I was shipped into the operating room for an emergency cesarean with no sympathetic person allowed to remain at my side. My doctor boastingly took all credit for saving my child who did manage to rate a healthy Apgar score of eight and ten, despite the assumed fetal distress.

—Laurie (Massachusetts)

Babies may just "arrive" as far as others are concerned. But from my point of view, the birth is like having a child going off to camp or to school . . . one at least wants to be able to see the child off. The most difficult thing about the birth was not the pain of labor—nor the pain of the recovery from the section—but the fact that she was born out of sight and touch, independent of my efforts.

—Judy (Massachusetts)

Once a Cesarean—Now What?

The baby inside me was fine
But I labored in fear and in pain
Cut off from all that I loved
Drugged, cut open, chained
"So your child won't die."

"Don't worry, you'll heal," they all say,
"Be a good girl, forget it!" they cry.
"A section's not bad, by the way—
And be thankful you both didn't die."

Not bad? For the doctor perhaps . . . .
And who sutures the wound in my mind?
I'll heal . . . in a lifetime or two
But the girl that I was I can't find
She was left all alone to die.

—Jami Osborne (Massachusetts; written four years after her cesarean section)

It is almost noon and I am visiting my friend across the hall. She is also pregnant but I am bigger and it is more difficult for me to climb the stairs. We are laughing as I leave for home to make lunch. As I step into the hall a warm stream of water goes down my legs and into my shoes.

It is two o'clock now and I telephone my husband at work. He has just started a new job and seems reluctant to come home. We have very little money and no medical insurance. I think thoughts like "Should we be having this baby now?" and "We never practiced our breathing."

My back hurts down in the sway. It does not go away when I stretch out on my side on the sofa. I have forgotten about lunch.

It is 3:30 now and we have arrived at the hospital. It is in a large city ninety minutes away from our home near the field of ripe cornstalks. The traffic and noise are frightening. It is rush hour.

As my husband signs forms and I sign a medical consent I think about my mother. She is frightened for me. She told me that she would never have had children if she had known then what she knows now.

Goodbye, husband. The elevator closes and I am taken away in a wheelchair. Why have I been given such a large enema? Why am I alone for such a long time in this treatment room? The nurse never talked to me except to tell me to position myself on my side. Why did she avoid eye contact with me? How will I get off this high, narrow table? Will I make it to the bathroom?

Another nurse brings me to a room with a bed. I get in (I'm supposed to, right?). She tells me I must be shaved now. My labor is uncomfortable but I must not move. She may cut something down there if I'm not good and quiet and still. She finishes and puts up the metal sides of the bed.

The window looks onto a brick side of a building. The ceiling light is bright and so white. There is no other bed in here. A large clock is on the wall in front of me.

Hello, husband. You have returned to see me transformed into a patient. I'm sorry the room is so ugly. Does it reflect me? "Don't let them take away my glasses," I say. Them. I have not made a friend.

A small tense woman, every hair in place, introduces herself as the head nurse. "Who was your Lamaze teacher?" she asks. I tell her. I am paralyzed by her reply: "No wonder you're doing it all wrong." She unflinchingly goes on, "Another woman came in from that class and she did it all wrong, too." I look away dejectedly. I am a failure.

It has been ten hours now. I am a beached whale. Many faces have peeked in the door. None acknowledge me. I have been catheterized because I could not let loose my bladder on the cold metal bed pan. I grip the metal bedsides with each contraction. I never cry out loud and stifle any moan that bursts into my throat. "I have been cruelly deceived," I think. My Lamaze teacher has lied. The contractions are pains!

"Please can I have ice, if not water?" "No" is the reply. The light is so intense. The clock is staring at my stiffened body.

"Then something more for pain," I beg. "Yes, of course." That's easy to get. The Demerol has "taken the edge off."

"No progress, very slow labor," I hear from the mouths of those who never look me in the eye. My God, it is eighteen hours now. I may die here. A moment of truth dulls me and I cannot even cry.

I look at my husband dozing. You cannot help me. You do not understand. You can go on living, but this is changing me.

I have not thought of my baby all this time. But now my doctor is speaking and *saying, "Your baby may be too large. We will give you six more hours. Then a cesarean will be done."*

I don't want my baby to be born here," I think. "This place is so barren."

My tongue is dry and swollen and I can hardly swallow. I have an I.V. taped to the inside of my elbow. My husband has left. A nurse inserts a catheter into my bladder for the third time. I have been here twenty-four hours in the same room, in the same bed, without food or drink, without eye contact (even you, husband). I have been confined alone, a curiosity for people to measure and poke at but never to caress tenderly. It is a place of isolation.

I am sedated and have been strapped in place, laid out like a sacrificial banquet. A spinal has left me detached from my body. I am awakened from my exhaustion and sense a tugging. A baby boy is pulled from my body. There is no moment of joy or satisfaction. He is cleaned and measured and wrapped. I fall in love with him when I see his face. We will be separated for more than a day.

Many hours later I am in a sunny room with voices of women around me. The light is like sharp steel blades and the voices peck at my head. I am having a spinal headache. I have no thought of my baby. I cannot eat the food they bring me.

At home I cannot stand up straight because I have a bladder and kidney infection. I can hardly hold my baby. I remember the bottle of Valium an intern has given me for the back pain.

My breasts are painfully engorged with milk—no one at the hospital had given me any advice for breastfeeding though I spoke of my desire and often made clumsy attempts. Now my hungry infant cannot grasp my nipple because of the engorgement. He screams and fights and turns red with frustration. I cry softly and decide not to have any more children.

Two months later my friend from across the hall has a "natural" birth. Her husband, filled with love for his baby and newly in love with his wife, tells me how his wife pushed out their baby. I am jealous and depressed but admit this to no one. After all, my baby is healthy and has a beautiful round "cesarean head." I have no right to be depressed, right?

—Jeanne (Massachusetts)

4 ❧ Grieving . . . and Healing

Just the Same Really
(Fantasies, 1979)

It's just the same, really.
The incision is so low it's
really almost the same. Just
in a different spot, that's
all. You just push in a different spot, at a different
angle, that's all. Something
like a dolphin giving birth.
It's quite simple, really.
Just the same. Really just
the same.

Cesarean, V

When they said We're gonna
hafta take the baby she
started screaming hysterically
She thought they meant
actually take the baby away
from her (Ya know, put it up
for adoption). So they
explained to her Oh no We
don't mean take the baby

Claudia Panuthos was a contributor to this chapter. (See About the Contributors.)

permanently We mean take it
temporarily Take it out of
your body But she wouldn't
calm down She just went on
screaming

They call it a Cesarean
birth instead of a Cesarean
operation They say I can be
awake with my husband
present and watching.
"Well, which is it?" they
smile. "Raven or Jordie?"
They are as joyful as the
other times. It's just the
same really. The only difference is the location, and
the baby being pulled
rather than pushed out.
Everyone is talkative. But
as I lie there, all I do is cry,
sob, cry.

May, 1979

Aw come on whatchu cryin' for?
You didn't get a hysterectomy
Just a Cesarean You haven't
been spayed Just sectioned
They didn't fix it so you can't
pull in more children Just so
you can't push them out Why
all the weeping?

I did not die in childbirth At least not for good
I did not die in childbirth But I also did not live!

*   *   *   *   *

(These poems by Marion Cohen are from a collection that appeared in *Mothering*, 16 (Summer 1980).

Why on earth would a woman grieve for the birth of a healthy baby? What difference does it make that the delivery was a cesarean? Isn't she overreacting just a bit? Oh, well, must be a touch of the "baby blues." She'll get over it . . . when she feels stronger . . . when the baby sleeps better . . . when she starts getting out more. You'll see—she'll be just fine.

Or will she?

The cesarean mother in our society is expected to trot cheerily out of the O.R. into her new role of motherhood. She is expected to remember with great sadness all her friends who couldn't conceive or who miscarried or who lost babies, and she is to feel extremely grateful to her doctor for giving her a living, healthy baby to cherish. While it is true that perspective can be useful, it is also true that ignoring or denying feelings can be defeating. No one seems to realize that having a cesarean is like being a baby rather than having one, that the cesarean mother sometimes feels as weak, helpless, scared, and weepy as a newborn, and that from the physical and emotional pain of an upsetting birth come many *other* issues.

Very few of the cesarean mothers who have written to us about their cesarean sections in the past ten years have felt peaceful about their births. Most letters are filled with bitterness, frustration, confusion, sadness, and pain. These women are all grieving, and no one is helping them to handle their grief productively so that healing can begin. In a song by Carol Hall we are told, "It's all right to cry; crying gets the sad out of you."* But for many women, the crying *doesn't* seem to get the sad out. It seems only to compound the hostile, depressed, numb, surprised, overwhelmed, tired feelings frequently expressed. Too often, the emotional scars heal far more slowly than the uterine incision.

We believe that all women grieve to some extent after their babies are born. However, the cesarean mother's grief reactions are generally stronger and longer lasting than those of the woman who has delivered vaginally. For some, the grief lasts but moments; for others, years. For some, the grief is mild, or merely poignant; for others, it is severe and painful.

In our country, grieving is discouraged. We are uncomfortable with it. We deny it. We push it away. We are a fast-food society, and we want our grief to be finished quickly. Cheer up! Don't rain on my parade! It was for the best! Get your act together! "For crying out loud!" we say sarcastically. We need to remember that grief is an inevitable part of life, and an experience that, however short-lived or painful, fosters growth.

We believe that coming to a place of peace about birth is vital. Unresolved feelings from a birth can weaken the relationships in the family involved. Peaceful, loving feelings about oneself and one's baby help cement family relationship,

---

*"It's All Right To Cry," by Carol Hall, in *Free To Be . . .You and Me,* produced by Carole Hart, Bell Records, New York, 1972.

but these kinds of feelings are often fragmented and splintered, in the aftermath of a difficult or disappointing birth—much like pieces of driftwood after a storm. We believe that recognizing, experiencing, and dealing with grief are essential. Grief's masked presence seeps into relationships and experiences like fog. It clogs up the drain, so to speak. Clouded vision distorts the new family relationships and the clarity needed for subsequent normal birthing.

Claudia Panuthos, childbirth therapist, and author of several books on "positive birthing," makes a plea for the acknowledgment of birth as an emotional, psychological event involving the body, mind, heart, and soul.

> As we would dedicate ourselves to the physical healing, so let us dedicate ourselves to the emotional healing, so critical to our relationship with ourselves and our children. Let us stay conscious and heal any birth-related emotional pain. The hurts that are present are not a sign of insanity but rather a testimony to aware, awake mental health. Childbirth is an opportunity for enlightenment and increased well-being, regardless of the external events of the actual birth. It is a chance to heal the past and create more positive thoughts and patterns for the future. This can be accomplished only by women determined to internally hold birth as a self-affirmation and as an expression of feminine competence and power. No woman who has conceived, carried and delivered a child deserves any less.

Until we begin to view birth as a psychological as well as a physiological process, we will have to continue "mopping up" birth's "debris": women's tears.

Grieving? For What?

Keep in mind that twenty years ago there was little difference between a cesarean section and a vaginal birth. All women were hospitalized for ten days or more, medicated, and separated from their husbands and babies. About the only difference was where it hurt. Cesarean women were cut on their bellies, while vaginally delivered women were cut on their bottoms. As prepared childbirth became integrated into our culture, couples began to be aware of the benefits and delights of active childbearing. Most want to be active decision-making participants in their infant's births. In a study on "Prepared Childbirth and the Concept of Control," L. R. Willmuth[28] questioned couples to determine the factors that made them feel most positive about their birth experiences. He identified control, a feeling of autonomy, as being most important. The extent to which couples were integrally involved in decision-making influenced how positively they viewed their births.

In many situations, the cesarean mother is not permitted, or is unable, to see, touch, or hold her infant. Some women are in such physical pain that they have no interest in the baby, which often leads to regret, guilt, and sorrow later on. When a cesarean is performed, months of planning go up in a puff of smoke; many decisions must be changed, rescinded, or abandoned by the couple. Choices are limited and sometimes impossible. Couples feel as if they are not qualified to make decisions about their own baby's life. They often become frightened, disoriented, and confused. The physician, not the couple, is "in control."

Cesarean women grieve for all the things for which every new mother grieves. They process all the same data. They grieve, for example, for the baby they imagined in their uterus, since the baby in their arms is often quite different. They grieve for the relationship that they had with their spouses before the baby arrived, even if the baby was planned. They grieve for the loss of attention from the pregnant woman to the baby. They grieve for a night's sleep or for a stomach with no stretch marks.

Woman grieve for their pregnancy: on a physical level, the body loses the baby. In *Positive Birthing*[20] we are told, "The inner sanctum that once housed a precious and beautiful life collapses and gives way as the body returns to its former state." In order for a mother to be born, a pregnant woman must "die"— and death, at least, is an accepted reason for grieving in our culture. Thus, grieving, even after having had a healthy normal baby, is normal, healthy, and appropriate. However, along with the "normal griefs," cesarean mothers have concerns unique to them.

A cesarean mother grieves for her healthy body, for in every cesarean—necessary or not, welcomed or not—the body is violated. (One woman wrote, "I've been physically *bisected* and emotionally *dissected*.") She grieves for the enforced separations from spouse, newborn, and other children. She grieves about the loss of control that Willmuth spoke about. She grieves for her self-esteem.* Bampton explains that cesarean mothers see other new mothers caring for their babies while they cannot, and they may feel inadequate and helpless. Deutsch[7] spoke about the importance of the delivery to the mother's self-esteem. She believed that having a baby is a task that a woman needs to master, as a child learns to tie his shoe. She stated that the mother's unconscious participation or nonparticipation in the delivery leaves something unresolved in her.

A cesarean woman grieves for her energy, stamina, and strength. She grieves for her femininity and for a feeling of trust and confidence in her body: "My body doesn't work the way it should" is a common feeling. Some women had little trust and confidence in the first place, and this may have been a factor leading to the cesarean.

Grieving can be completely independent of the health of the new baby. It may be delayed if the baby's well-being is in question, or it may begin with

---

*See "The Mother's Self-Esteem after a Cesarean Delivery," by Bonnie Cox and Elaine Smith, *Maternal and Child Nursing (MCN) Journal*, 7 (September-October 1982), p. 309.

feelings of guilt: "What did I do wrong?" It may not appear at first if the mother judges that it is *inappropriate* to grieve after having just had a baby, or that "It isn't *nice* to feel this way." Henrietta wrote, "I always thought that I shouldn't complain because I had had one wonderful birth and I did have four healthy children. But somewhere inside I have always felt ripped off and disappointed. Now, six years later, I am allowing myself to grieve. It feels so good!"

All this grief is compounded by additional guilt over not being able to accept the experience. (After all, some women can't even have children.) Cesarean mothers often feel jealous toward other women, or distant from them. "I know I'm not a man," said one cesarean mother, "But I certainly don't feel like a woman. Is there a third sex?"

Volumes have been written on grieving. Klaus and Kennell[14] describe grief in classic stages: shock, denial, anger, sadness, acceptance, and readjustment. Others describe the stages as numbness, searching and yearning, disorganization and disorientation, and resolution and reinvestment. We wish to add as the final stages peace and, beyond that, joy. *Joy.*

Factors Affecting Grieving

We think it is important to keep in mind that a woman's expectation of birth is a factor in how she will react to her cesarean. If you have always dreamed of a home birth with candles and soft music, it will be difficult for you to integrate the realities of a cesarean. If your mother and all of your sisters had cesareans, and your physician has told you that you have a small pelvis, the actual experience may be quite similar to what you envisioned. Vicki Shives writes, "The more the experience is wanted and hoped for, the greater the experience of loss."[25]

The support system and role models that a woman has in her life, before, during, and after the cesarean will influence the length and severity of her grieving response. If she is surrounded by understanding, supportive friends and family who accept whatever reactions she has, this will facilitate the process.

Past experiences, losses and surprises in a woman's life may influence her grief. Panuthos and Silva[20] tell us that birth is a "highly emotionally-activating experience that can trigger off feelings associated with personal birth memories, family childbearing traditions, body-related embarrassments and fears, unfinished sibling conflicts, previous abortions, miscarriages or births, our marriage relationship, and general health-related care." They explain that we file life events according to their emotional content and in so doing we create "files" or "stacks"—stacks for pride, stacks for fear, stacks for loss, etc. Every time we feel a loss, for example, we add to our loss stack. We spend a lifetime accumulating stacks without knowing it! For some women, the cesarean may be just the loss that prevents the file drawer from closing, or topples the stack, much like the straw that breaks the camel's back. If previous losses haven't been appropriately acknowledged and healed, the stack may be high: with this new "load" it is easily upset and toppled. One woman couldn't understand her tears until she realized that she was grieving not only for her cesarean, but for her mother, who had died several years before. "I wanted her present at the birth," she said.

If a woman has lost a parent or a child or has had other traumas in her life, having a cesarean may seem insignificant in comparison. For some women, the surgery is the first exposure to a difficult and frightening experience. It may be a first awakening to one's mortality. "Of course I knew I wasn't going to die, that was silly," said one mother. "Still, I thought I was going to die."

The circumstances under which the cesarean was done may influence the grieving. If a woman believes that the operation saved her baby's life, or her own, it may be easier for her to accept the experience and move on through it. Or it may not. If she believes that she was victimized and cheated out of the experience of giving birth, she may be angry for a long while and find it difficult to work through her feelings.

Cesarean Sections: Decisions of Love

Women in our culture are conditioned toward covering up negative feelings. We are also conditioned toward failure rather than success. It's considered "cute" when we can't balance a check book or fix a tire. If a man can't do those things, he is considered inadequate. So when we judge for whatever reason that we haven't been successful at having our babies, the "failure" may be a comfortable, familiar feeling within us. Many women "beat themselves up" after a poor birth experience. They need not do that! They made the very best decisions they could. They never once made a decision that put their babies' needs after their own. The "system" doesn't work that way.

A mother deer flees from danger. She knows that if she tries to fight a lion she will lose. The only time she will fight that lion is if she perceives that her fawn is in danger. She will distract, fight, offer herself as sacrifice if necessary. Survival instinct of the species is so strong that she will do anything to protect her fawn or give it time to run from danger—anything to assure that *it* will live.

Our selflessness and survival instincts are equally strong. If we perceive that our child is in danger, we will do anything to protect her. Millie said, "The pain was excruciating. I kept thinking that my baby must be suffering, too." We will permit ourselves *to be cut open* to save the life of our baby. What we applaud as courage and strength in our animal friends, we interpret as weakness in ourselves. In this context, cesarean mothers are not weak failures; they are courageous women who are willing to be cut apart for the lives of their infants! Perhaps it is time to congratulate yourself for your strength and courage. It is time to love yourself for what you did. What you did was *an act of love*. Not one of you would have permitted a cesarean to be done if the doctor said, "A cesarean would be dangerous for your baby, Mrs. Jones." You needn't punish yourself for acting in the very best interests of your baby, nor feel guilty for *protecting* your baby.

Some women do not perceive that their babies are in danger. When they are certain that their infants are fine, their own survival instincts surface. If the labor has been long, and the pain seems excruciating, self-preservation becomes all-encompassing. Having a cesarean signals an end to the ordeal. Relief from pain is an anesthetic away. Even this decision is made out of love for one's baby. When a woman is in *so much pain* that she is willing *to be cut open* in order to have it end, the thought that she must also be close to death is usually, if subconsciously, present. If an animal dies, she knows that her offspring will fall prey to other animals or starve to death. The human mother's thoughts about dying, whether conscious or not, are also thoughts about the survival of her infant. Seen in this light, allowing or begging for a cesarean is also a loving decision.

We believe that some cesareans occur when a woman is not ready to "grow herself up." Bearing a child is not a girl's experience, it is that of a woman. Some women perceive no danger, per se, to themselves or their babies, but are frightened to accept responsibility and "do it." They want someone else to "get the baby out" for them. Feelings of being overwhelmed, inadequate, and fearful surface. One woman said, "I was only 22. I wanted to be pampered. I wasn't ready to pamper a baby."

We ask you to look at yourself with respect, just as you'd look at that mother deer. You did your best. You acted out of love. You don't have to get down on yourself because you had a cesarean. You can forgive yourself: it isn't a crime to protect one's baby or to want to remain a little girl for a while longer. You can also begin to forgive your body, your baby, and your mate, if necessary. They did the very best they could at the time, too.

Grieving Responses

Each woman's response to her cesarean birth is unique. One woman said, "I was disappointed, but the birth was over; that was that." Another said, "It's been seven years, and every birthday of his, I still cry." A woman with a history of infertility said, "This may be the only baby I ever have in my life. I wanted this one chance to experience giving birth, along with becoming a mother. I guess I asked for too much." Another woman with a history of infertility said, "I wouldn't care if this baby came out of my eyeballs. All I wanted was a healthy baby, and that's what I got. It's a miracle just to hold her."

We are all unique, and we grieve uniquely. For example, our grief may have the appearance of anger. A woman may feel angry at her doctor, her husband, or her baby. Frequently, the anger is directed at herself or at her childbirth educator. "If only I had breathed correctly," she says. "If only the instructor had taught us better breathing techniques. If only the doctor hadn't insisted on a monitor. If only I had been coached better. If only this baby had weighed a little less than eight pounds. If only I hadn't eaten the whipped cream on the sundae. If only . . ." On the other hand, grief may look quiet and withdrawn. As one mother remarked, "We grieve in the same measure that we love."

Fathers' Grief

Fathers go through a grieving process, too. Fathers present at their babies' births grieve, and fathers denied the experience of their babies' births grieve as well. Fathers present for cesareans will have reactions to integrate, as will fathers who choose not to attend their baby's birth.

Some fathers berate themselves because they "stood by" while their wives were cut open. Perhaps they are grieving for lost competence and strength, since many feelings of helplessness arise as a result of a man's loss of control. One father was upset for months. "I couldn't believe that my own child had to be tugged and pulled out of a cut made into Jan's belly. It made me feel very sad." Another wrote, "I would have to see my wife dying before my eyes before I'd ever consent to surgery again." Some fathers feel totally positive and have little understanding for their wives' feelings. Others experience grief that matches their mates' in intensity and duration.

Eli's response to his wife's cesarean is typical of many fathers' responses: "I feel it was the right decision in my wife's case. I was very happy to become a father and relieved that my wife and baby were fine. I liked our doctor and feel that his judgment was sound. I would have liked to be present at the birth, but all in all, things went well. It doesn't seem that important to me how the baby came out, and I don't feel that I have anything 'heavy' to work out."

Norman's response to *his* wife's cesarean is also typical of many fathers' responses: "I had planned on being at our baby's birth. I just *assumed* things would go well. Instead, I watched from a doorway, unable to see very well, and much too far away to touch my wife or my baby or to comfort either of them in any way. I had such mixed emotions: overjoyed at seeing my child, very nervous that something might go wrong with the surgery, disappointed, angry, sad, you name it. A certain feeling of horror has increased as I realize that there is a very high probability that the operation was not necessary. I find it increasingly hard to believe that my wife benefited from the callous production-line atmosphere in the labor room. Within thirty minutes of entering the hospital, she was reduced from a proud woman in labor to a whimpering, terrified, shivering apology of a person. We are both in quite a state right now."

Often, the father and mother are at different stages of grieving. This is understandable and appropriate, considering that their experiences and perceptions about the baby and birth are different. However, the difference can complicate matters, especially if understanding, patience, and acceptance are scarce. The character of the marital relationship and the degree of communication and support present will influence the patterns and expediency of grieving.

Identifying the Symptoms . . .

How can we identify women who are grieving? Some signs, like tears, are clear. Although we should never pass up the opportunity to cry (crying is an "inside bath!"), many cesarean women's cries are not cleansing tears, but distress signals.

Physical exhaustion is another sign. We are bound to be tired after surgery and while caring for newborns. But some women are chronically exhausted for months after the operation.

In contrast, some women exhibit boundless energy or forced cheerfulness. We asked one woman what would happen if she stopped being so busy. "I'd begin to cry and never stop," she replied.

Irritability. Sleeplessness. Excessive house-cleaning. Overeating. Undereating. Difficulty functioning on a day-to-day basis. Colds. Headaches. Backaches. All of these can be camouflaged signs of grief.

Loss of creativity is a more subtle indication. Growing a baby and birthing are acts of creativity. If these are denied, other creative areas are often blocked. When Nancy discussed creativity at a lecture on cesarean grieving, one woman began to cry. Right after her cesarean, she had given away a beautiful painting. It was a pastel that she had painted when she realized she was pregnant, and it was to have been a gift in keeping for her child.

Difficulty making eye contact or physical contact with the baby is an important concern, which can further distort any other problems in the relationship. Nancy notes that while 99 percent of the VBAC women she has worked with name their babies within minutes of the birth, many cesarean mothers have not named their infants even days later. Along these lines, marital discord is also an issue. In a strong, loving relationship, the love acts as an arch; as the couple leans together, they unite in strength. When an arch or a relationship is stressed, the supports aren't centered and crumble easily. And women who have little or no support from any source often find the days and weeks following the birth intolerable.

Grieving displays many signs, many intensities. But grief is normal and healthy. It is our way of gradually integrating sadness or trauma, a way to move on. Lester Hazell, author of *Commonsense Childbirth*,[13] describes grief as "sorrow experienced over what might have been." Grief is working though the pain of loss. It is a process—a learning process—and, we hope, a healing one.

. . . And Working Our Way Through . . .

How can we facilitate each other's grief? Some people suggest that it is best to leave a woman alone to "work it out," claiming that time heals all wounds. This advice may be due to our inability as a culture to deal with grief; we are uncomfortable with one another's sadness, for it brings up all the unresolved sadness *we* feel inside. Time has its merits, but most often it merely acts as a bandaid: something that needs attention may be concealed.

We can help one another by listening, by accepting each other's feelings, by being patient and careful not to judge or impose our own values on someone else. We can support, hug, and love one another. We can help build self-esteem by pointing out how much our babies need and love us. We can help ourselves, by eating well and taking long walks (or short walks). Or by touching—a wonderful healer—and allowing time to give us a new view. We can look ahead, even as we continue to reflect. Helen Keller said, "When I look to the sunshine, I cannot see the shadow."

We can help by keeping humor in our lives. Laughter isn't medicine: it's an opportunity for the heart to dance for a few moments, for the child in each of us to come out and play. Grieving is hard work, and occasionally we *need* to dance and play.

We can help by opening up areas of creativity. Buy a box of crayons! Get out some modeling clay. Write poetry, or express your thoughts in a journal. Nurse your baby—producing milk is a creative process, and breastfeeding will deepen your attachment to your baby. Listen to music, play an instrument. Learn from your last birth, and welcome the next. As the poet Shelley wrote, "If winter comes, can spring be far behind?"

. . . To Healing

Having a purebirth can be a healing experience in itself. Jack wrote, "A normal birth was the only thing that could bring my wife back to normal, or close to what she was when we got married." His wife concurred. "I feel whole again," she wrote. "No loose ends." Healing may result from a positive birthing, or it may be a precursor to one.

Not all cesarean women go on to have the birth they desire. For some women, the joy of VBAC makes the pain of the cesarean more difficult to bear. It is good to know that a good birth experience is not a necessary prerequisite for healing, and that it is possible to return to a birth that took place long ago and feel healed and whole from it, too.

In order for childbirth to lead us to increased well-being, it is important that we know how to release and heal our bodies, minds, and spirits of any pain left over from the childbearing process. The following suggestions for healing are for women to use at home. Although these techniques can be highly effective in healing childbirth-related pain, there may still be times when outside assistance is needed.

Traditional therapy often aims at adjustment rather than healing. Adjustment, or coping, implies that a person becomes more equipped to handle the pain and is therefore less debilitated by it; she has found a way to live with her troubles. Healing implies that the pain is gone and has been replaced by a feeling of well-being. Coping with a headache means feeling better about having it; healing a headache means that the headache has gone away. So let us always aim for healing, and for health.

The three cheapest and most effective forms of healing are thinking, breathing, and touching. Thinking can heal our hurts by providing us with objectivity—an inner observer or witness who can review our birth experiences with a neutral eye and determine exactly which areas were painful or unsatisfying. In such observing, for example, one might discover angry feelings toward a particular nurse, physician, midwife, or birth attendant.

It would be useful to list on paper any persons with whom you are still angry and each specific act that upset you. Review these lists until you can honestly say, "I forgive (name) for (deed). I forgive (name) for everything." At first, such a task may sound impossible. When we are angry, we do not feel forgiving. However, if we are successfully releasing and letting go of anger, forgiveness is inevitable. Remember that forgiveness never implies that an individual or an act was justified or right, but rather that you value your own physical health and peace of mind enough to let go of anger, pain, turmoil, and the damage they can cause you if you hold on to them.

Such a review may also put us in touch with feelings of inadequacy or grief. The mind tends to zero in faster on our shortcomings than on our strengths.

If there is some sense of inadequacy, a process called affirmation can be helpful. This process reprograms the mind to think positively. Since we are not accustomed to positive ideas, we tend to experience them at first as overly idealistic or unrealistic. But, with practice, we can tolerate even our own goodness. Affirming yourself means thinking or listing or speaking into a tape recorder every *positive aspect* of your childbirth experience.

Affirmations (or good thoughts) might sound like this:

I, Denise, affirm myself for eating well and exercising throughout my pregnancy.

I, Denise, affirm myself for my ability to labor for so long.

I, Denise, affirm myself for choosing a birth attendant and a male partner who stood by me.

I, Denise, affirm myself for acting in the best interest of my child, for being willing to have a cesarean delivery in order to keep my child safe *in my view*, regardless of medical necessities.

I, Denise, affirm myself for being strong enough to handle a cesarean delivery.

The second cheap and effective form of healing is breathing. Most Westerners do not breathe fully. We tend to hold our breath under stress, and since we are a highly stressed culture this means we hold our breath most of the time.

Breathing provides a release for stored tension, hurt, or pain. We recommend a special breathing/releasing process that Leonard Orr termed "rebirthing."

Rebirthing is a form of yoga that involves long, slow, deep breaths. Each inhale is connected to the exhale, and each exhale to the next inhale. We tend to work harder releasing air than we do pulling it in. Actually, by reversing this breathing process we would gain more effective release, since gravity will take our exhale without effort. It is useful to breathe out the day's accumulation of tension, hurt, and upset, as well as childbirth-related feelings. In fact, breathing, crying, and laughing are the best forms of release available!

The third way to healing is through touch. A woman is extremely responsive and open to touch after childbirth, much as her infant needs and wants to be caressed. However, most touching between men and women in Western culture is in the form of foreplay to sexual intercourse, not a unique experience in and of itself. Postpartum women have experienced physical and emotional trauma and desperately need to be touched. Yet, so often, the touching they need doesn't occur until the infamous six-week checkup is past and the physician proclaims the woman ready to resume sexual relations. She and her mate may then be physically close; sometimes the only touching she receives is confined to the physical act of intercourse.

In cultures where women are touched and massaged after birth, women experience very little postpartum depression, as we know it. Depression in its natural form is a signal to the body, mind, and spirit to rest and recover, to take time for relaxation, for all aspects of the being to regenerate and make ready for the new challenges and responsibilities ahead.

In Western culture, women are not touched, held and stroked in ways that might heal natural postpartum depression, thus prolonging and exaggerating the symptom into a disruptive painful event. Simple holding, back rubs, foot rubs, massage—almost any loving skin contact—can heal the hurts of childbirth in ways that words can never change nor thoughts alter.

The technique of visualization can be an extremely effective tool for healing. Visualization (also called "guided imagery" or "guided fantasy") is merely using your imagination, picturing something in your mind. Sometimes the technique is used to create a vision of what a person would like in their life. Sometimes it is used to recreate a memory (without denying the actual experience), to affect the inner workings of the body, or to provide a sense of closure for an emotionally "unfinished" experience.*

Here is a shortened form of visualization exercise that we do in VBAC classes:

We ask those of you who have had cesareans to take your cesarean experience and imagine that you are painting it on a canvas . . . take plenty of time to create a really vivid mental picture . . . Use whatever colors you need, in whatever quantity, to paint the picture . . . You are all the artists and can paint whatever details need to be included in your design . . . Take your time . . . When it is completed, blow the painting dry . . . As you use your breath to blow it dry, imagine you are blowing out whatever anger, bitterness, frustration, and sadness you may be holding . . . Let the negative feelings or thoughts stream out from every nook and cranny in your body . . . Take a few moments to appreciate the loving decisions you have made . . . When you have done so, and the painting is dry, roll up the canvas . . . Keep rolling it up until it is small enough to fit somewhere in your home, out of the way . . . Find a place to store it . . . When you need to learn from it, or to remember who you were at the time, take it out . . . The learning, the absorbing, the healing may require lengthy, patient, and gently gazing at the canvas. . . When you want to review the joys and gifts you have as a result of it, you can also take it out . . . But when you are having your next baby, leave it in its special place, for if you bring any left-over paint from your last birth, any feelings of anger, sadness, or inadequacy, these tensions may stiffen the bristles of your brush . . . For your next birth, create a whole new painting with whatever colors and textures you need . . . Every design deserves a fresh canvas and a new brush. . . And every painting is a work of art.

Often, what is most painful for cesarean women is the hospital-enforced separation from their newborn babies and the intense sense of loss that accompanies that separation. A woman who suffers from this sense of loss can visualize the birth from the moment right after the delivery of her baby. This is her opportunity to recreate her first moments with her newborn baby. She has the right to redo these moments *her* way.

---

*For more information about visualization, about how it works and why it is so effective, you can begin by reading *Birthing Normally*, by Gayle Peterson; *Creative Visualization*, by Shakti Gawain; and *Getting Well Again*, by the Simontons.

Sometimes, during this visualization, a woman will imagine that she is holding her baby in her arms and talking to him. She can now tell her baby all the things that she wanted to say to him that she didn't have the chance to say before he was taken from her. She may then wish to share with him some of the thoughts and feelings she hasn't been able to express to him about his birth.

Some women go home and repeat some of their words directly to their children. Ruth took her eight-year-old daughter into her arms and said, "When you were a little baby I wanted to tell you how happy I was that you were here and that you were a little girl. I didn't have the chance to tell you that the very first thing after you were born and I want to tell you now." Ruth looked directly into Lisa's eyes and told her how much she loved her. She later told Lisa that she had been worried that perhaps she wouldn't be born healthy, and that she was so happy her daughter was born strong, fine, and perfect: "I missed you so much when you were in the nursery, but I thought that the nurses could take better care of you than I could at that time, and that's why I let them take you. Sometimes I feel like I made the wrong decision, like I wasn't a good mother. I feel very sad I let them take you." Lisa said, "Mommy, I missed you at that time, too, and I was happy when you took care of me all by yourself!" Ruth held Lisa in her arms and rocked her. "I wanted to hold you just like this right after you were born," she told her daughter.

Ruth later told us, "It was a very special moment. We pretended Lisa was a newborn and we replayed those first moments after birth. We both cried!" Ruth had told Lisa the truth about her sad and lonely feelings. The truth frees us and heals relationships.

A mother who has been separated from her baby can also imagine that before her infant is taken from her, she is giving him a special gift. This gift should symbolize all the love she has for her baby. She can imagine that her baby reaches out, takes the gift, and cuddles it close to his heart. We then ask the mother to believe that the baby has the gift with him and that he now feels totally loved, protected, secure, and content as he is taken to the nursery. Some women feel a need to go out into the world to find the gift, or some symbol of it. Some happen upon the perfect gift when they least expect to find it. The truth is that babies *do* have their mother's "gifts" with them during the time they are separated.

A cesarean mother can also imagine that her baby, in his infinite understanding, has given *her* a gift. This gift is something that symbolizes his love, strength, resilience, and forgiveness. She imagines that she has held this gift close to her during the painful separation. And the truth, again, is that the mother did have this gift. Nora said, "When I used to remember Chris' birth, it was with negative feelings—anger, blame, guilt, frustration, and sadness. Now when I remember it, feelings of joy, closeness, and peace mingle with those feelings. I know that these new thoughts are helping to heal my relationship with myself and with my son. In no way do I deny that my cesarean was the way it was, but I feel so much better."

Another suggestion: take the time to place in your mind a kind and loving voice—a voice that reminds you of your competence as a woman and your eternal right to self-love. This voice can be called upon at any time to speak to and nourish your heart and soul. Claudia tells us that any effort to heal childbirth-related hurt, through these suggestions or any others, is always useful—not only for women, but also for their partners and children. Birth is the beginning of family life, and positive emotional beginnings set the stage for positive family living.

Conclusion

Don't be afraid to be with your grief, there may be gifts for you to discover. Remember that, as we read in Claudia's book *Ended Beginnings*, grief is "natural, liberating, and enlightening—as long as it is expressed, understood, and supported."* Acknowledge its presence and use it as an opportunity to learn and grow, to tap strengths, to forgive, to appreciate what is good. (Paul Anka's song "Time of Your Life" reminds us to "reach out for the joy *and* the sorrow . . . ") To those of you who are grieving, we offer our understanding and support. We hope you will take responsibility and do whatever grieving and releasing may need to be done. Some day you will be able to look at your cesarean without anger or bitterness or blame. Some day you will be able to look into your child's eyes and *thank her*, not only for being born, but for the gift of her birth as well. In a letter we received from Minnesota, Susan wrote, "I have stopped chastising myself/ourselves for all the what-ifs and should-have-beens. I am more gracious about accepting the birth for what it was. We were as fully conscious as we could be, and we are allowing the possibility that it was what it was supposed to be. While looking forward to a VBAC, I am happy that I can claim my birth experience with pride." Love fully, grieve fully, and peace and joy will come.

---

*Claudia Panuthos and Catherine Romeo, *Ended Beginnings: Healing Childbearing Losses* (Bergin & Garvey, 1984).

5 ❧ Of Sound Mind and Belly: Uterine Dependability

It seems appropriate to review our previous beliefs and biases . . . [VBAC] would accord the following benefits: a decrease in postoperative and postpartum morbidity, in anesthetic complications, in wound infections, and in postoperative discomfort; there would be a faster recovery period with early participation in infant care. There would be a shorter length of hospital stay resulting in significant financial saving; there would be greater psychological enhancements such as bonding, embracement, and parenting; there would be an increased incidence of breast-feeding in those selecting this option because of an increased feeling of well-being; there would be present the normal silent psychological "high" which is missing in surgical patients because of the postoperative discomforts.[51]

The risk of "uterine rupture" is the excuse given for thousands of unnecessary repeat cesareans. In this chapter, we will share with you what we know to be true—that the risk of uterine instability is extremely small, that even when it does happen it is rarely catastrophic, that there is far more risk involved in repeat cesarean than in VBAC, and that an impressive amount of research has been done to support these claims.

In a poem entitled "Thoughts on Risk," midwife Judith Dickson Luce writes, "I love, and risk loss and pain/ I trust, and risk betrayal/I live, and risk death." She also writes ". . .the computers and statisticians tell us . . . they can reduce risk—and with it, our capacity for living and touching and caring." Judy's husband Tom adds, "It's very risky to be born, since very few people who are born avoid dying—although many avoid living."

Fear of risk makes us the victims of the outdated cliché, "Once a cesarean, always a cesarean." Many of us were victims of an initial unnecessary cesarean: must we add insult to injury (or injury to injury) by allowing a second or third? Even if your primary cesarean was unavoidable, the chances that a repeat will be necessary are remote. And if a repeat *is* called for, the chances that this will ensue because of uterine instability are even more remote. Furthermore, even if you are one of the rare cases in which the uterine incision separates, there is little likelihood that anything dangerous will happen to you or your baby as a result of the separation. You and your baby take a much greater risk by permitting an elective repeat cesarean to be performed. Cesarean women need not have their bellies reopened in order to safely deliver their infants, and it's time we put all the misconceptions about "uterine rupture" to rest.

In discussing "uterine rupture," we must constantly remind ourselves that we are not discussing a risky versus a safe procedure. Choosing a repeat cesarean is not avoiding risk; it is choosing different and, we believe, greater risks. Uterine separation, in the rare circumstance that it does occur as a response to labor, is rarely dangerous, especially in healthy, well-nourished women who have had good prenatal care. Cesarean section, as we explained in Chapter 2, is frequently risky. Danforth states that:

> Cesarean section is not an innocuous procedure unaccompanied by significant matters of fetal risks. A variety of complications, including unexpected fever, endometritis, wound infections, hemorrhage, uterine tract infections, aspiration, and thrombopulmonary embolism, to name a few, occurs 25–50 percent of the time. . . . The accepted maternal death rates are from one to two per thousand, and 25 percent of these deaths are related to anesthesia complications. The comparison of survival rates of infants delivered by elective cesarean section shows approximately a two-fold increase in death and neurological abnormalities due to cesarean section.[24]

Case reported that cesarean section carried out on a healthy mother is three to seven times more dangerous to the mother than vaginal birth, she noted that the mortality rate hasn't fallen in more than ten years.[18]

In a spoof of the medical profession, "Dr. Exacto" has his own answer to the question of maternal mortality:

> "There's one old saw I hear a lot that's always irritated me: a surgeon buries his mistakes. Now, I suppose that's true, up to a point, but did you ever stop to think that we bury lots of successes, too? We do. I'd estimate that half of the really first-rate jobs I've done have gone unnoticed and uncelebrated just because the weak-willed patient didn't have the stamina to make it through the rigors of the operation."*

National Lampoon, November 1978. Reprinted with permission of the publisher.

The problems associated with cesarean section have been stated and restated. Most of us seem unaware of the many dangers involved in cutting open a human being. Yet, even as Craigin's words were being broadcast near and far, others were proclaiming that many of the cesareans performed in the United States are not essential, and that better fetal and maternal results could be achieved by vaginal delivery. Throughout the literature, the risks of surgery are frequently identified. Any medical text alerts readers to the dangers and debilitating consequences of any major abdominal surgery: pneumonia, blood clots, shock, hemorrhage, infection, and death are just a few of the "complications" one might expect. All along, the safety of VBAC has been well documented. It is unfortunate for hundreds of thousands of mothers and babies that the documentation has been ignored, and that sound recommendations about VBAC have gone unheeded.

For example, in the 1950s, Donnelly noted that elective repeat cesarean does not guarantee a lower infant mortality rate than VBAC,[28] and Lawler stated that the fetal mortality rate is three times as great in cesarean section as in VBAC. Even adjusted statistics show that maternal mortality in cesarean section is ten to fifteen times as high as vaginal delivery.[65] In 1953, Eames and his colleagues concluded that repeat cesarean does not give the superior results its proponents expect, and that VBAC should be the method of choice in most circumstances. Cesarean section, they said, has a higher mortality and morbidity rate.[34] Much later, in 1966, Pauerstein reported that both maternal and fetal losses are far greater with repeat cesarean than with VBAC.[92] Even more recently, a report (1981) on repeat cesarean after labor stated that repeat elective cesarean sections arc associated with other risks of mortality that counterbalance the risks of uterine "rupture." In that study, a hypothetical model of ten thousand pregnant women was obtained from the literature. Trial of labor resulted in 37 fewer infant deaths and 0.7 fewer maternal deaths.[114] An article in the *New England Journal of Medicine* reported that the perinatal mortality rates associated with cesarean section are higher than those associated with vaginal delivery.[10] Pettiti's report further confirmed that increased cesarean delivery rates have not resulted in lower neonatal mortality rates.[96] The facts are all out there in black and white, but so few seem to be comprehending them! Women are scheduled for cesareans as casually as if they were being scheduled for hair appointments—and, as we have shown, cesarean section is hardly as safe as a haircut. Remember that the United States is one of the only countries where repeat cesarean is practiced. At a lecture in Boston in 1981, Dr. Michel Odent, from Pitheviers, France, was asked whether women with previous cesareans were permitted to birth in the birthing center there. He responded, "Why, yes, of course. Why not?" A woman who wrote to us was in Sweden when her second baby was born. Her physician and birth attendants seemed so relaxed that she thought perhaps they didn't know she'd had a cesarean. "I wasn't certain if my accent had been so bad that they had misunderstood when I told them I'd had a section. So I kept pointing to my incision and yelling, "Look here! *Ici! La* boo boo! *Une* ouch! *Une grande* ouch!' " Evidently, everyone knew she'd had a previous cesarean, and it didn't make a difference. It seems that neither her 8 pound 6 ounce baby girl nor her healthy, healed uterus cared any more than her physician that there had been a previous uterine incision.

Women in our country are cut open, supposedly to prevent us from tearing open. Having surveyed the abundant literature that exists on the subject of VBAC and uterine rupture, we cannot understand this blind adherence to Craigin's worn-out cliché. There is simply no logic to a policy of elective repeat cesarean sections.

Before we specifically address the issue of uterine rupture, it might be useful to briefly describe the uterus and cervix, how they function in labor, and the placement of the various cesarean incisions.

The Uterus and the Cervix

The pregnant uterus is shaped like an upside-down pear. The uppermost portion (called the *fundus*) and the body of the uterus (corpus) are made up primarily of muscle fiber that contracts during labor. As the fundus contracts, it begins to shorten, or "take up," the lower portion of the uterus. As labor continues, the retracted longitudinal muscle fibers in the fundus pull on the lower segment, causing it to thin out. The lower segment begins to develop prior to the onset of labor, although most of its development occurs as labor begins and progresses.

The cervix is a canal whose upper portion opens into the uterus and whose lower portion opens into the vagina. Through uterine activity, the cervix is shortened, drawn up, and merged into the lower uterine segment. The cervix is gradually thinned (effaced), and the upper canal widens. The lower opening, or mouth, also expands as the uterus contracts. This is "dilation."

Uterus and Cervix

Fundus

Cervix

Lower segment

Uterus and cervix with no effacement or dilation

Cervix completely effaced beginning to dilate

Cervix completely dilated

Uterine Incisions

There are several incisions that can be used to open the uterus during a cesarean section. It is important to note here that we will be referring to the *uterine* incision, not the *abdominal* incision, which opens the belly. The abdominal incision is usually made in the same direction as the uterine incision, but not always. Several women with whom we have worked have vertical abdominal incisions—referred to by them as "railroad tracks," "scars of honor," "battle scars," or "badges of courage"—from the naval to the pubic hair line, but the incisions on their uteri are lower segment horizontal. The *external* horizontal lower incision is referred to as a Phannenstiel incision, a "bikini cut" or a "smile."

The most commonly used uterine incision is the lower segment horizontal (or transverse) incision (also referred to as the Kerr technique) and most of our discussion will pertain to this type of incision.

Uterine Incisions

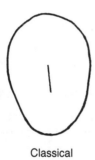 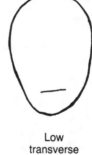 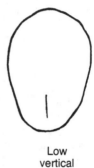

| Classical | Low transverse | Low vertical |

"Smile" Poems

1) Gently and casually, the nurse lays me back on
the bed and removes the bandage to check the
stitches, which are low because the doctor
thought I care about bikinis, rather than a
chance for another Lamaze birth.
She pats the incision and muses, "My, what
a nice Smile."
I lift my head to see, thinking, "From *my* end
it's a frown."

2) *I* couldn't, so my body did. ("Smile," i.e.)

3) Okay, so I finally get up the nerve.
Emerging from the shower, I face the mirror and
confront the Smile.
It's really almost comical, I reflect. My nip-
ples for eyes, naval for nose, and then the
Smile.
I Smile back, Smile and curtsey. "Pleased
t'meetcha." Shyly.
The Smile winks, and becomes a smirk.

4) Yes, it's really almost comical.
The thin black stitches, and skin puffing out
on top and bottom. How can such a thin line
hold me together?
It's really almost comical. Why, it looks just
like a dolphin. Just like a dolphin's Smile
Which is really not a Smile at all.

5) Praying that the Smile
Will not become a Laugh.

6) Plenty of women have episiotomies, but it isn't
everyone who has a Smile lurking beneath her
pubic hair.

—*Marion Cohen*

However, lower segment vertical incisions (Sellheim incisions) or vertical classical (midline) incisions are occasionally used. Infrequently, a J-shaped incision is made. It is generally the result of an attempt to perform a transverse lower uterine segment incision when the lower segment is too narrow. A T-shaped incision may also be made for the same reason, "or on the hasty management of the unexpected finding of placental implantation beneath the area of the incision."[24]

Popularization of Repeat Cesarean Section

As we have mentioned, when the odious phrase, "Once a cesarean, always a cesarean" was coined in 1916 by Dr. Edwin B. Craigin, cesarean section had been approached cautiously, since maternal and fetal morbidity and mortality associated with this procedure were extremely high. Women labored for many hours before a section was considered, and when the decision was made, the operation was performed with trepidation. Physicians were apt to be called before their obstetrical superiors to justify having resorted to the knife. Craigin himself wondered if the fundamentals of obstetrics were being neglected in the enthusiasm for radical obstetrical surgery. He worried that routine precautionary methods that could prevent such surgery were being overlooked.[23] At that time, classical cesarean section was the rule. The uterine incision was often extended toward the top (fundus) of the uterus, the portion that contracts most energetically during labor. Many an OB breathed a great sigh of relief when the mother and/ or infant came through alive, since a goodly number did not. Once labor was established and membranes ruptured, the maternal mortality rate associated with classical cesarean section was 10 percent, rising to 30 percent if several vaginal exams had been done or if there had been an attempt at vaginal delivery. Many women had a "one-way ticket" only to the O.R. For subsequent pregnancies, physicians were concerned that if they didn't "get to" the woman before she went into labor, her uterus would begin to contract and rip open. The precautionary policy of performing cesareans two weeks early caused a number of serious problems in itself, not the least of which were premature babies who often did not survive.

The custom of resectioning cesarean women, which began during Craigin's reign, can be attributed to several factors. Most women who were originally sectioned were assumed to have a pelvic obstruction, since prolonged labor had not produced a child. This being the case, it seemed useless to permit another labor. The rate of classical uterine rupture was high, and reported associated catastrophes staggering. Unperfected suturing materials and techniques, and unsterile conditions, were partly responsible, especially in emergency situations. In addition, there were no blood banks or antibiotics, and the results of anesthesia were unpredictable. All of this contributed to the threat of a weakened uterus and, therefore, supported the adoption of Craigin's dictum.

Craigin himself reported that many exceptions occur. He cited a patient in his practice who had delivered vaginally three times after a cesarean section. Yet, in spite of his own openmindedness, his edict became medical dogma. Picture a mob of obstetricians congregated in the town square. A man with a long, white, George-Washington-style ponytail and velvet waistcoat unrolls a parchment scroll: "Hear ye, hear ye! A proclamation! From this day forth . . ."

The Transverse-Incision Revolution

In the early 1920s Monroe Kerr pioneered the adoption of the transverse incision, made in the lower portion of the uterus. The technique of lower segment cesarean section had been developed in the early 1880s, but it was Kerr who was responsible for the general adoption of this operation by the English-speaking world. A paper by St. George Wilson on lower segment cesarean section appeared in Great Britain in 1931,[126] further convincing obstetricians. Lower segment cesarean section revolutionized obstetric practice because it made abdominal delivery safe even when performed late in labor or when the uterine cavity was infected. It was this technique which resulted in the whole concept of trial of labor and vaginal birth after cesarean. Ironically, the relative safety of the lower segment operation was also responsible for the rise in the incidence of cesarean section.

There are many advantages to the transverse or lower segment horizontal incision. When an incision is made in the lower segment, it is made through a thinned-out uterine wall (especially if the woman has been in labor), rather than the thick uterus. Healing takes less time and there is less patient discomfort. ("It still hurts plenty!" remarked one cesarean mother.) There is less blood loss, because the lower segment is relatively avascular, and massive hemorrhage is extremely rare. Repair is easier, and because the low transverse incision is wholly covered by the bladder, any "discharge" has no direct entry into the peritoneal cavity—a definite safeguard.

For our purposes, the most important advantage of the low transverse incision is its dependability in subsequent labors. Because of the proportionately low ratio of muscle fiber in the lower segment (compared to the fundus), it does not contract nearly as powerfully during labor. You might say it is "less involved" in labor than the body of the uterus. Kerr himself perfected the low segment technique so that women and babies would not have to be subjected to the risks and dangers inherent in cesarean section. He noted its strength and urged physicians to use it and then think toward vaginal delivery.

When you consider that we now have efficient blood transfusion services, blood volume expanders, effective and widely available antibiotic agents (which help prevent infection as well as cover a multitude of sins), more complete attention to antenatal care, more dependable suturing techniques and materials, and safer anesthetics than were available to Kerr—with all this, it seems extremely unfortunate that repeat cesareans have continued to be the law as the lower transverse incision gained in popularity. In the rare event of a medical emergency, we have far more back-up than Kerr ever dreamed possible.

According to several articles, Craigin's rule has been expanded to embrace the lower segment operation, which is an entirely different procedure from the classical incision. Leslie Williams, associate professor of obstetrics and gynecology at the University of Miami, is reported[104] as remarking that Craigin's dictum has been invested "with the sanctity of biblical truth. . . . [But] I cannot share the philosophy. The benefits of vaginal delivery far outweigh the slight risk of uterine rupture."

The Specter of Uterine "Rupture"

"RUPTURE." What feelings does that word elicit? What images, what colors, thoughts, sounds, smells, expressions? The use of this word in connection with c/section, and the dire images it conjures, have been responsible for hundreds of thousands, thousands of thousands, of totally unnecessary operations. We are programmed to believe that if we dare to even consider VBAC, we will rip open, bleed profusely, and die on the spot. This is an unmerciful, unforgivable deception. The term "uterine rupture" is a despicable abuse of the English language.

"Rupture" conjures up thoughts of bursting, blood, and explosion. In Craigin's day, uterine crises of that sort did happen on occasion. As we've mentioned, some of the reasons for such catastrophes were the conditions under which cesareans were performed. In the stacks of recent American obstetrical articles we surveyed on VBAC, there are *no instances of catastrophic lower segment uterine rupture.* Several articles had no incidences of uterine rupture. In the infrequent references to "uterine rupture," rupture was generally *benign.* Yes, benign.

Rupture implies recent tearing with consequent bleeding from the newly torn tissue.* At the time of repeat cesarean, most obstetricians have seen a hole in the old uterine scar. This opening is called a "window." It occurs with some frequency and is considered to be a result of healing. *It is not a rupture.* A window shows no recent tearing of tissue. Case states that windows can be present throughout pregnancy and that they represent a response to healing rather than a response to labor.[18] However, only a few of the studies differentiate between windows and rupture, or between complete and incomplete ruptures. In most studies, windows are recorded as ruptures and included in rupture statistics, *even though they are of no serious consequence!* In an editorial comment in an obstetrical text, we are told that a woman can have a VBAC even if there is a defect in the lower uterine segment. "On finding such defect, many obstetricians would find it difficult to resist operating for a ruptured uterus . . . [However,] the patient is not in jeopardy." (Incidentally, we refute the term "defect" as well as the term "rupture.")

Another situation that is included in "rupture" statistics is called "dehiscence." Dehiscence refers to an area on the incision in which not all the layers of the uterus are together—a separation. We're reminded of paper doilies, which separate cleanly in layers, or the pastry baklavah. Dehiscence, like a window, is

---

*The 14th edition of *Williams Obstetrics* defines rupture as "separation of the old scar throughout its entire length, rupture of the fetal membranes with connection between the uterine and peritoneal cavities, usually accompanied by massive bleeding, and all or part of the fetus is extruded into the peritoneal cavity." Hellman and Pritchard, editors. New York: Appleton-Century-Crofts, 1971, p. 937.

a result of healing rather than a response to labor. *It is not a dangerous circumstance for mother or baby,* yet it is included in the statistics for "uterine rupture."

It is important to remember that no uterus is immune to rupture. Rupture in an unscarred uterus is far more catastrophic for both mother and baby. In an intact uterus, the point of least resistance and most powerful contractility opens. This is the uppermost portion of the uterus, and a ragged, sorry tear occurs. It is much more catastrophic than weakness in an incised uterus. A 1980 study by Golan reported 93 cases of uterine rupture during a five-year period. Sixty-one ruptures occurred in normal uteri, while thirty-two were found in women who had had a previous cesarean. There were nine maternal deaths, *all in the group of women who had not previously had cesarean surgery.*[40] In the rare circumstance that a uterus with a previous cesarean does separate, the incision generally opens gently and neatly, like a seam or a zipper. **We found no reports of maternal death associated with the lower segment incision in all the studies we surveyed; the incidence of fetal death associated with VBAC is agreed to be less than that with elective repeat cesarean even by the most reluctant VBAC skeptics.**

In 1953, Harris noted that there is a distinct difference between rupture of a normal uterus (we ask, does a *normal* uterus rupture?) and a rupture through a poorly healed section scar. In the former, he said, there is profuse bleeding and rapidly advancing shock. The fetal and maternal mortality rates are high. However, in cases of rupture through a weakened scar, hemorrhage is minimal, and both fetus and mother have an excellent chance of survival, particularly if the scar is located in the lower uterine segment. He stated, "We have demonstrated both clinically and experimentally that the strength of a well-healed scar is as great as the uterine muscle itself."[48] Mason and Williams also showed experimentally that the area of the incision is more resistant to rupture under tension than intact uterine muscle.[68]

A veterinarian friend shared with us his experience with surgery on dogs. He knows each dog that has been operated upon, since he's the one who performed the surgery, but he often cannot find the original incision when he needs to operate again. We know physicians who have been unable to find the original incision on a woman whom they have previously sectioned. *This is because our bodies heal!* That's what our bodies *do* when they get cut! Williams[98] states that the site of the previous operation may not be recognizable by gross examination or even microscopic study!

According to *Williams Obstetrics,* little information has been garnered from studies of cesarean section scars. Williams himself was of the opinion that the uterus heals by regeneration of the muscle fibers, not by scar tissue. He based his conclusions on examination, and also on his observation that inspection of the unopened uterus usually showed no trace of a former incision. If present, it appeared as an almost invisible linear scar.

Schwartz et al. theorized that healing occurs mainly by the proliferation of fibroblasts (branched cells found throughout connective tissue). They concluded that as the scar shrinks, the proliferations of connective tissue become less perceptable, requiring special stains for demonstration. If the cut surfaces are brought in close apposition, gradually the normal relationship of smooth-muscle and connective tissue, as in the uninjured uterus, is reestablished. The authors remark that this accounts for the fact that sometimes there is no trace of a former incision, while at other times a definite scar is seen.[111] Douglas remarks that "neatness of [the] operation decrease[s] the incidence of uterine defects."[30]

Iatrogenic Causes of Uterine Instability

Uterine dependability and the safety of VBAC have been demonstrated for years! Iatrogenic (physician-induced) causes of uterine rupture are finally being exposed, and we assume *many* more problems with uterine incisions to be directly associated with physician interference than are reported. It is well documented that oxytocic agents, used to stimulate uterine contractility, can result in hyperstimulation of a uterus which may then rupture even when there is no obstruction to labor. Many "ruptures" cited in the literature are associated with the use of these dangerous agents. Bhattacharya and Dutta reported seven cases of iatrogenic uterine rupture from obstetric manipulation or administration of oxytocic agents.[7] Additional iatrogenic factors may predispose a uterus to rupture; these include drugs, damage to the uterus during insertion of an intrauterine contraceptive device, and perforation of a uterus during performance of an abortion. C.P. Douglas states that untrained or overambitious use of instruments for delivery; unskilled, clumsy, or difficult manual removal of the placenta; oxytocic drugs in combination with conduction anesthesia; and roughness on the part of the obstetrician can also lead to rupture.[30] Researchers from other countries note that the cause of rupture in the United States is shifting because of more aggressive management of labor.

It is intriguing to speculate about the few incisions that do separate: what was the level of skill of the operator? The amount of pride in his work? The time of day the cesarean was performed, and the technique used for suturing? "Uterine rupture" is often the fault of the operator, not the uterus. A recent rupture in Boston, for example, occurred when a suture used to prevent cervical incompetence was not removed prior to labor.

Signs of "Rupture"?

Many of you must be wondering, "If I am in that zero-point-five percent of lower segment uterine separation, how will I know?" A little message on positive thinking, which we believe has merit: with better than a 99.5 percent chance of things going well, and with most problems occurring in improperly nourished, unmotivated, oxytocin-augmented labors, it doesn't seem likely that you will have a problem. But women in our culture are conditioned for disappointment rather than success. A little reconditioning is definitely in order.

First, pain and tenderness are unreliable indications of impending rupture. Meehan and others[73] report that many patients with a history of cesarean section will complain of tenderness over the lower abdomen in late pregnancy or during labor, but when a cesarean is performed, or after the baby is born vaginally, the scar is intact. Many labors are halted because of complaints of pain over the lower uterine segment, although pain is quite notorious for its inaccuracy as a diagnostic tool! Most separations are unaccompanied by pain or tenderness.

In the rare circumstance that a uterine incision proves unstable and there *is* the signal of pain, alcohol, drugs, and conduction anesthetics will mask this. There are many other reasons not to use alcohol, drugs or anesthetics during labor, although all were used to some degree in VBAC labors reported in the literature. Many physicians *threaten* women who want a VBAC: "You won't be able to have any medication, you know. Not even a little." Some have actually seemed excited about that, as if to say, "Let's see if the lady freaks out."

Many women are sectioned because the staff has paranoid suspicions of rupture, only to find an intact uterus at the time of surgery. McGarry noted that many repeat cesareans are done for inadequate reasons, particularly out of fear for the scar. Several articles noted that most obstetricians have found an intact scar during repeat cesarean for suspected scar rupture. Also, women who have written to us were sectioned because their physicians were convinced that their incisions had ruptured, only to find a perfectly healthy uterus going about its business safely and efficiently.

So symptoms of uterine separation may include all, some, or none of the following: abdominal pain, vaginal bleeding, shock, swelling over the lower segment, a rise in pulse followed by a drop in blood pressure, fever, or a boardlike uterus which does not contract. In 173 labors that we have followed, none of these has been a problem.

When Instability Does Occur—Sterilization or Repair?

Does "Rupture" mean instantaneous death for a woman—or at the very least hysterectomy, as we are so often told? *No!* In 1969, Pauerstein reported that in properly equipped hospitals (are there actually *un*-equipped hospitals out there!?), death from lower segment uterine rupture should be nil, and that the infrequent uterine and infant losses caused by rupture are preventable.[93] Browne and McGrath[13] reviewed 566 VBAC women. The three cases of rupture (.53

percent) were "uneventful." Smith also disagrees that rupture of the uterus always means loss of the mother's ability to have future children. In his study of ten ruptures, six women had their uteri repaired, and four went on to have subsequent pregnancies and healthy babies.[118] Merrill and Gibbs reported four "uterine ruptures" in 634 women. Two were from classical incisions found at the time of section; both were repaired. The other two were VBAC women. Neither exhibited hemorrhage.[76] (Were these latter two really "ruptures," or—more likely—*windows?*) In another study by Merrill and Gibbs, with 526 women, the "uterine rupture" rate was 0.5 percent. The complications were not serious; hemorrhage and shock were absent, and only one hysterectomy was performed.[76] It is not clear if the hysterectomy was necessary as a result of the "rupture."

Hills believes that choice of repair or hysterectomy depends on the character of the tear, the condition of the patient, and the philosophy of the operator.[49] We certainly hope those "operators' " philosophies match ours—or at least those of the women on whom he might operate.

Other articles on repair vs sterilization seem to follow this principle: use whatever technique gets the patient off the table in the best condition. We hope this takes into account the patient's *emotional* condition also. Murphy (1976) reported on forty-one ruptures between 1965 and 1974. Twenty-nine separations occurred in 2,479 women (1.2 percent) following previous cesarean section. Nine were found at repeat cesarean before labor. No hysterectomies were required as a result of these "ruptures."[83] A Ghana medical journal reports that of 444 women, 269 (60.6 percent) had VBACs. Ten (2.3 percent) had scar ruptures, four of which were lower segment scars. There were six hysterectomies. One rupture occurred during labor in a woman who had had four previous sections, and required a hysterectomy. Her 8 pound 10 ounce baby was fine.[60]

Pauerstein pointed out in his study that it was especially significant that fertility was returned in all but two of over 634 cases of uterine separation that he studied. Commenting on a study by Morley, Pauerstein created a hypothetical model of 10,000 women with lower segment incisions. Maternal mortality, if rupture occurs, is 0.1 percent, he said. Therefore, it would take 1000 ruptured uteri of 400,000 patients with lower segment scars to yield one maternal death from this cause. The twenty-five ruptures in 10,000 scarred uteri would theoretically yield 2.5 percent fetal deaths. "As we have seen, in cesarean section both the maternal and fetal losses are considerably greater."[92]

Again, how exasperating that windows and dehiscences are included in the rupture rates, and that these benign separations are often sutured! Saldana reports that the probability of gross rupture of the transverse uterine scar and maternal consequences are largely exaggerated. In most studies the patient is found to have a "uterine rupture" at the time of elective repeat cesarean.[107] A rupture that was *undiagnosed* until repeat c/section? Could this be true? But we've all been taught that ruptures are dangerous, explosive, *catastrophic!* Obviously, most of these "ruptures" were windows or dehiscences.

Our own experience with 173 women with previous cesareans who planned VBACs has shown two separations thus far. These two openings were found *at the time of repeat cesarean* and at no time posed a problem for mother or baby. How can 98 percent of the authors writing on the subject of uterine stability get away with calling these benign separations ruptures? Lawler reported that often ruptures are found when the abdomen is opened at the time of section. These windows, he said, are only discovered if a cesarean is done.[65] Windows are not ruptures! Why is this distinction not made? Murphy said that all the dehiscences in his study were incomplete and repaired.[83] Dehiscence is by its very definition incomplete, and does not need any repair. It may even provide "give" to the incision, if left alone.

As you may already have gathered, most of the separations that are not windows or dehiscences occur prior to the onset of labor. Thus the practice of sectioning women at 38 weeks in an attempt to prevent rupture is absurd. Any incision that is going to separate is likely to do so before the 38th week, and taking babies early exposes them to needless risk. In Donnelly's study, four separations occurred prior to 37 weeks; one occurred at 33 weeks.[29] Lawler advised that repeat cesarean cannot forestall uterine rupture because many occur several weeks before the section is scheduled.[65] Douglas agreed, claiming, "Fifty percent of 'ruptures' occur prior to the time elective surgery would be considered."[31] They occur through an avascular portion of the uterus and are not catastrophic. Donnelly states that VBAC is generally safer for mother and child than elective repeat cesarean at 38 weeks,[29] and Case argues that it is pointless to advocate a trial of scar. If a scar is going to rupture, or a window extend, it is likely to do so prior to or at the onset of labor. She goes on to say that, except by avoiding all intrauterine manipulations, there are no available means of protecting the scar.[18] Most of the studies report "silent, incomplete" ruptures (we're still having trouble associating these unthreatening terms with the specter of rupture) that are no more dangerous than Winnie the Pooh's blustery friend Tigger. Since we now know that most incisions that separate do so prior to the onset of labor and rarely cause a problem, if your incision is intact at term, the chances are that it has proved its integrity. Being overdue does not cause added stress on the incision. We'd like a penny for every woman who has been told she can't be overdue if she wants a VBAC! "On Friday, I was a great candidate," said one woman. "By Monday, my doctor was hysterical." When she was three days overdue, she changed doctors, and one week later had a 9 pound baby by VBAC.

Some authors insist women go into the hospital at 38 weeks, to await their fate. McGarry, for one, believes this practice is unnecessary. His opinion is that the temptation to deliver patients once they have been admitted has proved irresistible on a number of occasions.[70]

Scare Tactics

Study after study, from the 1930s until the present, substantiates the fact that "uterine rupture" is rare. Rarely, if ever, is fetal loss related to the rupture or mode of delivery. We have been collecting and surveying articles for ten years, and *there is not an article written on the subject of VBAC since the 1930s that says that VBAC is so risky that it should not be permitted.* Although some articles are more conservative than others, every one of them points to VBAC as a reasonable alternative. Most are *overwhelmingly favorable.* We are frustrated by the multitude of doctors who have obviously done no reading on the subject of VBAC, and who confront women with absurd statements such as, "It's too great a risk; I can only guarantee you a healthy baby if you agree to a cesarean . . ."; "Sure, we'll try it—what difference does a hysterectomy make?"; or "If your uterus ruptures, it means instantaneous death for you and your baby." *These are all actual quotations,* and now that all the votes are in and we have the envelope, we'd like to announce three more winners. The most popular phrases used to frighten women away from VBAC are (drum roll): *"If you were my wife. . ."; "In **your** particular case . . .";* and *"We have to be concerned about what is best for that baby!"* No article among the scores we've surveyed has discouraged VBACs with a lower segment incision, and many have supported VBACs even with a classical section.

Please remember that many of these studies were done on medically indigent women. One article states that it is reasonable to assume that results would be even more favorable if studies were done with patients who received adequate prenatal care and good nutrition. We can only concur. Nutrition and good health play an extremely important part in any labor and delivery. Motivation also plays a crucial role, yet, with the exception of one study,[107] there is absolutely no acknowledgment of this fact in the VBAC obstetrical literature.

In spite of the good results described in most studies, we wonder how many *more* of the women in these studies would have delivered vaginally if they had been walking around, taking warm showers, and getting lots of hugs instead of internal exams! How many were sectioned needlessly because a time limit was placed on their labor? How many times was the fetal monitor inaccurate, leading to an unnecessary section? How many times did it contribute to a section by immobilizing the woman? How many women were required to be on their backs during labor? We know that induction of labor and instrument delivery are associated with uterine rupture, yet how many women were given oxytocin and delivered by forceps before rupturing? How many women were deprived of the comfort of friends or relatives who could have created an atmosphere for safe and normal birthing? The studies leave out all these details that would help us understand why the rates of VBAC aren't much, much higher than they are. Saldana's study mentions that eight women were apprehensive about labor, "probably on the advice of previous physicians."[107] We suggest that at least 99 percent of the women in the American VBAC studies were probably apprehensive about their labors, and we *know* that apprehension lowers the potential for natural birth, while loving, confident support raises it. It's hard to be relaxed when people are standing around watching the clock and waiting anxiously for your uterus to burst.

In "Studying Childbirth: The Experience and Methods of a Woman Anthropologist," Brigette Jordan suggests that research on birth is most easily and appropriately done by women. She believes that women are much more likely to achieve the involvement, reciprocity, and trust which an event "as intimate, emotion-laden, and delicately sensitive as birth requires. For that very reason, they are likely to produce less disruption in the process than men, so that we can expect more valid data from investigations by female researchers."[53] We, too, find it most disturbing that research about women is most often done by men, and we suggest that VBAC would have been encouraged far sooner, and there would have been even greater success statistics, if women had designed and assisted in the research.

Perhaps we ask too much, but we'd love to see expressions of elation in accounts of women scheduled for repeat cesareans—because they had been categorized as poor candidates for VBAC—who delivered naturally and without complication while the cesarean room was being readied for them. No comments like: "Hey terrific! Gee, that was a wonderful surprise! So glad you can leave the hospital right away! Thanks so much—I wasn't really in the mood to cut anyone open today!" And out of more than 60 articles we surveyed, only one— one!—mentioned that there was a cosmetic reason for considering a low horizontal abdominal cut. Some call it vanity, but we wonder how many men would be delighted with a long, red, raised scar on their torsos. Those physicians who patronizingly assure us that we needn't worry, we'll still be able to wear a bikini, may be thinking more of their own concern about what is visually pleasurable to men than about the violation of a cesarean incision to the body of a woman.

Another objection we'd like to raise about the studies we reviewed concerns inappropriate and misleading language. While we cannot change all this terminology, we can be aware of words that subtly affect behavior and thought patterns, contributing to a lower-than-acceptable VBAC rate. For example, healthy, normal, birthing women are called "patients." As far as we are concerned, a patient is a person who is sick, and birthing women are not sick. In "What Every Pregnant Woman Should Know about Cesareans," Lynn Richards (Browne) says, " . . . We are informed *clients*, not *patients*."[14] In most studies, however, "patients" are "allowed" or "permitted" a "trial" of labor, and their labors are always "managed" by the obstetrical team.

The concept of "trial" of labor is inappropriate. A trial conjures images of a judge and jury. At any moment the gavel may come down—bang! Sentenced!

Off with you to the OR! Another cesarean by order of the court! Case dismissed! Several articles state that a VBAC labor not only "tries" the scar, but also the obstetrician's ability to withstand peer pressure and stress. We do not use the term trial of labor. You aren't on trial, nor is your incision.

The word "attempt" is also over-used. The patient *attempted* labor. Does an obstetrician *attempt* a cesarean? We don't like the word "candidate," either. Candidates have to prove themselves in order to win. Sometimes excellent "candidates" are not even put on the ballot; it depends on who is setting the standards. A good candidate in one study would not even be considered for VBAC in another. A woman should not be excluded from VBAC because of the rigid and inappropriate standards in her area. We know that potentially *excellent* candidates were unjustly excluded from VBAC in most of the studies because of certain unfounded and biased criteria.

Never do the articles speak of women *delivering* their babies. One study says, "Thirty-two of the women *were delivered* by the vaginal route" (as if there were *several* routes). Another states, "Our study demonstrates the safety of allowing women who have had previous cesareans to go into labor to determine whether they can be delivered vaginally." Still another says, "A woman should be allowed to demonstrate her capacity to be delivered vaginally." To *be delivered* vaginally, by us, the obstetricians of the world! *We* will determine if you can be delivered. If you can, *we* will then *deliver you.*

The term that is most difficult to bear is "uneventful." If a woman's uterus does not rupture, the delivery is "uneventful." Has there ever been a birth that was uneventful? Can *any* baby's entrance into the world ever be called un-eventful?

As we have noted, many articles and most obstetricians refer to vaginal de-liveries as birth "from below." Cesarean sections, by contrast, are births "from above!" We find this distinction offensive. Delivering "from above" sounds more glorified and heavenly, and it shouldn't. Cesarean section is major abdominal surgery. (True, more women get to Heaven by being sectioned than by delivering vaginally, but we don't consider this a reason to glorify the procedure.)

The total lack of respect for birthing as a normal, safe, natural process is evident throughout most of the obstetrical literature. The lack of respect for women is even more striking. Indeed, we are vessels from which a product must be removed. We constantly wondered as we reviewed the obstetrical journals where the feelings had gone—the awe, the joy, the faith. Of course, there's probably no room for any of that when you are sitting around waiting for a uterus to produce or rupture.

Language is important! For example, using the term "cesarean birth" rather than "cesarean section" adds to the complacency with which our country views a major abdominal operation. We shudder when we think that women them-selves were initially responsible for many of the word changes. Perhaps there was a way to humanize necessary cesareans without contributing to the callous attitude about surgical delivery. We are in total agreement with Marion Thompson, former president of La Leche League International, who says, "For a long time we have put acceptable labels on procedures which might otherwise not be so acceptable. . . . I wish that 'cesarean birth' had the same kind of physiological and psychological outcome as a natural delivery. But it doesn't, and changing the label won't make it so." On the other hand, changing the label "uterine rupture," to "uterine dependability" or "stability" may take us a long way from elective repeat cesarean section.

Growing Support for VBAC: The Studies

As the lower segment incision became more widely accepted and replaced (for the most part) the classical incision, the maxim, "Once a cesarean . . ." began to have its critics.

The 1940s

In the 1940s Craigin's dictum was challenged independently, by such researchers as Schmitz and Gajewski,[110] Waters,[124] Hindman,[50] Adair,[1] and Burkons.[15] In 1949, Lull and Ullery stated that the stress and strain *on the obstetrician* during a VBAC labor was one of the factors that caused physicians to become advocates of repeat cesarean.[67]

The 1950s

By the 1950s, interest in VBAC had begun to grow. Dewhurst reported a .53 percent rate of "uterine rupture" (8 out of 1,530).[26] Harris reported that VBAC was a rational procedure, and made a plea to discard the old dictum. He reported a 74 percent VBAC rate and urged physicians to test the natural possibilities.[48] Cosgrove stated that cesarean section once employed does not always necessitate its repetition at a subsequent delivery, and that he preferred vaginal delivery whenever possible. He reported 179 VBACs (35.8 percent), 12 "ruptures," 6 of which occurred prior to labor, and no deaths. Six deaths occurred in the repeat section group.[22]

Zarou echoed Lull and Ullery and stated that VBAC strained the obstetrician more than the scar.[129] McLane reported 43 VBACs with no ruptures and no maternal mortality.[71] Eames,[34] Lawrence,[66] and Dewhurst[26] concluded that the dictum did not give the superior results assumed and implied by its proponents, and that VBAC for a nonrecurring reason should be the method of choice. Women's Hospital in Sidney, Australia, reported a 67.5 percent VBAC rate.[30] Lawler stated that the possibility of "rupture" was by no means to be disdained, but neither was it to be viewed with "abject terror."[65] Douglas reported that of 1,957 cesarean women, 737 had VBACs. He believed it significant that there was *not a single maternal complication, nor a single infant lost* as a result of a defect or rupture of a lower segment scar in this large sample.[31] (Indeed, when infants are lost, it is because of situations unrelated to the VBAC, such as anesthesia-related consequences. When a uterus does separate, there are often predisposing circumstances, such as a severe congenital abnormality or previous manual removal of an adherent placenta.)[118] A five-year study in Dublin (1952–1957) proved that "cesarean section does not mar a woman's future obstetric career."[3]

The 1960s

In 1963 Allahbadia stated that a 97 percent VBAC rate was possible. He stated emphatically, "Once a cesarean is NOT always a cesarean!"[3] Douglas reported a 40 percent VBAC rate of 317 women. Observations on 2,377 women led him to believe that this figure could be higher. "This dictum does not apply to current obstetric practice. We need not be hampered by a policy enunciated nearly one-half century ago," he said. He went on to say that emergencies during labor for VBAC are rarely more urgent than any other situation encountered in obstetrics. He noted that in 3,000 cesarean women, there had never been an emergency as a result of rupture of the lower uterine segment, and that *no fetal losses due to rupture or that mode of delivery should be expected.*[31]

In 1964, Salzmann echoed Douglas. Rupture of the lower segment scar, he said, occurs very rarely and is almost never explosive. "It is safe to permit a trial of labor."[108] In 1966, O'Driscoll reviewed 2,170 VBACs in Dublin and stated that VBAC was safer than repeat cesarean.[89] In an article printed in 1966, O'Connell stated that VBAC was neither unique nor experimental. The medical profession as a whole, he said, "exhibits a profound reluctance to accept the fact."[88] In 1966 Pauerstein stated that approximately four-fifths of cases can deliver vaginally. He said that the presence of the lower segment scar adds "little maternal and fetal risk to that inherent in labor and delivery."[92]

In 1967, Notelovitz and Chrichton reported a .27 percent rate of "uterine rupture" (21 of 7,645).[86] In 1969, McGarry stated that many repeat cesareans have been done for inadequate reasons, in particular for fear of scar "rupture." He said that uterine rupture of the lower segment scar is too uncommon to justify repetition of the cesarean for that reason alone; a repeat cesarean that becomes necessary during a "trial" of labor does not carry an unacceptable risk to mother or fetus. "VBAC is frequently possible and certainly desirable. Cesarean section may be required in less than 12 percent." In his study 114 (80 percent) had VBACs.[70]

The 1970s

In the 1970s, more studies substantiated the safety of VBAC; *yet women were still being sectioned more than 99 percent of the time.* Still, the winds of change were blowing. In 1974, Nancy coined the term "VBAC," and by 1975 she was hearing the acronym being used all over the country and was seeing it in medical articles as well.

In 1972, Meehan et al. stated that when no recurring indication exists, and the vertex presents, VBAC should be anticipated. "We consider elective repeat cesarean meddlesome obstetrics."[73] In 1973, Morewood et al. asked if all patients needed to be subjected to repeat cesarean. They answered their own question: "We think not!"[79] In 1973, Ruiz-Velasco et al. reported 1,112 women who had VBACs, including nine women who had had more than one cesarean, and many who had been sectioned for CPD. "These results disprove the saying, 'Once a cesarean . . .' "[106] In 1978, Merrill and Gibbs said, "The policy of once a cesarean, always a cesarean is now outdated, and that such a plan (VBAC) is safe has been documented previously."[76]

In a paper written in the mid-1970s, Dr. Victor Berman stated that from 21 to 91 percent of patients selected for VBAC can deliver vaginally. He reported on a study at New York Lying-In Hospital in which, of 2,094 women, eight cases of lower segment "rupture" occurred. All "ruptures" were incomplete, and there was no maternal perinatal mortality associated with the separations. He cited two other studies. One, the Margaret Hague 1948–1961 study, reported a 51 percent VBAC rate (2,904 women). The other was a 1949–1964 report from thirteen teaching hospitals in Great Britain. In 3,429 previously sectioned women, the VBAC rate ranged from 85 to 91 percent.[6] In a 1979 article entitled, "Should All Previous Cesarean Sections Be Sectioned Again?" Yoram Sorokin, M.D., concluded that to anticipate a VBAC for nonrecurring conditions is very reasonable. With individualization and a selective approach, he said, VBAC is in the best interests of both mother and baby.[120]

In 1979 Saldana wrote, "There appears to be no rational or scientific basis for a 99 percent repeat cesarean rate, and this practice should be abandoned." There were no uterine ruptures in his study of 145 women, and 38.6 percent delivered vaginally.[107]

The 1980s

In a 1981 "Cesarean Controversy Update," it is stated that "the theory of 'once a cesarean' has been seriously challenged. . . . [Consumer] groups have caused physicians and medical institutions to reevaluate their thinking and policies regarding cesarean sections."[19]

In 1981, Silfen and Wilf reported a 78.5 percent rate of VBAC at Booth Maternity Hospital.[115] A 1981 report by Shy et al. used hypothetical cohorts of 10,000 pregnant women, 6,623 of whom "were delivered" vaginally. Trial of labor resulted in 37 fewer perinatal deaths and 0.7 fewer maternal deaths than elective repeat cesarean.[114]

A 1981 report by Meier on VBAC states that it is reasonable to expect between 60 and 70 percent of mothers allowed to labor to deliver vaginally. "Uterine scar separation is rarely encountered . . ., often asymptomatic, and occurs with equal frequency in patients who are allowed to labor or who are electively delivered by repeat cesarean."[75] Dr. Charles Mahan from Florida persuades his clients to have VBACs. He reports that Shands Teaching Hospital, where he works, has an 83 percent rate of VBAC. Dr. Mahan believes that within ten years, VBAC will no longer be considered high risk. We appreciate his efforts and hope it doesn't take that long for his colleagues to shape up.

The 1980s have brought additional support for VBAC. The October 1, 1981 Obstetrics and Gynecology News, bastion of U.S. obstetrical opinion, remarked that "Once a cesarean . . ." may be true for some patients, but that many former cesarean section patients should at least be offered the option of a "trial by labor."[84] Dr. Mussenden-Jackson reported to the National Medical Association that healthy patients with uncomplicated pregnancies should be allowed a trial labor.[84] In the October 1981 *Research Resource Reporter*, it was stated that the number of cesareans could be reduced if doctors did not steadfastly follow the old dictum.[101] Dr. M. Rosen, Chairman of the NIH Task Force, conceded that the idea of performing routine repeat cesareans made sense years ago. Now that surgeons cut nearer the cervix, however, the scar that forms is stronger—"reason enough to try a normal birth."[101] Dr. C. Hobel, professor of obstetrics and gynecology at UCLA, contended, "It is safe to deliver vaginally, even when the patient has had a cesarean. There is less morbidity and less cost in a vaginal delivery than repeat cesarean."[101] Kaiser, in San Diego, reported an 83 percent VBAC rate. Kaiser protocol is now to consider every cesarean mother for VBAC, with only compelling medical circumstances as exceptions.[101] In a 1982 article by Lavin et al., we are told that a previous vaginal delivery improves the prognosis for a successful VBAC, but a "substantial percentage of those without such a history will deliver vaginally when allowed a trial of labor."[64]

As information about and demand for VBAC increase, a growing number of obstetricians have begun to support VBAC. Dr. Gerald Cohen from Framingham, Massachusetts, remarks, "It is not only gratifying to the woman to have a VBAC, but satisfying to the obstetrician to be able to share in this experience." Richard McDowell, an obstetrician from Stoneham, Massachusetts, writes as follows:

> Since there are few contraindications to VBAC, the routine repeat cesarean section seems unnecessary. A woman previously delivered by cesarean section should be informed that the complications of repeat cesarean are generally greater than those of vaginal delivery. . . . Her parturition should be approached as one with an uncomplicated vaginal delivery. . . . She needs to believe that she will be successful in her efforts, and she will have a real sense of achievement in VBAC.

He adds, "It is a rewarding experience to attend a VBAC." In another letter, Dr. Robert Margulis writes:

> My initial variation from common practice was to allow all women with previous cesarean births to go into labor. Then a cesarean could be done on an unscheduled basis. This ensured that the baby was not born "before its time." Inevitably, some of these women progressed so well that at first examination in the hospital it was obvious that a vaginal birth was not only possible but imminent.
>
> In the past three or four years I have treated more than fifty VBAC aspirants. Previous indications were mixed. I have not officially analyzed the data, but over 75 percent of these with previous "failure to progress" have delivered vaginally, and over 90 percent of those with previous breech presentation or fetal distress have delivered vaginally.

Dr. Charles Mahan of the University of Florida believes that VBAC will make one of the biggest differences in the decrease of cesarean sections in our country. The hospital with which he is affiliated has been encouraging VBAC for over six years and has "an 83 percent success rate."

Don Creevy, an obstetrician at Stanford University in California, has a 90 percent VBAC rate. This is higher than many obstetricians' vaginal rate.

Lynn Borgatta, an obstetrician and herself a VBAC mother, writes, "Sometimes I forget what all the fuss is about."

And a physician who wished to remain anonymous gave a classic response when questioned about the chances of encountering a uterine rupture in VBAC: "There's a better chance a flying saucer will land in my driveway."

"The Experts" Speak Up . . . Sort of

A recent and long-overdue announcement of a policy change by the American College of Obstetricians and Gynecologists (ACOG) caused many cesarean women to feel hopeful and relieved. In cautious tones, the college decreed that "an attempt at vaginal delivery after cesarean childbirth appears to be an acceptable option." The specific data used by the committee suggested "that the risk of maternal mortality from uterine rupture is almost nonexistent, and the risk of perinatal death is relatively small." Despite that finding, the "Guidelines for Vaginal Delivery After a Cesarean Childbirth" distributed by ACOG are so restrictive, so discouraging, that they allow only a tiny percentage of cesarean mothers in our country to be candidates for VBAC. (For example, the fetus must weigh under 8.8 pounds in order for the mother to "qualify." We wonder if a fetus with an estimated birth weight of 8.9 pounds would be rejected as a potential VBAC.) It is obvious that physicians are going to be slow to change and that the ACOG Committee Statement will add little impetus to that change.

VBAC: Getting Down to Specifics . . .

"What If My Pelvis Is Too Small?"

We have heard from hundreds of women who have been told they are not candidates for VBAC because their cesarean was done for cephalopelvic disproportion (CPD). We have mentioned the bugbear of CPD in Chapter 2. Many women are told that they must have had a previous vaginal delivery in order to have a VBAC. Otherwise, they have not proven that they can accommodate a baby. Nonsense! In our own sampling of 173 VBAC women, only 4 had had previous vaginal deliveries. In the studies we have cited, a previous vaginal birth was not a prerequisite for a VBAC. In fact, most of the thousands of women in these studies had never delivered vaginally prior to their VBAC. We'd like to acquaint you with the literature on VBAC/CPD. We would also like to state here that we do not condone the use of x-rays as a tool for diagnosing pelvic size (see Chapter 8).

As you will read time and time again in our book, the diagnosis of CPD is quite subjective and usually inaccurate. Riva and Teich note that CPD cannot be properly assessed without a trial of labor with ruptured membranes.[104] Kaltreider and Krone believe that CPD is actually uterine inertia, "which is a problem of the first pregnancy and seldom repeats itself." The diagnosis of CPD must be made, they say, after full dilation of the cervix.[54] Many of the women with whom we work were sectioned for CPD long before they had the opportunity to reach full dilation, or were sectioned without an adequate amount of time to push their babies into the world.

Some physicians tell a woman that if she has had a cesarean for CPD, there is a greater likelihood of rupture during a VBAC labor than if she was previously sectioned for a different reason. The physicians who use this scare tactic generally believe that CPD is a repeating situation. CPD is a nonrepeating reason for cesarean section.

In 1969, McGarry wrote, "Cesarean section with an incorrect diagnosis of disproportion, even supported by x-ray pelvimetry, may be followed by vaginal delivery of a larger infant."[70] In Saldana's study, 22 out of 30 women with a previous diagnosis of CPD had VBACs. Some had had x-rays that diagnosed a contracted pelvis. Six delivered infants larger than the ones for whom they had been sectioned.[107] Pauerstein reported that 12 out of 23 women who had cesareans for "x-ray substantiated CPD" delivered vaginally,[93] and Salzmann wrote that "contrary to popular belief, it appears more reasonable to permit a trial of labor in those patients whose original section was performed for CPD after an adequate test of labor."[108] Peel's study reported 51 out of 66 women, or 77 percent, delivering vaginally with no difficulty after having been sectioned for CPD.[95] Silfen and Wilf reported eleven VBACs in women who had been sectioned for CPD, *all of whom delivered larger babies at the time of the VBAC.*[115]

We've lost count of the number of women we have worked with who have had VBACs after a diagnosis of CPD. It is well over a hundred by now. Most have had larger babies, some significantly so. In more than one situation, a physician permitted a "trial" of labor based on his predictions that the baby would be smaller than before. When the babies were born weighing *pounds* more than had been predicted (or with a head circumference much larger than the previous baby), many physicians stated that they would not have permitted a trial of labor had they suspected the baby was that size. The baby's size is only one of *many* factors that determine its ability to be born normally, and certainly not the most important factor. A determined mother and healthy pelvis can safely birth a healthy baby of almost any size.

Studies support the claim that among women who have had a previous cesarean section for CPD, over half can have a subsequent successful vaginal birth.[128] Our success rates are much higher than that, with 85 to 90 percent of the women who have been sectioned for CPD going on to have VBACs, often with larger babies. According to the *British Medical Journal*, "Cesarean section with an incorrect diagnosis of disproportion, even supported by x-ray pelvimetry, may be followed by vaginal delivery of a larger infant."[12] ("And he told me I couldn't give birth to a 5 pound baby!" one VBAC mother recalled with delight. She had just spontaneously delivered an 8½ pound baby girl.)

A woman from Colorado received the following letter from her obstetrician:

Yes, I have delivered many patients of a second or third baby vaginally after they've had a previous c/section. In your case, however, you were born with a small pelvis. You are smaller than normal in two of six diameters, but the critical one is the bispinous, which is very narrow in your case. Your birth canal is absolutely compromised. The pushing of a normal sized baby against a narrow spot leads to a high incidence *of rupture of the old scar, that leads to instant death for the baby and sometimes maternal death. If you want to come to Denver, I'll be glad to help, but if you were my wife or sister, I'd try to get you to have a cesarean section.*

The woman had a 7½ pound VBAC at home. Another woman who received a similar warning from her doctor birthed a 10 pound 6 ounce baby two years after being sectioned for her 7 pound baby. "My original doctor was publically embarrassed when I had a VBAC," wrote a third woman. "He had used my case to demonstrate to other physicians what a truly contracted pelvis looked like."

Failure To Progress

What if your original c/section was "necessary" because of "failure to progress"?

McGarry states that 60 percent of women previously sectioned for inefficient labor, failed induction, failure to progress, or uterine inertia ("slow uterus") can be expected to deliver vaginally, and 80 percent in nonmechanical situations.[70] We believe the statistics can be much higher. According to Peel, the degree of dilation prior to the section has "very little bearing" on subsequent VBAC success.[95] Since most physicians put an arbitrary time limit on VBAC labors, it is reasonable to assume that many more women would have delivered vaginally if they had been given more time. Salzmann reported that it is not true that more common occurrence of rupture following cesarean section is due to a longer trial of labor[108] (and, as you will see, limits on labor as well as other factors limit the woman's ability to relax, which can adversely affect progress in labor).

More Than One Cesarean

Can you have a VBAC if you've had more than one cesarean? Absolutely! Wolfson and Lancet[127] and Jerusun and Simpson[52] reported success with women who had had two previous cesareans. Browne and McGrath reported 22 VBACs after two previous cesareans, 2 with three previous cesareans, and 1 patient with *five* previous cesareans followed by three subsequent VBACs.[13] Riva and Teich, too, cite many examples of VBACs after two and three previous cesareans.[104] McGarry sums up: "It is acknowledged that delivery by cesarean on two previous occasions does not constitute an absolute indication for elective repeat cesarean."[70] Camillieri[16] and Klufio[60] support VBAC after two cesareans. Armon described a woman who delivered vaginally after three previous cesareans, and supported VBAC after more than one cesarean. "She desperately wanted . . . [VBAC] and I reluctantly agreed . . . . She proceeded to deliver a seven pound baby . . . without assistance."[4] Donald stated that the dictum could be rephrased to, "Twice a cesarean, always a cesarean."[27] Armon remarked that even that dictum need not be absolute.[4] Waniorek's sample showed that 62 of 63 cases with two previous cesareans could deliver vaginally.[123] Most studies note VBAC after more than one cesarean.

We've worked with 24 women who had had more than one cesarean: 21 had VBACs. One woman with four previous cesareans had a VBAC homebirth with her fifth child, and two others with four previous cesareans had their fifth babies vaginally in the hospital. We recently learned of a woman in California who had her sixth baby VBAC after five cesareans (the first was for CPD, the rest repeats). All of these women and their babies have been fine. We have also recently been contacted by two more women who have had five previous cesareans and who would like to deliver vaginally. At a lecture at Boston City Hospital in 1982, Dr. Irwin Kaiser, who has been attending VBACs for 30 years at Albert Einstein Medical Center in New York, stated that he believes that a woman with a low segment is a candidate for VBAC even if she has had several previous cesareans, "although, unfortunately, the data base upon which we can be reassuring is limited." The data that do exist are clear and inspiriting. Lavin et al. state flatly, "There is little objective evidence to support the widely held view that multiple cesarean sections predispose to an increased risk of uterine rupture in a subsequent pregnancy."[64]

VBAC after a Previous Uterine Infection

Many women are told that if they had an infection following their cesarean, they are not candidates for a VBAC. And *who didn't* have an infection? Have you checked the infection rate in hospitals? Robert Mendelsohn tells us the germs in hospitals aren't just ordinary ones, either. Hospitals harbor a variety of germs that could keep an army of bacteriologists busy for a lifetime, he says. He assures us that hospitals are so germ-laden that many patients contract new infections they didn't have when they arrived.[74]

However, it has never been established that infection weakens a scar. Back in 1951, Wilson wrote, "It might well be that if infection encourages more fibrosis, it strengthens rather than weakens the scar."[125] McGarry, too, noted that infection has not been shown to make scar rupture more likely in a subsequent pregnancy or labor, and that infection does not predispose to improper healing.[70] Obviously infection *prevention* is important; but if an infection did occur, you can still have a VBAC. Lavin et al. (1982) report that there is little objective evidence to support the relationship between infection and uterine rupture.[64] Donnelly reported that "even the breakdown of the abdominal wound requiring resuture does not adversely prejudice the ultimate state of the scar."[29]

Breech VBAC

Breech VBACs are reported in the literature. Several external versions have been done. McGarry states that there is no reason to consider that a version (or turning of the child in the uterus) carries a substantial risk of scar rupture. "It is illogical to submit to the strain of labor a uterine scar considered unable to bear an attempt at version," he has said.[70] The *Ghana Medical Journal* reported 10 breech VBACs with no ruptures in any case.[60] Allahbadia reported 22 breech VBACs,[3] and the *Central Africa Journal of Medicine* reported 3 breech VBACs that were "surprisingly uneventful."[4] We have worked with several women whose babies were breech late in pregnancy. Most did breech tilt exercises, and their babies turned prior to labor. One had an external version. One woman delivered an 8-plus pound breech baby after two previous cesareans, and was home by the time her baby was five hours old, and two other women delivered their breech babies without any complications.

VBAC Twins

VBAC twins are also reported in some studies. Allahbadia reported three sets,[3] Browne and McGrath noted thirteen sets,[13] and Booth Maternity one.[115] Our own contacts include four women with twins, three sets birthed vaginally and one by cesarean.

A Time Limit for VBAC Labor?

Assuming the baby's heartbeat is good and strong, there is no reason to put a time limit on labor, and we can think of many reasons not to. One article suggested that the maternal morbidity rate is higher in groups of women who had a cesarean after many hours of labor. We would like to know the number of vaginal exams performed in this study and how many internal monitors were used, since the infection rate with these procedures is high. The general consensus is unavoidably that *automatic repeat cesarean is far more dangerous than labor.* Labor isn't supposed to be dangerous—it is our bodies' healthy work to deliver our babies. Besides, labor is the only way to avoid a cesarean!

Shearer (1982) remarks, "For VBACs, many doctors set arbitrary time limits on the length of labor, or require a woman to go into labor by 40 or 41 weeks.

Why? Just because she has had a cesarean before—should she be expected to deliver early or have a short labor? If she did not reach five or six centimeters in her first labor, I consider her a primipara for *labor*, even though it is her second child."[113]

How Many VBACs?

How many VBACs is it safe to have? As with all related issues, there is controversy about how many vaginal deliveries a woman should be "permitted" after a cesarean. Donnelly and Franzoni stated that successful accomplishment of one or more VBACs does not lessen the need for continued precaution with all later pregnancies.[29] In Lawler's opinion, once a woman has had one successful VBAC, her outlook in future pregnancies is much improved. "She is not as much the obstetrical cripple," he said. Twenty-four women in Lawler's sample had two VBACs.[65] Harris stated that after a VBAC, the patient and physician can be lulled into a false sense of security. "There is a limit to the abuse an old scar should be expected to take."[48] We consider his suggestion to sterilize a woman after a reasonable number of successful VBACs illogical and *un*reasonable. Consider the woman cited by Cosgrove who was "delivered of" eleven babies vaginally after an initial cesarean.[22] Allahbadia reported a woman with nine VBACs and believed the greatest risk was during the first VBAC labor. "The first labor, as far as we're concerned, would cause rupture if the scar is defective. If it is sound, it will withstand repeated labors."[3] Schmitz and Baba maintain that a successful vaginal delivery on one occasion does not guarantee against rupture on a future occasion,[109] but Schmitz and Gajewski believe that the greater the number of vaginal deliveries, the less the likelihood of rupture.[110] Lavin et al. agree that an intervening vaginal delivery is unlikely to influence the risk of uterine rupture in subsequent pregnancy.[64] As far as we're concerned, if you want a whole *slew* of VBAC babies, why not?

How Long between Pregnancies?

How much time must you allow between pregnancies to assure a well-healed scar? There are many factors that influence healing, including, for example, proper nutrition and hygiene. Guttmacher believes that the incision is as well healed after three months as it will ever be,[45] although Camillieri and Busittil believed that a woman's chance for a VBAC was increased if two years or more had elapsed since the section.[16] It is curious that some physicians refuse to consider VBAC because "it hasn't been long enough" since the cesarean, and at the same time discourage VBAC because "it's been too long; your cervix won't dilate quickly enough and that will cause the uterus to rupture."

We have worked with many VBAC women whose babies are under sixteen months apart. Our experience leads us to believe that it makes little difference what the interval is, *in terms of the scar*. We have a basic belief that nature expects us to have approximately an eighteen-month to two-year wait between births. This is demonstrated in other cultures where breastfeeding is used as a natural means of birth spacing. Our bodies were designed to conceive, carry a child, deliver, breastfeed (La Leche League-style), and return to fertility some-where after the first year. Some couples, however, deliberately space their babies closer than two years. For others, an unexpected pregnancy results in a shorter span between children than anticipated. We know from our work that many women become pregnant soon after their cesarean, not so much because they are ready for another child, but because they want another chance to "do the birth right."

Is It Ever Too Late To Decide on a VBAC?

It's *never* too late to decide to have VBAC (not unless your uterus has already been cut!). We were once introduced, in the library, to a woman who was 38 weeks pregnant and scheduled for a c/section in five days. The woman had had two previous cesareans. She asked for information, changed doctors, and had an 8 pound VBAC baby boy two-and-a-half weeks later. Maybe we should hang out at the library more often!

If at First You Don't "Succeed" . . .

One supportive physician offered the suggestion that perhaps in some rare circumstances the uterus has been damaged during the previous cesarean (or birth), and that this prevents it from contracting. "Rather than rupture, it rests," he says. Some women with whom he has worked have not had a VBAC on the first "try," but have had one with a subsequent birth. He believes that each new pregnancy can offer an opportunity for vaginal birth.

Forceps

Many VBAC women have been told that forceps must be used at their labor to extract the baby quickly so that there will be no undue pressure on the scar. In our opinion, this is unproven, unnecessary, and even dangerous. Case states that forceps are not justified,[18] and Allahbadia believes there is no need for prophylactic forceps.[3] However, other studies seem almost casual in their prescription of forceps for VBACs. Remember that instrument interference is associated with uterine rupture and infection. We'd like physicians to consider what could be done to enhance a vaginal birth and make forceps unnecessary. The dangers of using forceps for delivery are discussed in detail in Chapter 9.

"Your Uterus Is Paper-Thin!"

Women are rushed into operating rooms and expected to be grateful that a cesarean was performed. *After all*, they are told, *your incision was paper thin.* It has never, as far as we know, been proven that the thickness of an incision gives information about its well-being. Silk is a thin material, but it is very strong; styrofoam is thick, but can be torn by a child. Our healed incisions, like elastic, may be thin but flexible and stretchable at the same time. Several articles, including one entitled "Rupture of the Gravid Uterus,"[58] state that the risk of uterine rupture in subsequent pregnancies cannot be predicted on the basis of the incision's type or thickness. Lawler wrote that an anatomically "weak" scar does not predispose inability to withstand the distension caused by pregnancy or labor,[65] a claim we know to be true. Joanne T., Eileen G., and Susan S. know it, too. Along with *countless* other women, they were told that their uterine incisions would not hold up during subsequent labor. And, along with countless others, their incisions never caused a moment's concern.

What about Hysterography?

Hysterography, a risky procedure that utilizes radiological examination to provide direct visualization of the scar, is of questionable benefit, since "defects" are noted even in patients who undergo uneventful vaginal delivery. However, hysterography has been employed frequently, and Morley used it to identify well-healed scars in two patients after five cesareans and in one after six.[80] Another procedure, called amniography, detects dehiscence. This dangerous technique involves amniocentesis *in addition* to fetal exposure to radiation! (See Chapter 8.) Results are of little use since dehiscences are known to be present in absolutely nonthreatening scars. How many women have been needlessly subjected to these procedures? How many were inappropriately classified as poor risks for VBACs? How many two-year-olds were needlessly separated from their mother for seven days while she recovered in the hospital from surgery—surgery made necessary by her *alleged* inability to survive normal birthing intact?

Some doctors will not attend VBACs unless a woman has had ultrasound to determine the location of the placenta. If the placenta is located near the scar they will not permit a VBAC. Kaltreider and Krone[54] speculate that if the placenta is located beneath a uterine scar that ruptures, there will be more bleeding than when the rupture is in an area where the placenta is not attached. What has not been documented, they said, is that rupture is more common when the placenta lies beneath the scar, and they alert us to the fact that the methods used to locate the placenta are inaccurate. Our concerns about ultrasound are discussed in more detail in Chapter 8.

Donnelly reported a case where rupture occurred under the placenta—and there was no bleeding.[28] Lavin concludes that the effect of the placental implantation site on the incidence of rupture is unknown.[64]

Fibroids

We have worked with several women with pelvic adhesions or fibroids who have gone on to deliver vaginally. There have been no problems, even when the fibroids were in the lower segment and were described as "extensive." One local physician remarks that he'd be loath to cut into a uterus with fibroids unnecessarily, and that a "wait and see" attitude is kindest. With the increasing use of sonography, more fibroids are being discovered (or uncovered); we are certain that before sonography many women had perfectly normal deliveries *in spite of* fibroids.

Besides, fibroids often shrink; yours may well do so, or may even disappear prior to birth.

"Management" of VBAC Labors

In *Birth and the Family Journal*,[113] Elizabeth Shearer writes, "Most obstetricians use technology defensively in VBAC labors, in spite of the fact that there is no more justification for routine intervention than in any other labor." She reminds us that if a horizontal scar separates, it does not cause massive hemorrhage, "so there is no need for prophylactic I.V. The uterus continues to contract normally, and an electronic monitor will not pick up a scar separation." She believes that there is no reason to deny the use of sedation or anesthesia, if it is necessary, "since there is no pain if the scar separates." Shearer adds there is no reason why a woman cannot deliver in a labor or birthing room after a previous cesarean, "since there is no evidence that the scar is more likely to give trouble at the last moment." She cautions, "Such restrictions may well make it more likely for a woman to require a repeat cesarean."

Later in our book, especially in Chapter 9, we discuss interventions into the birth process. Each interference has potential risks. We firmly and unequivocally agree with McGarry, who tells us that a VBAC can generally be managed "as if the scar didn't exist."[70]

At many hospitals, VBAC women are hooked to every piece of apparatus available. In one local hospital, for example, an internal observation monitor is required for VBAC women. An indwelling catheter with a pressure gauge is inserted into the vagina and cervix after the woman's bag of waters has been ruptured by the physician (another interference). During the latter part of the dilation phase of labor, sometimes referred to as "transition," the readings from the gauge are solemnly observed. If the woman's contractions become "too strong," she is immediately whisked into the operating room for a cesarean section. If her contractions are too weak, or "inefficient," she is also wheeled into the O.R. "Yet another unnecessary implement of torture for VBAC mothers," remarks disheartened VBAC childbirth educator Jami Osborne. As you will see in Chapter 9, the disadvantages and dangers of electronic monitoring devices are numerous, and we shake our heads along with Ms. Osborne when she asks, "What will they think of next?"

Manual Exploration of the Uterus

Must the old incision be examined after a VBAC? Many so-called ruptures in the literature were found after a woman had delivered vaginally. When the baby and placenta were birthed, the operator put his hands up through the cervix and examined the inside of the uterus. If he noted a hole in the uterus, he reported a "rupture."

Most of the articles we surveyed recommend a manual exploration of the uterus following VBAC. *For the life of us, we can't imagine why, and we do not recommend this procedure.* If your baby has been born vaginally, if your blood pressure is fine, your temperature is normal, and you are not bleeding profusely, there is no reason to suspect a problem. You run a high risk of uterine infection from manual exploration of the uterus after birth. "No one's grubby—or un-grubby—paws are going into my uterus after *my* VBAC!" announced one mother. You know by now that any hole found may well have existed before labor, and that it presents no danger. If you've had a VBAC, you have every reason to believe that your incision held up. Whether or not there was a previous window or a dehiscence is immaterial.

If a new separation has occurred, some doctors insist on suturing. Others leave it to heal on its own. The extent of the separation, the amount of bleeding, and the woman's future childbearing plans are factors to consider. Gun reported that routine exploration may be fallacious and is not necessary.[44] Lavin et al. concede that postpartum uterine examination is generally advocated, but claim that its prognostic significance is uncertain.[64] Why, then, is it advocated? we ask.

You have the right to refuse to have your uterus manually explored. However, if you should decide to permit this unnecessary examination, you do not need to be anesthetized. One woman had a completely natural VBAC, only to be wheeled into the O.R. for a spinal so that her scar could be explored. Another was told she needed anesthesia for the pushing phase, because as soon as her baby was born and the placenta delivered, the doctor had to reach in and examine the scar before the cervix closed. Smart cervix to close immediately after the placenta births, before anyone can disturb it! The doctor told her the pain of the examination would be excruciating and impossible without anesthesia. This is just not true! After you've experienced the contractions to deliver your baby, another moment of discomfort won't overwhelm you. It's to be hoped that the physician will be *gentler* if no anesthesia has been given. Most women who have had their uterine incisions checked have noticed no discomfort whatever. The examination, if performed, should take no more than a few seconds. To repeat— *we do not recommend exploration of the incision.* Outer space is for exploring; the insides of our uteri are not.

VBAC with a Vertical Incision

The rate of uterine instability with a horizontal lower segment incision is approximately .05 percent, and rarely problematic. Even this figure can be reduced, as we will see. But what of other types of incision?

We must begin by asking why vertical incisions are done in the first place, given that lower segment transverse incisions are the method of choice. Perhaps it is the only technique known to a particular operator. Obstetricians trained early in this century may have had no experience with a lower segment horizontal incision. Many articles urge caution in resorting to vertical section on the grounds that it will permit easier or quicker delivery. Inexperienced physicians sometimes do classical incisions, especially under emergency conditions, although a lower segment can be done with almost equal rapidity by an experienced operator. Residents often do the suturing. Obviously you should be asked whether this is acceptable to you, and you need not grant permission. Although we have faith that our bodies heal even when the suturing is less than perfect, each of us has the right to be "worked on" by the technician of her choice. In some of these cases, an unskilled or inept operator performed the incision. The incision may extend too far upward. According to Case, the importance of placing an incision in the lower segment is often overlooked by modern obstetricians, who "rather perfunctorily make an incision at the most convenient place and hope that antibiotics will cover any deficiency in surgical technique."[18]

Lower Segment Vertical Incision   As we have shown, lower segment vertical incision is a vertical incision in the lower part of the uterus. It is also called a low vertical or a Kroenig incision and is used most often for a breech presentation. Its disadvantage is that it may extend up into the upper segment a bit, making it less desirable, to a nervous obstetrician, than the Kerr incision. Medical records generally do not indicate the length of the lower segment vertical incision, so some physicians will regard it with the same fear they have of a classical incision. However, many women, including Lois, have had this kind of incision and had no problems at all with a VBAC.

Timonen et al. reviewed 2,000 section patients and could find no significant difference in the perinatal mortality of patients with transverse and low vertical incisions.[122] Case et al. reported that even when a vertical incision is made, if it is in the lower segment, the morbidity rate is greatly reduced.[18] We have worked with several women who have had low vertical incisions. They all had VBACs. As far as we are concerned, a lower vertical incision poses no problem. More than half of the women had been in labor before their cesarean was performed, so a lower segment had formed, and the incision was made through a thinned uterus. Others were not in labor, so it is debatable whether their reported lower verticals were truly lower vertical or more centrally placed.

Midline Classicals   Because traditional classical incisions are made vertically on the portion of the uterus that contracts most energetically during labor, some physicians are terrified to see a woman labor following classical cesarean section. They fear that as the uterus contracts, the incision will rip open, causing severe distress to mother and infant.

The projected rate of rupture for a classical incision is between 1 and 3 percent. We believe it can be closer to 1 percent than 3 percent, a significant difference. To look at it another way, if someone told us we had a 99 percent chance of winning the million dollar lottery by buying a large number of tickets, we'd probably sell all our earthly goods and go for it. With good nutrition, good health, proper prenatal attention, and appropriate observation during labor, risks in these cases can by minimized. According to an impressive study done in Germany, "wound closure by one row of interrupted sutures" provides optimum healing conditions, cutting down on scar formation. "The risk of classical section is lowered by this technique," it was stated.[62] When we learned the many dangers of cesarean section, they were far more frightening to us than the 1 percent possibility of uterine separation, even with a classical incision.

We have been told that medical students are shown a film of an explosive classical rupture. One picture of this type may be worth a thousand words, although we wonder who the photographer was and how he happened to be there. Yet *most* doctors admit that they've never been involved in a problem of that magnitude, nor have any of their colleagues. We can only wonder what circumstances precipitated the rupture in question and whether, indeed, the woman had actually had a previous cesarean.

We must bear in mind that all the medical advancements since Craigin's day outlined in our discussion of rupture in general apply to an emergency for classical rupture as well. MacAfee believes that if the classical incision is intact at term, it should withstand labor, since those with questionable integrity usually separate prior to the onset of labor, if at all.[69] Schmitz and Gajewski believe that the number of successful vaginal deliveries reported after previous classical section indicate that the site of the incision does not preclude an attempt at vaginal delivery.[110] Lawrence agrees with the condition that "close observation is essential."[66] In a series from Rotunda Hospital, twenty-one patients with a history of classical section had vaginal deliveries. Twelve had one vaginal delivery, six had two vaginal deliveries, and the remainder had three, four, and six deliveries without rupture.[13] Drew-Smyth stated that classical section scars have been given an undeservedly bad reputation for subsequent labor.[32] Lane and Reid believed the classical scar was more likely to withstand the forces of labor than the lower segment.[63] However, Douglas echoed most of the researchers by asking that a classical incision be avoided if at all possible in a woman anticipating a subsequent pregnancy.[30]

Although Lavin et al. concluded that the probability of uterine rupture is greater with a classical incision, "the precise magnitude of the increased risk can not be accurately determined."[64] The risk to the fetus is increased, but again, many factors must be considered. Whenever possible, classical cesarean section should be avoided, although it does not totally rule out future VBAC.

A woman from Pennsylvania with a classical wrote, "I was having constant lower abdominal pain, so they feared a rupture. However, when they did the cesarean, the incision on my uterus was perfect. My obstetrician said he could hardly see the scar. I was disappointed, to say the least. My constant lower abdominal pain was *active labor*, not a problem with my uterine incision!"

Our contact with midline classical incision has been eventful: seven wonderful, healthy VBAC events. One woman with four previous cesareans delivered vaginally: she had had two lower segment incisions and two classical incisions.

A resident who was to attend one woman until her physician arrived left the room abruptly when he learned she had a classical incision. He mumbled something about checking to see if he had to be "a witness to this insanity." Meanwhile Jeanne just rocked in her rocking chair, the one she had carried into the hospital herself. Several hours later, she delivered her daughter vaginally.

Inverted-T Incision

Infrequently, an inverted-T incision may be used. Allahbadia explains that a very difficult delivery through an inadequate transverse incision may necessitate a supplementary classical incision.[3] There are only a few mentions of T incisions in the literature we surveyed. Our experience with an inverted T is limited to a woman who, after four cesareans (two classical, two lower segment), delivered her fifth child vaginally.

Hysterotomy

Along with classical incision, we should mention a procedure called hysterotomy. This is a cesarean performed during the second trimester, either for abortion or to remove a dead fetus after a failed induction. We have worked with three women who have had hysterotomies, all of whom have gone on to deliver vaginally. C.P. Douglas reported that hysterotomy scars have an uncertain potential for rupture, but the consensus is that the risk is smaller than after cesarean section.[30] As for other surgical procedures performed on the uterus, the nonpregnant uterus is less active and therefore healing can be relatively uncomplicated. Several women we know who have had uterine surgery apart from cesarean have had VBACs. Some with cervical adhesions or scar tissue as a result of previous suturing have gone on to deliver vaginally, as well. Many were told that their cervices would not dilate: the cervices dilated normally.

We have worked with three women who had septa in their uteri and had VBACs.

Our Statistics

We have worked with several hundred women who have had previous cesareans and who are planning to deliver their next babies vaginally. Some of these women have taken Nancy's VBAC classes or have attended her workshops or seminars. Others have been counseled on an individual basis—in person, via long-distance telephone, or through correspondence. A number of these women are not yet pregnant: they are using the time before they conceive to read, collect information, educate themselves, and find support.

Thus far, 173 of the women with whom we have worked have had their babies. Of these, 157, or 91 percent, have delivered vaginally. *Ninety-one percent of a group of women whom physicians generally insist upon sectioning delivered their babies vaginally with no complications whatsoever.* (One baby with chromosomal abnormalities died moments after birth. The problem was not related to the fact that he had been born VBAC. The baby's mother was grateful that she did not have to recover from major surgery, and for the experience of having given birth naturally to her child.) We believe that this percentage could and should be higher: at least a 93–95 percent rate should be possible, and we trust that our own percentage will continue to climb. We consider anything less than an 85–90 percent VBAC rate unacceptable.

Of the women we worked with who had repeat cesareans, several lived in communities where they could not find physicians who would agree to their requests. Frequently, their position in labor was restricted and food was forbidden. Often, fetal monitors were required, but warm, soothing showers were prohibited. I.V.'s were promptly put into place, but labor assistants or friends were not allowed into the labor rooms. Many of the women who wrote us felt little positive support or encouragement during labor, were given inaccurate or misleading information, and suffered a variety of scare tactics. All these factors cannot help but contribute to the outcome of any labor experience.

There were no complications among any of the mothers or babies whose labor for a VBAC resulted in a repeat cesarean. (As we have already mentioned, there were two uterine separations noted at the time of the cesarean; neither posed any problem.) One cesarean was performed because of a prolapsed cord, and one because of placenta praevia. Other reasons given for the sections were PROM (premature rupture of membranes), CPD, failure to progress, or a combination of factors. Two of the cesareans were done because of physician distress, and in a few cases the woman's limits were ultimately defined by a long and difficult labor.

Because we had no idea when we began counseling for VBAC almost ten years ago that we'd someday need information for statistics, we did not always collect, and cannot now provide, data compiled from all 173 women. The following data represents information we gleaned from 105 (60 percent) of the women we worked with. A few women did not return the questionnaires we sent, and many of our questionnaires were returned with no forwarding address. However, additional information about our ten years' experience has been included within the text of this chapter, and throughout the book. What follows are some outstanding statistics—highlights, if you will—compiled from our work with VBAC women.

Out of 105 Women . . .

- Four had had a vaginal delivery prior to their cesarean.
- Twenty-four had had two or more previous cesareans; twenty-one of these delivered vaginally.
- More than half the women were "overdue," several by two to three weeks, and one by five weeks.
- Twenty women had VBAC homebirths, including five women who had had more than one cesarean.
- Six women had more than one VBAC.
- Fifteen women had VBACs within eighteen months of their cesareans.

- Three women had VBACs more than eight years after their cesarean sections.
- Six with midline classical incisions (including three previous hysterotomies) had VBACs.
- Ten women had had low vertical incisions.

. . . And out of 105 Labors . . .

- Shortest VBAC labor—45 minutes.
- Longest VBAC labor—44 hours of strong contractions every three or four minutes (another woman, with two previous cesareans, delivered a 10 pound 7 ounce baby after *ten days* of intermittent active labor!).
- Five women had Pitocin (a synthetic uterine stimulant) and three of these women were delivered with forceps.
- Three women had forceps deliveries without Pitocin.
- Four women had medication during labor.
- The shortest second stage (pushing phase) was ten to fifteen minutes: the longest was six and one-half hours (with a classical incision, incidentally, and no complications).

. . . Came More than 105 Babies!

- Over 85 of VBAC babies were larger than their cesarean sibling.
- Two were breech VBAC babies (one followed his two cesarean-born breech brothers).
- There were three sets of VBAC twins.
- The largest babies were:
  —11½ pounds (a homebirth VBAC).
  —10 pounds 6 ounces (a homebirth VBAC).
  —10 pounds 7 ounces (after two previous cesareans).
  —9 pounds 4 ounces (with a previous classical incision).
- The smallest babies were: 3 pounds and 2½ pounds—a set of premature VBAC twins whose 4-year-old brother and 2-year-old sister had been born by cesarean section.

Many women from all over the country who have had VBACs heard about the preparation of this book and wrote to share their stories. We know that these women, as well as those with whom we have worked personally, are well motivated and eager to avoid a cesarean. Most women, given the opportunity, and the support, become willing and eager candidates.

A number of midwives, labor assistants, and childbirth educators have also written to let us know that they support VBAC and have worked with women who have given birth vaginally after a previous section. The voices of VBAC began with a whisper. Soon, they'll be a deafening roar!

Healed and Healthy

Perhaps it was a VBAC mother who noted, "Those who say it can't be done are usually interrupted by others doing it." VBAC is safe and has been well-documented. It is safer than repeat cesarean. Why, then, isn't it done more often?

O'Connell summed up the issue when he wrote that the medical profession as a whole seems to exhibit a profound reluctance to accept the safety of VBAC.[88] The truth is avoided, ignored, resisted, and maligned for the same economic, political reasons Marieskind stated in her report. Uterine rupture is merely an *excuse* for refusing to support VBAC. We find it interesting that the serious risks of amniocentesis (a procedure in which a needle is inserted through the mother's abdomen into the amniotic sac to withdraw fluid) are between .05 and 1.5 percent—higher than VBAC—yet amniocentesis is fast becoming routine, while VBAC is scorned! And, too, some women themselves have a fear of labor or of "failing," or they find it "appealing" to choose the baby's date of birth ahead of time. Most notably, most physicians are ignorant about the safety and desirability of VBAC and have little investment in helping women avoid surgery. Why be awakened and have to wait for a woman to deliver her baby when you can schedule a cesarean for 10:00 A.M.? In a summary about VBAC, Meier states that patient acceptance of a trial of labor depends on the attitude of the attending physician.[75] Many "attending physicians" are not overjoyed, to say the least, at the prospect of a VBAC.

In an article entitled, "Debate: Are Repeat Cesareans Necessary?" in *Childbirth Educator*, October 1981, one physician stated that any information about VBAC is pure opinion since "there are no definite studies."[99] We hope this physician will check our bibliography as well as the VBAC literature survey and reference list available through C/SEC, Inc.* In the same article, a professor of obstetrics from New York remarked, "I have serious doubts that vaginal delivery after cesarean saves money or improves the outcome of delivery. A trial of labor can tie up many people for a long time, making it an expensive option. . . . If women want VBAC and are willing to take the risks involved,

---

*Available for $2.00 from C/SEC, Inc., 22 Forest Rd., Framingham, Mass. 01701.

however, they should be permitted to do so, provided they know there is a small but distinct possibility of losing their babies or their fertility or their lives." **What of the distinctly greater, well-documented possibility of losing these with a cesarean?**

When a lecture on VBAC was scheduled at a maternity hospital in Massachusetts, one doctor wrote an irate letter to the hospital administration. He said, "Really, who cares or gives a damn about previous sections being high risk or not? The physician is the one who has ultimate decision responsibility. The paraprofessional, nurse, and childbirth educator are hurting rather than helping by according this kind of nonsense an audience. Thank you, but I will not attend."

Elizabeth Shearer, a member of the National Institutes of Health Consensus Task Force on Cesarean Childbirth, reported in *Birth and the Family Journal* in 1981, "When I pointed out that the first draft recommended no change in existing policies of routine repeat cesarean, it produced a violent negative reaction on the part of all but one of the obstetricians, including table pounding and swearing *never* to recommend vaginal delivery as a safe choice."[113] Although the final draft supported VBAC, Ms. Shearer pointed out that it was enormously difficult for these obstetricians to admit that cesarean rates were too high, and they took a very roundabout way to come to the new conclusion. Some physicians continue to perform cesareans inappropriately. They placate the woman by telling her that now that VBAC is safe, she shouldn't be upset: maybe she can have a vaginal birth *next* time. Others, eager to *appear* progressive, give lip service to VBAC.

A woman from Pennsylvania reported that when her original physician learned of her subsequent VBAC, he sent a message through a friend. "Tell her that was a stupid thing to do," he said. Another woman changed physicians when her original physician did not support her VBAC. Her new doctor reviewed her situation and was enthusiastic about VBAC. He then learned that the original physician had been one of his medical school instructors who now practiced at the same hospital. He asked that she return to the original doctor and have another cesarean. "He's a wonderful doctor," he said. Loyalty within "the clan" and resistance to VBAC are high.

We are told we are too young, too old, too short, too small, too nervous, too weak, too high strung, too overconfident to have a VBAC. What we really are is *just right*. When confronted by a physician who is anti-VBAC, ask for the references that have influenced his thinking. One obstetrician looked through the literature for articles that supported surgery as less risky. "You were right," he said sheepishly, "I couldn't find any." Fortunately, even the most conservative articles recommend individualization in decision-making and care. Those who familiarize themselves with the wealth of supportive VBAC literature rarely even think about the scar during labor or delivery.

Do you feel better? Can you get a picture of all your healthy red and white blood corpuscles getting excited after your cesarean and coming out in numbers to rally round and get things fixed up? Do you cringe because this habit of cutting women persists in spite of a wealth of literature that substantiates the safety of VBAC? Do you wonder why the "care givers" in our country haven't read any of it? Are you angry that your health and vitality were zapped by an unnecessary repeat cesarean? Do you wonder why physicians are worried about "uterine rupture," but frequently and nonchalantly rupture your membranes themselves? You are in good company. We have received almost 40,000 letters asking the same questions.

You now can understand why we will no longer use the term "rupture" for the almost nonexistent instance of a uterine incision gently opening or separating. We will not continue to foster the intense and irrational fear that exists in this country about the status of the uterus and its inability to heal appropriately. We ask you to join us. We ask you to educate physicians, childbirth educators, and nurses who continue to perpetrate the myths, to educate friends and family as well. From now on, we ask that you *refuse* to use the term "rupture," and that you *refuse* to be cut open unnecessarily in the name of uterine unreliability. Most uteri will hold up through rain, sleet, snow, hail, and labor. You might even want to take a minute out to respect and appreciate the one in your body. It's the only one you've got, and it's healed and healthy and strong.

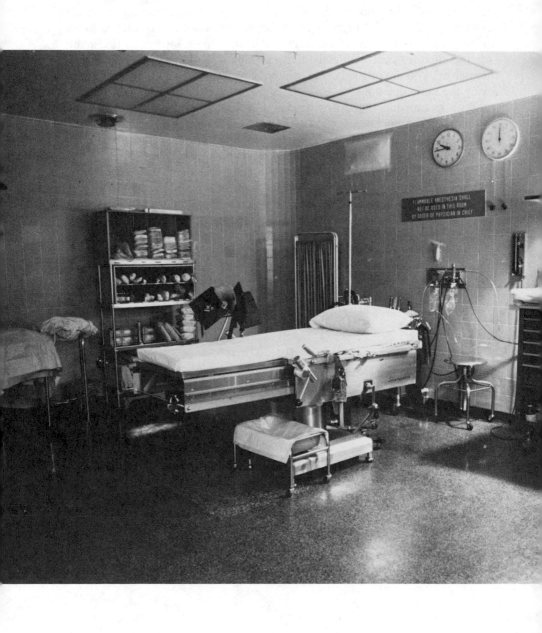

6 ᑌᕼ *The Fallacy of Natural Childbirth*

How Natural Is Natural Childbirth?

Cesarean section is probably the ultimate *unnatural* birthing experience. What then is the ultimate *natural* birthing experience?

It seems that natural childbirth in America today has as many definitions as it has advocates. For some, a natural birth is one without any medication whatever. For others, a natural birth is one in which the mother is awake—that is, any birth without general anesthesia. Increasingly, as the cesarean rate continues to climb, natural birth is becoming synonymous with vaginal birth.

Suzanne Arms remarks that "natural childbirth in America today may mean anything short of a cesarean section."[1] We fear that natural childbirth may soon include cesarean section!

The photographs that Arms uses to illustrate her "Natural Childbirth?" chapter of *Immaculate Deception* are worth ten thousand words apiece. The first three show a woman in various stages of labor and delivery in a hospital setting. The pictures are in black and white, but we intuitively know that we aren't missing much in the way of color. Shelves of towels, jars, and labeled boxes adorn the walls. The I.V., waving gaily on its pole, adds a festive touch. The three masked and capped figures hovering busily over the "patient" are so indistinguishable that we wonder if even the mother knows which one is her husband. The woman is lying on her back, her behind hanging precariously over the edge of what looks like a dentist's chair without the leg rest. Her ankles are up in stirrups, giving her the appearance of a trussed turkey about to be stuffed. There is ample room under her voluminous drapes for herself, her baby, and all three masked strangers. It is clear that she is having "natural" childbirth—we can tell by the expression of agony on her face.

Arms ends the chapter with a fourth photograph. This one shows a woman lying on a flat table (her head bisected by the I.V. pole in the foreground), trying valiantly to nurse the slithery newborn squirming around on her chest. "A Determined Mother Tries to Nurse on the Delivery Table," the caption reads. Although another masked and capped trio tries to keep the baby from sliding off, the mother is obviously much too uncomfortable to have much success in breastfeeding. We wonder why her three attendants didn't help her to sit up so that she could hold her baby herself.

It's no wonder that less than 2 percent of cesarean mothers choose the option of "natural" childbirth over elective repeat cesareans! If we accept the current definition of "natural" childbirth as birth without anesthesia, then a woman can have an enema, a shave, an I.V., a fetal monitor, Pitocin, an episiotomy, and all manner of interventions while still considering her birth to be natural. We are amused by statements like: "I did it natural! I didn't even have anesthesia when they ruptured my membranes and started the Pitocin!"

"I had natural childbirth. All I had was a little Demerol at the beginning because the I.V. was hurting me."

"It was completely natural! All I had was a local for the episiotomy!"

Natural? Must we accept births such as these as natural? Is this the dream of the thousands of American women who dutifully attend their childbirth classes and diligently practice their breathing exercises? Was this in fact the dream of Dick-Read in England, of Platanov and Nicolaiev in Russia, of Lamaze and Vellay in France, of Chabon and Bradley in America? We think not.

Yet a brief historical perspective of "natural" childbirth shows us that the method had its problems from the start. First of all, "natural" childbirth was the invention of men; as such, it could not help but become another way for men to manage and manipulate women. This is not to say that the method was designed with malicious intent. On the contrary, the physicians who worked to improve childbirth conditions were probably kindly men who sincerely wanted to help their women patients escape from what they saw as the terror and pain of childbirth.

Where they went wrong was that their techniques were diversionary rather than confrontational. While encouraging us to distance ourselves from the birth experience through controlled breathing, hypnosis, or Pavlovian responses to stimuli, they overlooked our intrinsic need to confront and assimilate our birth experiences. No doubt acting from their own male conditioning, they convinced us that we needed to stay in control during labor. Phrases such as "childbirth without fear," "childbirth without pain," and "prepared childbirth" fooled us into thinking that we could master the uncontrollable forces that work within us during labor.

"To stay in control," says Lynn (Browne) Richards, "is only our human fallacious attempt of gaining power over the all encompassing force of nature—of staying in control of our own mortality." She suggests that instead of seeking to stay in control, we must choose to "let go—to let go of our fears, our egos, and our very desire to control."[4] Rather than screaming in terror at the approaching waves, rather than trying to stoically withstand their force, we can choose to welcome them and ride them in to shore. Like body surfing, labor can be and should be a way of "going with the flow."

A second problem of "natural" childbirth is that it continues to submit us to medical intervention. Only anesthesia was eliminated, and labor remained a medical event in a hospital setting. Grantly Dick-Read himself greeted laboring women with enemas and then put them promptly to bed. Numerous studies have shown that when women are allowed to choose their positions in labor without any outside direction, the supine position is absolutely last choice. We also know that enemas are generally unnecessary and often disruptive. Dick-Read's patients may have achieved childbirth without fear, but they didn't achieve childbirth without intervention.

A third problem with "natural" childbirth is that it often denies the intensity of labor pains. In many prepared-childbirth classes, the word "pain" is avoided altogether. "Contractions" are what we have, and we are seldom prepared for how much they are going to hurt. Our "coaches" pinch our arms, and we easily "breathe through" the pain. It is irresponsible to give women the impression that these labor rehearsals prepare them for actual labor.

In *Birthing Normally*, Gayle Peterson warns that ". . .to not deal with the issue of pain in depth is to not address the source of much of the fear and struggle for 'control.' " Five or six couples giggling uncomfortably on the floor as they pinch and breathe their way through class is hardly a realistic re-creation of a childbirth. How each woman will relate to "the incredible energy of the life force she is creating within her as she gives birth to physical form"[13] remains unknown right up to the time that labor begins. However, realistic preparation will at least eliminate some of the mystery.

Purebirth

How do most women in our country give birth? Are unmedicated, uncut birthing women becoming extinct? We have already seen that 20–30 percent are delivered abdominally, by surgery. Of the remaining 70–80 percent, few manage to avoid any intervention at all. If we assume a 25 percent cesarean rate and a 75–90 percent episiotomy rate (actually the latter is 100 percent in some hospitals), then less than 8 percent of birthing women avoid being cut in some way during delivery. Though many women claim to have had "natural" childbirth, we estimate that less than 5 percent of birthing women experience an entirely pure birth, or "purebirth."

Purebirth is birth that is completely free of medical intervention. It is self-determined, self-assured, and self-sufficient, without necessarily being solitary. For most women, purebirth requires loving support, comfort, and guidance from people who have positive energy to contribute to the birth environment. Where "natural" birth is a system designed and perpetuated by physicians as a medical event, purebirth is childbearing as an act of mother love, a way of thinking and feeling about birth that allows us to take responsibility for the experience in whatever way we choose.

Purebirth precludes management and manipulation by others. A woman can experience purebirth in a hospital, but she is not a "patient." Robbi Pfeuffer says, "Practice, not fact, has made the hospital a necessity for childbirth and has transformed a woman in labor into a hospital patient."[14] We suggest that practice and consumer pressure can transform the laboring patient back into a birthing woman, that hospital birth can be achieved with dignity, respect, and pride. But women who feel only negative energy in the hospital environment will not be able to experience purebirth there.

Purebirth has no rules, only suggestions. Anything that makes the laboring woman more comfortable is acceptable, as long as it is nonmedical. Some women choose to walk through early labor, while others prefer to sit and rock. Some women need food for energy; others are too excited to eat. Some women need lots of friendly faces for comfort and support, while others want to be alone with their thoughts. The important ingredient is flexibility. Each woman must be free to labor in her own way, uninhibited and undisturbed. There is no breathing, no position, no method of relaxation that is right for every woman at every "stage."

In fact, purebirth has no stages. Rather, it is a continuation of a creative energy that began with conception and will grow through years of nurturing. "The point of birth becomes a meeting ground of intuitive body knowledge and conscious, logical mind process," says Peterson.[13] This transformation that occurs with the passage from unconscious to conscious mothering is what we should see as transition—not a phase of labor to be dreaded and overcome, but rather a place where the continuous flow of labor narrows into an intense stream of life-filled birth.

Purebirth is not a cry or demand for perfection. There have been enough demands made of women already. Purebirth can be long and loud. It can be painful, and it can withstand pain as well as periods of tension and impatience. But it is pure because it is our own. It is not Pitocin's labor or Demerol's labor or the doctor's labor. It is something that *we do ourselves*, for ourselves, and for our babies.

Finally, purebirth has its own time. It can't be induced, and it can't be hurried. Like fruit ripening on a tree, birth takes time. If we start too soon or try to rush, it will be like picking unripe fruit: harder work, longer hours, and possible damage to the crop. Purebirth requires patience and a respectful attitude toward labor. It requires complete trust in the woman and in the process.

Purebirthed babies enter the world the way Nature intended—what a gift this is! They are born to fully conscious mothers who can welcome them, hold them, and nurse them immediately. They are free from any interference that can dull their senses and color their first impressions of the world. They are peaceful and loving, yet filled with energy—able to nurse well, open, alert, and trusting. This first experience of life outside the uterus may influence their development in many ways; soon-to-be born babies are not "unconscious blobs," as we have been led to believe, and their passage into life may affect them for longer than we imagine.

Purebirth is what cesarean mothers mourn and what VBAC mothers seek. Having had their prior birth experiences shaped by medical intervention, women planning VBACs are often particularly determined to experience purebirth. When purebirth replaces "natural" childbirth as the goal of all pregnant women, when we begin to see routine medical interventions as intrusions into the birthing process, when medical personnel learn to save their skills for those who truly need them—only then will we have reclaimed our birthing rights.

Knowing how desperately many of you want to be able to create your own purebirths, we would like to help. In the following chapters, we will demonstrate how you can increase your potential for a purebirth experience.

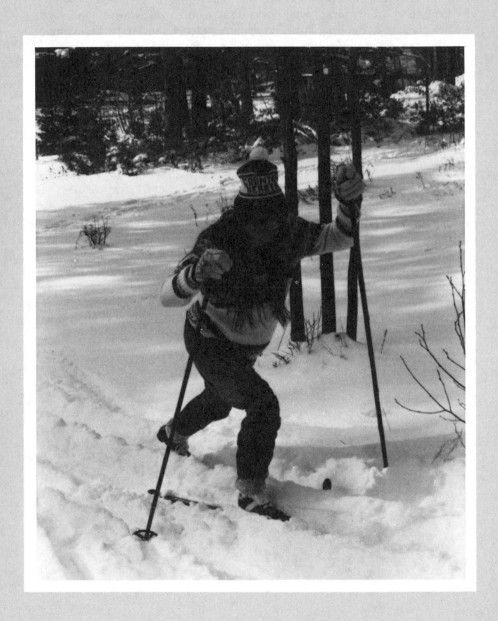

7 ❧ Increasing Your Potential for Normal Birth: Nutrition and Exercise

The role of malnutrition during pregnancy in causing human reproductive pathology remains in the Western medical-surgical culture the best kept "secret."

—Thomas Brewer, M.D.

We want to help all women increase their potential for safe, normal, pure-birthing. Every woman owns that potential. We are told in the book *Natural Health and Pregnancy*[51] that there is a great deal we can do to minimize problems, avoid distresses, resist hazards, and emerge from pregnancy and birth as healthy mothers of healthy and happy children.

We offer information and a variety of suggestions throughout this book. It is each woman's responsibility to create the optimum environment—physically, spiritually, and emotionally—in which to birth safely. Each of you can set the stage for actively giving birth or for having your baby delivered. Ultimately, the choice is yours.

How wonderful it would be if we were all so well nourished from the start

"Hey Mom, What's for Dinner?"

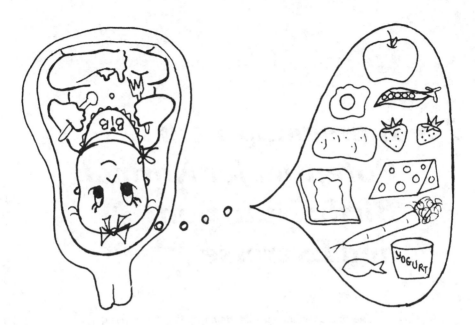

that we did not have to think about a shape-up program during pregnancy. But many of us are not well nourished from the start.

Most of us were not breastfed. We were brought up on processed foods with artificial flavorings and colorings, as well as additives, chemicals, perfumes, nitrates, and hormones. Much of what we ate was filled with sugar. Even today, the majority of people in America have a diet that is high in calories, low in nutrition. In fact, the practice of invading bodies with "junk" foods begins right in the hospital nursery with bottles of glucose water. It is followed soon after by the pediatrician's advice to begin cereals by three months so the baby will sleep through the night, and it is reinforced every time a child is rewarded or bribed by dangling a cookie in front of her nose. How young bodies can grow to be strong without the proper nutrients is beyond us. How can deficient bodies produce healthy pregnancies, labors, births, or babies?

It has been predicted that the cesarean rate will rise as our children's generation births. Our own bodies seem increasingly incapable of delivering and we are only one generation away from whole, natural, unprocessed foods grown right on one's own farm or nearby! Each generation has gotten further and further away from good nutrition; although there is an abundance of food in our country, much of what is consumed is less than adequate for maintaining good health. (We understand that a popular chocolate candy is even being eaten for *breakfast* by some children these days.)

It is fairly common knowledge that farmers will not breed their livestock unless the animals are in excellent health. They know that if you breed what isn't healthy, you are bound to get offspring that aren't healthy either. They take time to condition their animals before allowing them to conceive and bear young. It is a fact that how we eat prior to conception influences the health and well-being of our developing babies. Yet most of us spend little if any time getting ourselves ready to conceive in the best possible state.

Good nutrition affects how we eat, sleep, act and think. It affects everything about us—our work, our moods, our ability to relax, our sex lives, our patience with our children—everything. It affects how well we grow our babies and how well our uteri contract. It affects the elasticity of our cervix, and our stamina during labor. However, many physicians pay little or no attention to a woman's diet, past chastising her for gaining too much weight or telling her to restrict her salt intake (*harmful advice* on both counts). Most physicians we have questioned admit that they know very little about nutrition and that their training in this area was less than adequate. Additionally, many of them have little interest in the subject.

People are often sensitive about their eating habits. The foods we choose, the way we prepare them, and the way we eat them are bound up in feelings about our backgrounds, our childhoods, our memories, our homes, our friends, our roles, and our mothers. We ask women to make a list of what they have eaten in the course of a week, and a separate list for weekends (since it has been our experience that weekend diets differ markedly from midweek meals). We ask them to take a lovingly critical look at what they have eaten and to make a list of what improvements could be made and what improvements they are *willing* to make. We know that what constitutes "healthy" varies from person to person, from culture to culture. For our own well-being, and for that of our unborn babies, we must begin thinking about our food styles and choices, making some changes, and finding alternatives to empty calories. Our bodies do so much work when we are pregnant! It may not look as if a women is doing anything, but even when she is sitting quietly, SHE IS GROWING A BABY!!!

To grow a baby well, a mother needs a lot of really good, healthy food. Most women are amazed at the volume of food they consume during pregnancy. "I've always had a healthy appetite," said one woman, "but this was phenomenal." Many women ask how much weight they should gain. For some, 30–35 pounds are enough. For others, 35 pounds are not nearly adequate. To us, the best rule of thumb is to eat whenever you are hungry (so move all of the furniture into the kitchen and camp out there—who cares?), but eat only nutritious foods. That means, if you are unable to sleep in the middle of the night because you are hungry, you need to get up and have something to eat. Right at that particular moment, your baby may be growing her toes or ear lobes. She may need nourishment *at that very moment* in order to do so! Once again: listen to your body, eat when you are physically hungry, and eat a variety of whole, natural foods. Although we live in a culture that values "thin," we must leave that look to models and actresses, and make sure that we take care of our nutritional needs during pregnancy.

Some women lose their appetites when they are pregnant. If you haven't eaten for many hours, your baby has no way of obtaining what she needs for her rapidly growing and changing body. "Hey, Mom, could you send down an orange? And while you're at it, how about a big bowl of granola, smothered with fruit and topped with yogurt? You see, I'm growing some new organs today, and that's hard work. Wait until tomorrow! Then I'm growing *legs!*" We know that for baby, growing arms, or legs, is easier on *good food* provided at *regular intervals* throughout the pregnancy.

Some women who are planning to have their babies vaginally after a cesarean are told by their physicians to keep their weight down. Other women, concerned about the size of their pelves, eat sparingly during their pregnancies. They are told, or they believe, that if they grow small babies, they will have better chances of delivering "from below." This is dangerous nonsense! If you grow a small baby, you may also grow a baby that will not be strong enough to withstand the energy of labor. Your uterus will become malnourished, not having received all that it needs to contract strongly and powerfully. Your placenta will not function properly. You may become weakened yourself. All of you—you, your body, and your baby—must be healthy and strong. The size of the baby is not the most important factor in whether or not you will be able to deliver vaginally, and you *must not* try to keep your baby small. Babies' heads are designed to mold, and your pelvis is designed to open and change shape in order to accommodate your baby. Your baby and your body can only do the things they were designed to do if they are healthy and strong. Birth weight is only partially determined by heredity; good nutrition is what tips the scales to health. It is true that larger babies have a better chance of being born safely and of living well, and you owe it to yourself, your body, your baby, and your family to eat well.

Father's Nutritive Role

It is also fairly well known that you can't breed a healthy cow with a sick bull and come out with a top-notch calf; that in order to insure that the calf will be healthy, *both* parents must be strong and healthy. We are still amazed at the number of men who tune out information on nutrition, thinking it is the woman's concern and has nothing to do with them. You men contribute to *one-half* of that baby! Men who drink, smoke, take drugs, and freak out on sugar must take responsibility for the fact that much of that baby's well-being depends on what they have contributed. In addition, how well you can support your wives in labor will depend on your health and well-being. Men are often stressed during pregnancy. They work late so they can take time off when the baby comes. They grab a bite to eat here, a candy bar there. They drink extra coffee or sugared beverages.

It is extremely important for the man to come to the birth as well-rested and relaxed as possible and in as good health as possible. We believe that some cesareans become necessary because of exhausted husbands who are in such poor health that they cannot withstand the stress of a labor that lasts fifteen or twenty hours, and many perfectly normal labors last far longer than that. Their tired, cranky, poorly-nourished state manifests itself in an inability to give quality emotional support to their wives, or even physical support for any length of time. One husband, on being awakened at 2:45 A.M. to help his laboring wife said, "Oh, no. Not tonight. You *can't* go into labor now."

Some husbands are in such poor nutritional shape that psychologically they go out to lunch. Without realizing it, they are not emotionally *there* for their wives in labor. The communicative relationship between a woman and a man at the time of birth is important. A woman's senses are highly charged by labor; she quickly picks up other "energies," although not always on a conscious level. In her new state of consciousness she is sometimes vulnerable, impressionable. She may pick up her man's exhaustion, his need to have her hurry and have this baby so that he can relax, get home, and get to bed. She may interpret those signals as a lack of support and begin to feel pressured and abandoned. This anxiety can hinder her ability to relax and give birth. So husbands, take note: you, too, are helping to birth your baby!!

We've noticed that during pregnancy some men watch like hawks over what their mates are eating. There's got to be some psychological stuff involved in this—we haven't figured it all out yet. Is his paternal instinct coming out? Is he worried that his woman will be fat and unattractive to him afterwards? Is it an issue of control? Some men lose weight as their wives gain it, others gain right along with their partners.

A Few Nutritious Tips

We are not authorities on nutrition. We won't claim to be. We'd just like to make a few points and then we ask that you check our reference list for books, pamphlets, and articles that can help you. We hope that you will educate yourself about good nutrition and learn how vital it is at each stage and to all aspects of your life.

- Eat foods in as complete and natural a state as possible. Whole wheat over white, fresh fruit over cooked, frozen vegetables over canned (and fresh, of course, over frozen), for example.
- Read labels. Learn about the things that you are putting into your body. *The Supermarket Handbook*[17] by Nikki and David Goldbeck is an excellent guide for grocery shoppers. It is interesting and well researched and can help you decipher those four-syllable tongue-twisters on the backs of packages. You'll be surprised to learn *what else* is in the peanut-butter jar, for example, besides peanuts.
- Eliminate sugar from your diet or cut down as much as possible. Use honey, molasses, or pure maple syrup as a sweetener instead. In *Sugar Blues*[9] we learn that sugar wreaks havoc with the body's glucose-regulating system. It's like a drug in many ways, altering moods, affecting sleep, and ruining the appetite. In an article called "The Sugar Pushers," Jackie Hyland[18] tells us that women push sugar on other women. "I should know," she says.

  I'm an addict, and my best connections are hostesses of any social event given by or for women. What I want to know is, why do women have this great compulsion to ply everyone with sugar? Don't they care that they're turning their husbands and friends into arteriosclerosis victims? Doesn't it bother their consciences that they're ruining their looks and causing diabetes? It's high time women stopped thinking in terms of sweets when they want to be creative or to express good will or solace.

- Watch out for caffeine (coffee, tea, diet sodas, chocolate)—it depresses the blood sugar and acts as a diuretic. For nursing mothers, it can contribute to a diminished milk supply. Excess caffeine consumption has been linked to birth defects.
- Create new menus! Pregnancy is a time of great change, and it's easy to feel bored with the same old stand-bys. Pregnancy is also a creative process, so *create*! We have included a few (of many) excellent recipe books in the bibliography for this chapter.
- Get as many of the necessary nutrients as you can from your diet. Vitamins are *supplements* to a good diet, not *replacements* for one. Since synthetic vitamins usually have artificial colorings, perfumes, and additives, those of you who do take supplements might wish to take a natural brand. Some women who have had cesareans take vitamin E as a result of research done by Dr. Evan Shute on its effects on the healing of scar tissue. To prescribe the same vitamin for all pregnant women, across the board, seems inappropriate. Dr. Kamran S. Moghissi, Professor of Obstetrics and Gynecology in Detroit, remarks that for some women, the only nutritional

supplement necessary during pregnancy is iron. "For others, more extensive therapy is indicated."*

- Some herbs may be useful during pregnancy and birth, but many are potentially very dangerous. Don't use them unless you are fully informed about them.

- If you indulge in something you know to be less than ideal for your developing baby, why not make up for it by eating it with something of value? For example, a woman who called herself "the original Cookie Monster" made certain that she always had a large glass of milk or juice and a piece of fruit with her cookies. That way, she filled up sooner, ate less cookies, and provided her baby with some wholesome foods, too. Another woman began to add wheat germ, bran, and fresh strawberries to her ice cream.

- Be flexible. We know, for example, that the decision to eat eggs and meat was not easy for two pregnant women (one a vegetarian, one macrobiotic) who contacted us, but they listened to their bodies and decided to make some temporary changes in their diets. Rigidity in the diet is of concern to us, because steely rigidity in general is of concern to us. A byword of normal birthing is responsive flexibility.

- If you eat meat, perhaps you'd be willing to shop in a store that provides beef that has been organically raised. Most cattle in our country raised for consumption grow up on chemically treated feed, antibiotics, and stilbestrol, a controversial chemical hormone and potential carcinogen. Liver, by the way, being the detoxifying organ, collects residues from the feed as well as the chemical from the fertilizers sprayed on the pastures where the cows graze. Organically raised beef liver will be more pure, since the meadows and feed are not chemically treated. Be careful, too, about foods containing nitrates (bacon, ham, hot dogs, luncheon meats, for example); these are controversial, potentially dangerous carcinogens.

- Eliminate alcohol during pregnancy. Alcohol's damaging effects on a developing fetus are well known and documented. Even moderate drinking can result in minimal brain dysfunction, since alcohol is now known to prohibit a baby's developing brain cells from differentiating. Fetal alcohol syndrome is no joke, and no one knows how much *or how little* alcohol can affect a particular fetus for life.† One woman, who loved wine and

---

*Moghissi, Kamran, "Risks and Benefits of Nutritional Supplements during Pregnancy," *Obstetrics and Gynecology*, 58 (Nov. 1981), no. 5 (supp.).

†In an article entitled "Fetal Alcohol Syndrome," Dr. Henry Rosett writes, "Pending further study, the effects of light or occasional drinking during pregnancy remain relatively unclear." (From *Symposia Reporter* (May 1981), no. 4.) See also Rosatt, H., et al., "Strategies for Prevention of Fetal Alcohol Effects," *Obstetrics and Gynecology*, 57 (Jan. 1981), no. 1.

missed it during pregnancy, says, "Whenever I get in the mood for a glass of wine, or a drink, I remember a PBS special that stated that many of the world's fine wines are stomped by feet. I just close my eyes and picture that the *dirtiest* of all the feet was responsible for the grapes in my glass— and the desire disappears!"

- About smoking: it robs your baby of many nutrients, including vitamin C, not to mention *oxygen*! Smoking mothers produce more birth com- plications (such as placenta abruptio and praevia, intrauterine growth retardation, premature labor, hemorrhage) than nonsmoking women.* Nicotine is an addictive drug. Numerous studies support the conclusion that "second-hand smokers"—those exposed to the polluted air caused by another's smoking—are exposed to equal or greater dangers. Children brought up in homes with smokers have a significantly increased incidence of respiratory ailments. (There's nothing as offensive to us as baby clothes that reek of cigarette smoke or doctors' offices with ash trays.) Love yourself (and your baby) enough to stop smoking or to cut way down, and when you do stop, take the time to revel in the knowledge that you've risen above something that temporarily had controlled or conquered you.

- Remember that, with few exceptions, everything crosses the placenta. Alcohol, cigarette smoke, diuretics and junk food are all harmful. Aspirin (which can have an adverse effect on the fetus and which can interfere with blood-clotting mechanisms during labor)† and dental analgesics (such as Novacaine) have also been implicated as dangerous during pregnancy.[5,6] Any drug that *you* take will find its way to your unborn child. Ronald Glasser tells us that now that we are aware that drugs used during pregnancy can and do cause gross physical congenital defects, the deeper concern is the subtler and more difficult-to-evaluate effects of the drugs on the developing child's personality, his intelligence and mental abilities, as well as his motor coordination and psychological growth. "If drugs can cause arms not to grow and faces to be left open, then they can certainly get into fetal brain cells . . . not enough to kill the cells but enough to affect their functioning, leading to seizures, hyperactivity and decreased intelligence."[16] Be careful about *anything* you put into your body!

You owe it to yourself and to your baby to begin your pregnancy with the healthiest body you can have. You owe it to yourself and to your baby to come

---

*See Finnegan and Leifer, "Effects of Caffeine and Nicotine on Pregnancy and the Newborn," *Symposia Reporter* (May 1981), no. 4, as well as other articles listed in the bibliography to this chapter.

†Collins, E., "Non-Narcotic Analgesics during Pregnancy," in *Symposia Reporter*, 4 (May 1981), no. 4.

to labor and delivery well rested, strong, and hearty. We urge you to make decisions that will foster your good health, for in so doing, there is much to be gained.

Anyone for a snack?

Exercise during Pregnancy

If you knew that nine months from now you had to represent the United States in the Olympics, we imagine you'd start preparing immediately. Well, you aren't going to represent the country in an athletic event, but you are going to have a baby, and the better you feel, the more confident about your body you become, the better your chances for a positive outcome. If you are already quite pregnant, we'd still recommend that you begin now by taking walks, for example, or dancing or swimming. You can start out gradually, and do a little more each day.

Many of the women with whom we have worked believe that one of the reasons they were able to have their babies naturally was that they were well prepared for labor physically.

Last week, when we were talking about exercise in class, Marilyn pointed to her enlarging uterus and commented, "Surely, I must be ready for the Olympics by now: carrying this around all day must be equivalent to at least eleven miles of jogging!" While carrying your growing baby around can be as tiring as exercising, it is not the exhilarating kind of aerobic exercise that thrills every sagging muscle and wakes up all those eager-to-be-alive cells all over your body.

There are a number of excellent books available on the benefits of exercising during pregnancy, some of which are listed in our bibliography. We'll let them give you "the specifics," but we'd like to share a few of our views about exercising, as well as some personal experience.

Although change is in the wind, we are basically a sedentary culture. Our bodies just don't get the amount of physical exercise they need, and we, in turn, have no understanding of or appreciation for what our bodies are capable of doing. The most important reason for exercising is the confidence and pride you feel after you have begun to see the amazing capabilities of your marvelous body!

While you exercise, you sweat, your muscles ache, you might feel tired, discouraged, or cranky—you may even swear. Often it's not until the exercising is over that you feel terrific and proud and glad you made the effort. When you are having a baby, you sweat, your muscles ache, you might feel tired, discouraged, or cranky, and you may even swear. But when that's all over, you feel equally terrific and proud and very glad that you did it.

Natural Health and Pregnancy tells us that lack of demanding daily activity is one of the many reasons why modern woman has to "groan and struggle in the obstetrics wing."[51] Lack of physical exercise in combination with our modern diet contributes significantly to the degeneration of contemporary health. Over the course of time, the amount of stress women experience during labor hasn't changed, but our ability to withstand it certainly has.

As young girls growing up in the fifties and sixties, many of us got messages that physical exercise was for the boys. We rarely knew what it felt like to have sweat dripping from every pore, a refreshing shower at the end of a rugged workout—these were experiences known almost exclusively to males. As one woman said after she had made the decision to take up an exercising program, "I'm out to find you, sweat glands!"

Each of you has to assess your own body and life-style and come up with the activity that is right for you. (In addition, Elizabeth Noble[34] provides specific exercises to prevent or improve pregnancy-related complaints, such as chronic backache, leaking urine, or weak abdominal walls.)

Nancy began to swim during her third pregnancy. Her first day at the Y, she barely made it to the other end of the pool, gasping for dear life. She couldn't even swim back. The next day wasn't very much better, except that she promised herself she'd make it back. Day by day, things improved. At the end of two weeks, she could swim several laps with a rest in between. Finally, she made ten laps without stopping. She figured ten laps was practically swim team material, right? So she stuck with that for a little bit. She began to notice that on the days that she didn't swim, she felt tired, achy, and full of complaints. On the days she swam, she felt energetic, happy and more even-tempered.

One day, as she was doing her seventh or eighth lap, a little old lady bumped into her and yelled, "Watch yourself, girlie. I gotta finish my laps." The woman proceeded to *zip* across the pool. Nancy continued to watch in amazement. The woman was old, really old, but she kept zipping back and forth. Twenty minutes later she hopped out of the pool and into the sauna. That same morning, Nancy saw her riding her bicycle—what incentive! Nancy pushed harder. On days when she didn't think she could possibly swim another stroke, she continued swimming. She talked to herself the whole time: "You swam this distance yesterday, you can swim it today." She'd sing songs, think up the week's menu— anything she could do to distract herself so that she could make it.

And, surprise! She didn't turn into a prune. She didn't kill herself. She began to feel terrific every time she came out of the water. She really knew what people were talking about when they said they felt like a million dollars. Nancy says:

> Some days I loved swimming, some days I hated it. I only knew that I felt better, slept better, and had more energy than I had in years. My pregnant body felt lighter and more easy to carry than ever before. After a while, I no longer had to distract myself to get through each lap. I began to relax, even as I continued my pace, and to think about my body. I'd focus on different parts of my body, and concentrate

on how each felt when I swam faster or slower. Sometimes I'd listen to my breathing. I'd imagine each breath carrying oxygen to the parts of my body that needed it. I also began thinking almost exclusively about the baby growing inside me. I wondered what it felt like to have Mommy swimming and kicking her legs. I'd try out names: I'd swim up the lane with one name in mind, and back to the other end with another. By the way, in the earlier months when I was feeling some queasiness, I found that swimming in the pool completely eliminated it.

Thinking about what my body was doing, really concentrating on the work that it was doing, made swimming easier. I found that thinking about the baby also seemed to make the time pass more quickly. I used the time in the water, which was just about the only free and quiet time I had each day, to think about my life and to clear my head. I'd "speak" to my baby and listen to what my baby wanted me to know. Swimming became not only a physical exercise, but an important mental one as well. It was fun to see people's reactions when I was swimming in the pool just days away from my due date. It was even more interesting to see their reactions when I was overdue. Everyone gets nutsy around very pregnant ladies. I even went down for a swim in early labor. It helped me feel refreshed and revitalized, instead of cranky and impatient waiting for labor to pick up. I went right back to swimming very soon after Andrea was born.

When Lois learned of the benefits of squatting, she decided that she would get her leg muscles in shape for this unaccustomed position. With a mid-August due date, she chose gardening as a good way to practice squatting. For the May planting she squatted and kept falling over like one of those little wooden play family figures most of our children have around the house. By June she was more like a Weeble, rolling a bit from side to side, but managing to stay upright for most of the weeding. By July she was squatting comfortably for all her gardening, and did so right up until the day she gave birth.

Lois also raised a few eyebrows by riding her bike around the neighborhood, with a 38-pound, almost-four-year-old in the tot seat, right through her pregnancy. The exercise paid off—soon after her very quick labor and birth, she was able to take up jogging with a fair amount of ease.

We are concerned about physicians who ask women to stop exercising two to three weeks before their due date. After a week or so of not exercising, you begin to lose the strength and stamina that has been built up over the course of time. And what if you're two weeks late? It would then have been more than two months without exercise! Also, most women find they sleep much better when they have exercised, and certainly, during those last weeks, it's wonderful to be able to sleep well and wake up refreshed and relaxed.

It's important to find out why a physician wants you to stop exercising early, and to determine whether the reason is valid. We have noted that the physician who encourages a woman to continue exercising is apt to be an athlete himself, who understands the benefits, while those who insist that a woman stop are often not involved in any exercise program themselves.

We have known many women who have had wonderful births without having exercised a finger the entire pregnancy. You know our belief is that women's bodies were designed to have babies. Exercise is one way to gain—or regain—feelings of confidence and trust in one's body. We recommend that some of your exercise be a private experience. Taking a walk with your toddler is wonderful for both of you. Attending a prenatal exercise program can be fun and beneficial. But our thought is that exercise should be at your own pace, free from distractions. You deserve a quiet time for yourself, a time to focus on your pregnancy, and some private time with your growing baby. Whatever exercise you do, get in touch with the flexibility, stamina, strength, endurance, and beauty of your body. Honor it. It will not let you down.

Dr. Charles Kimball tells us that "prenatal physical activities that provide enjoyment and recreation help endorphin mechanisms to dominate the autonomic nervous system and to suppress depressive anxiety producing catecholamines."[24] Translated, that means that exercise increases your endorphin level, which increases relaxation and reduces pain.

So let's get moving!

Reaping the Rewards

In *Spiritual Midwifery*, Stephen says:

> If all your life you never do anything heavy, there's certain passages in life that are heavy. Having a baby, for instance, is one. If you be a total paddy-ass all your life, they're going to have to knock you out when you have your kid, because you're going to be too chicken to have it. And if you do something that builds character ahead of time, you'll have enough character that you'll have that kid, and it will be a beautiful and a spiritual experience for you.[14]

Making responsible, caring, positive decisions about your body and your health is just one of many ways to build character.

When you are in labor thinking that you'll never be able to get through another contraction, you can remember that extra lap that you thought you couldn't do—but you did. You can remember all the good food you ate, which created a terrific baby, a great uterus, a yielding cervix, and a stretchy perineum. You can call upon all the feelings of pride, confidence, and accomplishment that you have found in yourself as a result of eating well and exercising. Knowing that you have developed a strong, healthy body that works well under stress and strenuous activity will help you to feel ready, willing, and able to work with your body and actively give birth to your baby.

8 → Diagnostic Time Bombs?

Pregnancy as Pathology

There may be a correlation between acceptance of routine tests, adherence to hospital "policies," and cesarean section. A woman who seeks out or passively agrees to various tests and procedures during pregnancy obviously trusts medical technology over and above her own body's ability to produce and birth a normal baby. If she uses technology for reassurance about her own and her baby's well-being during pregnancy, we wonder whether she'll then *labor* without medical devices or "expertise" to "help out."

All women would like reassurance that their babies are fine. Believing that the tests can provide this makes the procedure seem very appealing. However, your baby may "check out" fine from an amniocentesis, for example, and still have problems not detectable by the procedure. Jane M. said, "I worried that my baby was defective, so I agreed to an amniocentesis. Now I'm worried that my baby will be defective *because* of it." Other women like Jane are bitter when they find out how many serious potential complications can result from various prenatal tests and procedures. No one told them about any of the problems before the procedures were done.

Informed Consent?

Greta wrote and told us that when she was on the operating table, her physician asked her what type of incision she wanted for her cesarean. "I didn't know that

135

there was more than one kind. I asked him, 'Which one is faster?' and he told me that the classical was. I thought, 'Good! I'll see my baby sooner!' " Greta *consented*, but she certainly wasn't at all well *informed*. Only later did she find out the potential problems associated with classical cesarean section.

Most of us depend on and trust in the knowledge and expertise of our physicians. We don't always have the time or the resources to fully educate ourselves about problems which could occur during labor and delivery and possible solutions. In the event of a problem, we rely on our doctors to inform us about the various courses of action and the appropriateness of each alternative.

There is a great deal of literature on the issue of informed consent in law and in medicine. Simply stated, a person giving her informed consent agrees to the doctor's recommended procedure after receiving sufficient information to make an intelligent decision. Most of us depend on obtaining this "sufficient information" from the physician, since he is the recognized and trusted expert. But what if the doctor doesn't *give sufficient* information? What if he is not aware of all the information necessary to help you make an informed choice? What if he withholds information that he feels is irrelevant but that *you* feel is vital to any decision you must make? There are many issues around informed consent that are not quickly settled.

Hospitals require that consent forms be signed in both emergency and non-emergency situations. Most forms are worded in favor of doctors and hospitals: they contain language that in effect authorizes any further procedures that the physician deems necessary. The consent forms themselves do not contain specific information upon which informed consent can be based, so that information must be obtained prior to signing the form. Even if you do sign, the consent you give is not unalterably cut into stone. You can get a second opinion, change your mind or invalidate the form verbally. You may refuse treatment until you feel fully informed of consequences and alternatives, and you may still refuse, even then.

David Stewart, founder and director of NAPSAC,* makes the following remarks about informed consent:

> All [drugs or medical procedures] have risks. Medical intervention should, therefore, never be done unless the risk of the intervention is less than the risk of the medical problem itself without intervention . . .

> Weighing such risks can only be objective up to a point. In the end, subjective choices are always made—sometimes for medical reasons, sometimes not. Sometimes there are no real reasons, only "traditions" or "accepted practices." And sometimes, such judgments are controlled by unknowing ignorance—on the part of either or both the health care provider and health care consumer.

---

*National Association of Parents & Professionals for Safe Alternatives in Childbirth, P.O. Box 267, Marble Hill, Mo. 63764.

. . . There is usually room for disagreement as to the best course of treatment to follow in any given medical situation. Authorities may disagree with each other. Authorities may disagree with consumers. And consumers may disagree with other consumers.

While physicians and hospitals fear malpractice suits from patients charging 'uninformed consent,' consumers fear the risks of medical procedures they do not understand. Both patients and providers stand to benefit from informed consent. . . . Professionals do not always have the best answers. This is not a criticism of professionals, but a simple recognition of a fact. It serves neither professionals nor patients to disregard this fact. All have limited experience and limited education. It is important for both professionals and patients to realize and accept these limitations. The best health care is available to consumers who participate in the medical decisions pertaining to themselves and their families. Informed consent is essential for good professional health care.

How can "Informed Consent" be accomplished and insured? Who bears the responsibility for such education? How does one become 'informed?' Is it entirely the duty of the professional? Or is it all up to the consumer?

If you rush to a hospital in an emergency and are given 60 seconds to read and sign a "consent release" form, can such consent be truly informed? If you, as a consumer, base your consent only upon what information your doctor gives you, are you truly informed? The answer is "no" in both of these instances. Informed consent about an unfamiliar medical crisis at the time of the emergency is impossible.

. . . To be fully informed requires preparation and education *before* the emergency. Doctors and medical institutions have a clear obligation to *assist* patients by providing unbiased pros and cons of policies and procedures. They do not have the obligation to be a patient's sole and complete source of education. Even if doctors and hospitals wanted to educate their patients completely, it would be impossible. Truly informed consent is only possible by *consumer initiative*. Personal education is a personal responsibility.[4]

Stewart reminds us that most medical situations are not emergencies, or at least do not begin as emergencies. In most situations there are at least a few minutes to do some quick phone calling, reading, or consulting. He tells us that although truly informed consent is not possible in all situations, it can be achieved in most situations in direct proportion to the effort you are willing to make to educate yourself. His suggestions for improving your chances of being an informed health care consumer include: reading; acquiring a working vocabulary with which to communicate to health professionals; subscribing to consumer health periodicals; taking short courses such as first aid, CPR, nutrition; finding doctors and hospitals who like informed patients; being discriminating in your choice of classes; finding an advocate for yourself; asking questions and asking about alternatives; getting other opinions; not feeling that you always have to take the doctor's advice.[4] In addition, we recommend *The Rights of Hospital Patients*, by George Annas;[2] "The Pregnant Patient's Bill of Rights and Responsibilities," available through ICEA;[7] and membership in Children in Hospitals,* a consumer group that seeks to "educate all concerned about the needs of children and parents for continued and ample contact when either is hospitalized."

In the following chapter, we discuss procedures inflicted on newborns. Your baby cannot give informed consent, so you, as legal guardian and official spokesperson, will have to make decisions for her. No test, examination, or procedure can be performed without your informed consent. One woman wrote us, "Right after I took a shower, I walked into the nursery to get my baby. A dozen medical students were standing around her. I heard the pediatrician say, 'Look here, we have a congenital hip abnormality.' It was the first I had heard about the problem, and to make things worse, the students were all lined up to feel her hips! I scooped up my daughter and screeched at them that they couldn't touch her. They were aghast." Babies deserve the same protection from unnecessary and callous examinations and procedures that women deserve during labor.

Every day we make decisions affecting the quality and direction of our lives and the lives of our children. When we do so, we must then accept the responsibility for those decisions. (Remember your folks telling you: "You make your bed, you sleep in it.") In order to be an active decision-making partner in the birth of our babies, and to make responsible choices, we must see that we have adequate information. Gathering and integrating this information should begin long before we begin our labors.

Women as Lab Rats

For a long while, women have been subjected by the medical profession to unproven and inaccurate tests, procedures, and drugs. The practice of treating and exposing women to unwarranted medical interventions, inconclusive and unnecessary examinations, and an assortment of dangerous chemicals continues during pregnancy, in labor, and during birth, and affects the birth process. These numerous acts are a result of the medical profession's general attitudes about women. Unfortunately, *women have become medical science's guinea pigs.*

For example, women are often administered drugs without their consent or knowledge of the effects. They are the most medicated of all Americans, and

---

*CIH, 31 Wilshire Park, Needham, Mass. 02192. (Send a SASE.)

are admitted to the hospital more frequently. They are given the Pill and expected to believe it contains the same things that our bodies produce. Over five million women take drugs to treat symptoms of the menopause, although less than a third of that number are estimated to be menopausal. More than four million women used intrauterine devices on the basis of studies that "charitably, can only be called inadequate."*

We are strapped to operating tables with alarming frequency. By the time a woman in the United States is 70 years old, she has nearly a 50 percent chance of having undergone a hysterectomy. In the book *Hidden Malpractice*, Gena Corea remarks that the physician's greed as well as his casual attitude toward the removal of female reproductive organs endangers women.[9] In *Gyn/ecology* by Mary Daly, we are told that well-known gynecologists resort to describing the uterus as "a possible breeding ground for cancer" and as "a potentially lethal organ."[10] Larned tells us that one-third of all hysterectomies in the United States have been performed on women with *normal* uteri.[14] Daly remarks that "if some gynecologists have their way . . . it will soon be abnormal for a woman over fifty to have her own uterus and/or breasts."

We are the repositories of a variety of twentieth-century laboratory creations that are being used in spite of their dangers (and in spite of the "unknowns" about each). Kay Weiss writes that the FDA has approved a women's "morning-after " pill contraceptive even though it contains 833,000 times the amount of DES banned for human consumption in beef.[18] The fact that birth-control pills, intrauterine devices, and chemical spermicidal agents cause cancer, cramping, infections, or bleeding in some women seems of little significance to many physicians. According to an article in *Science*,[12] lactation contraception,† probably has a statistically higher rate of protection than has currently been achieved by chemical or mechanical methods. Yet women are still discouraged from breastfeeding, and are encouraged to use technology's "improvements" instead.

Tests during Pregnancy: Help or Hindrance?

Before we discuss the interventions women are subjected to during labor and delivery, we'd like to alert you to some of the tests done during pregnancy.

There are several tests that have been designed to assess the baby's well-being in utero. The rationale for the use of these tests is that the maternal-fetal-placental unit must function properly in order for the baby to survive. If part

---

*Katz, Barbara, "The IUD: Out of Sight, Out of Mind," *Ms.*, July 1975.

†For information on lactation contraception, read *Breastfeeding and Natural Child Spacing: The Ecology of Natural Mothering*, by Sheila Kippley (New York: Penguin, 1975). For a list of natural planning resources, see *Mothering* magazine, Winter 1981.

of "the unit" is insufficient, doctors warn us, the baby may have to be removed from the malfunctioning system. Labor may have to be induced and/or the baby may have to be born by cesarean section. (When women are "overdue," for example, doctors are concerned that the aging placenta may not be able to sustain the baby in utero, or provide enough oxygen during labor.)

Of course, *we* believe that in healthy women "the unit" knows how to function. However, if a cesarean is to be performed, it must wait until the fetal lungs are mature enough for the baby to breathe on its own. If tests to determine well-being show that the fetus is in trouble, additional tests must then be made to determine whether its lungs are sufficiently developed to withstand life outside the mother's body. According to "The Obstetrician's Dilemma," most methods of determining fetal maturity are either inaccurate or test only a partial aspect of fetal maturity.[42]

Estriol Testing

Estriol production increases as pregnancy advances. Taking measurements of estriol levels in the mother's urine or blood is one way that fetal maturity is determined. By measuring and interpreting the estriol level, we are told, one can determine whether or not the baby is "ready" to be born, and how well the baby will fare outside the uterus. A gradual but continual fall or an abrupt drop is considered dangerous. According to Edwards and Simkin, however, estriol counts are not accurate enough to determine if a pregnancy is ready to be terminated.[36]

If all the women who were a week overdue were requested to bring in a 24-hour urine sample ("Honey, should I rent a U-Haul?"), there wouldn't be enough room on all the shelves in all the laboratories in the country to hold it. Most women with whom we work give birth many days after their "due date." Many have been more than two or three weeks overdue, and one VBAC woman who knew her exact conception date was five weeks overdue. (She delivered a robust 9 pound 2 ounce daughter and left the hospital a few hours after the birth.) Most of the women with whom we work do not begin estriol testing until at least two weeks "overdue." They make certain that their diet is superb and that they are taking wonderful care of themselves. We have had no problems with any of the "overdue" pregnancies. We'll talk about "overdue" several times during the remainder of our book.

Ultrasound

If the only tool you have is a hammer,
you tend to see every problem as a nail.
—Abraham Maslow

Ultrasound is "seeing with sound," a complex technique for studying the inner organs of the body. Although it has not been proven safe, it is being used with increasing frequency in American obstetrics. In simple terms, high-frequency sound waves are beamed into the body. They bounce back from the different surfaces and densities of various body organs. The "echoing" waves are duly measured and recorded.

A diagnostic ultrasound scan, or sonogram, utilizes a moving probe connected to a "black box." The box houses a screen where the sound echoes are reflected as a series of bright dots. A technician sees the dots form into moving pictures of internal organs. In pregnancy, an image of the fetus and all its tiny developing parts can be obtained (sometimes the sex of the baby can be determined) and then measurements of the organs and judgments of their health can be estimated. Accuracy of interpretation is greatly dependent upon the skill of the technician.

Diagnostic ultrasound relies on a "pulsed" or intermittent sound wave. A continuous wave of ultrasound is the medium of the Doppler unit, or Doptone. Routinely, in physicians' offices across the United States, mothers hear their babies' "heartbeats" with the use of the Doptone "amplifier." No one bothers to tell these women that they are actually hearing the echoes of a continuous wave of ultrasound directed toward the fetus's moving blood. The sound waves are apparently felt by the fetus; one study indicates that fetuses responded to a routine five-minute exposure of the Doptone with greatly increased activity. Both Joan and Robin said, "I noticed my baby jumped every time the Doppler was used." How does it feel to the fetus? We don't know.

Doptones are freely used with no thought of potential harm to the fetus; indeed, parents assume the Doptone to be merely an electronically amplified, perfectly harmless stethoscope. They are so commonplace that few physicians can still locate their once essential, and totally safe, fetoscopes. The Doppler principle is also the basis for the external fetal heart monitor. An ultrasound transmitter-receiver is placed on the woman's abdomen to provide a continuous recording of the fetal heart tones.

The reasons usually cited for ordering diagnostic ultrasound during pregnancy include: confirming a viable pregnancy in the presence of staining or bleeding; locating the position of the fetus and placenta before amniocentesis; confirming ectopic pregnancy; confirming the presence of twins; determining the position of the placenta before birth; and, most commonly, estimating gestational age and due date. With the exception of determining fetal position, however, results of ultrasound diagnosis are *often* inaccurate! In several situations, a twin pregnancy has gone undiagnosed by ultrasound, and in one case, a triplet was undiagnosed.

Doris Haire, who is the director of the Association of Maternal Child Health in New York, has called ultrasound "the DES of tomorrow." DES was given to mothers up until the early 1970s to prevent miscarriage. It has since been proven that it did not prevent miscarriage. But, much worse, twenty years after DES was first administered we all learned that it is associated with numerous reproductive abnormalities, high incidence of infertility and very high rates of cancer in the children whose mothers took it.

Diagnostic ultrasound has been around for decades, but has been widely used in pregnancy, birth and medical diagnosis for only the past seven to ten years. Children who were bombarded with ultrasound as fetuses are just now reaching the ages of reading readiness and mental/neurological evaluation. In fact, a current study funded by the FDA at the University of Colorado Medical Center, under the direction of Dr. Albert Haverkamp, is examining 1,600 children for reading or other learning disabilities as well as physical abnormalities that may be traced to ultrasound. Another study in Winnipeg, Canada, is following ten thousand exposed subjects.[30]

We won't know those results for years, but we already have results from short-term studies utilizing laboratory animals as test mediums. A 1979 commentary published in the *Federal Register* by the Department of Health, Education, and Welfare, entitled, "Diagnostic Ultrasound Equipment," stated:

> The possible risks associated with diagnostic ultrasound are not fully understood . . . Because human studies of adverse effects from ultrasound have been inadequate, there is no direct way at this time to establish the exposure limits that assure safety in the use of this modality. Thus, the Commissioner believes manufacturers should not state . . . that diagnostic ultrasound is unequivocally safe.[22]

In available literature,[24,27,30] a variety of effects of ultrasound on laboratory animals is reported, including genetic alterations described as chromosome damage and a breakdown of DNA materials; decreased clotting time in blood and other circulatory changes in primates; liver cell damage in mice; dilation of blood vessels and corneal erosion in the eyes of rabbits; brain enzyme alterations in dogs; alterations in electrical activity (EEG) in the brains of nonhuman primates; delayed reflexes and emotional reactivity in rats; and disruption of the spleen's ability to produce antibodies resulting in reduced immunology. This last effect has been documented in a study of human infants by at least one researcher, who followed exposed children through their first year of life. A number of the studies adjusted "doses" of ultrasound to those used on pregnant women. The results all spell danger. The thought that thousands of healthy women and unborn babies are unnecessarily subjected to these potentially horrifying sequelae is mind-boggling! Liebeskind remarks that all ova are present in a female child in utero, so not only are her cells being exposed, but all her eggs for the next generation as well. She says, "If we asked more questions on the benefits of ultrasound exams, we'd sonocate a lot less."[24]

Perhaps the most common use of diagnostic ultrasound is for gestational age determination. A determination of dates is possible with some accuracy only between the fourteenth and twentieth weeks of pregnancy, by measuring the bi-parietal diameter of the fetal head with ultrasound waves. However, *most* questions about dating seem to arise during the third trimester of a pregnancy, and as the weeks pass, measurements become increasingly inaccurate and useless because of variations in growth rates. Thus, all the ultrasound scans that are being done on third trimester women for dating purposes are in our opinion inappropriate, unnecessary, wasteful, improper, and worst of all, *potentially harmful to the fetus.* A Massachusetts woman wrote that her doctor urged a diagnostic ultrasound for the purpose of "confirming dates." When she protested because she wasn't sure it was safe, he responded, "You're probably right, and ten years from now we'll know what's wrong with it, but right now it's the best we have."

Another woman wrote of her anguish after learning some of the potential harmful effects of ultrasound exposure:

> My doctor insisted that it was safe, perfectly safe. In fact, he told me that the ultrasound technician was so confident of the procedure that he scanned his wife monthly during her pregnancy just to keep tabs on the growing fetus! Nonetheless, I just didn't feel comfortable with it; but he was worried about the seemingly small size of our baby—told me that maybe she was defective, with no brain, and that he couldn't support me if he didn't know for sure whether my dates were accurate. So I consented to an ultrasound scan in my 39th week of pregnancy. The "results" were fine, my dates seemed right on target. He relaxed, and I then waited three weeks longer before delivering a small but healthy baby girl.
>
> Since then, over a year has passed, and I've read what I can find on ultrasound. I now know that the scan was totally pointless at that stage of my pregnancy because it could not then give accurate dating information. . . . Whenever women tell me now how completely they trust their doctors, I cringe. "Trust yourself, too," I say, "because you *have* to live with the decisions you let your doctor make."

Why aren't doctors aware of the inaccuracies of ultrasound? If they are, why are they still ordering them? Even if a baby's "due date" is calculated in the sixteenth week by a sonogram, that baby still could arrive three weeks early or three weeks late. "Gadgets," said one woman:

> They get a gadget and they have to play with it. This time I decided just to let my baby choose its birthday, not the ultrasound. The first time, when I went three days overdue, my doctor insisted on inducing me. He said the baby was getting too big. I ended up with a section for my 6 pound 9 ounce baby! This time my baby was "overdue" by 2½ weeks and weighed 8 pounds 4 ounces, born vaginally. I know my first baby wasn't ready, ultrasound or not. By the way, I also had an x-ray last time, and I have since heard that if you have ultrasound and x-rays during pregnancy the effects of the two procedures are worse than either procedure alone.

Some doctors order ultrasound scans routinely to determine if there is a low-lying placenta. If this situation is present, they often insist upon a cesarean. The incidence of low-lying placentas seems to be on the increase; according to Esther Zorn, president of the National Cesarean Prevention Movement, it may be that a low-lying placenta is something that exists fairly often and that it is just being discovered because of the use of ultrasound. Given time, she notes, the placenta often migrates up and away from the cervix.

Another inappropriate use of ultrasound, we believe, is for determination of the viability of a uterine pregnancy. If a woman begins to bleed or stain in her first trimester, she may miscarry *or* she may carry a healthy fetus to term and deliver a perfect baby. The FDA has cautioned against the use of diagnostic ultrasound in the first trimester because of potential harm to the developing fetus. Yet many doctors choose to ignore the warnings and suggest scans to women who are staining, "in order to put their fears to rest." Submitting to an ultrasound in order to put "fears to rest" is like jumping into the ocean because your boat has a small leak. Suppose the pregnancy proceeds normally, and a healthy baby is born. We don't know, and we won't know for twenty more years, at least, whether children exposed to ultrasound *are* healthy or whether they have suffered long-term impairments. Women who have had ultrasound scans indicating a "troubled" pregnancy have gone on to deliver healthy full-term babies; on the other hand, some scans have shown viable, secure implantations, but miscarriage occurred anyway. Thus, ultrasound is unable to completely dispel anxiety, since the results may mean little or nothing in the overall scheme of that pregnancy. It should be carefully limited to such uses as early diagnosis of a suspected tubal pregnancy.

So, when you visit your physician, refuse the Doptone. Patience is a virtue, so they wisely say, and you will be able to hear your baby's heartbeat at about the twentieth week with a stethoscope or fetascope. If diagnostic ultrasound is recommended, ask for full details: Why is it recommended? Would the results be absolutely accurate at this point in your pregnancy? Would the scan provide essential information that can not be gathered any other way and which would then determine resultant care? What difference does it make if you already know your "due date"?

Amniocentesis

Another procedure used to determine fetal well-being is amniocentesis. Amniotic fluid is drawn from the uterus through a hollow needle inserted into the abdomen. The procedure is used for several reasons, including the detection of chromosomal abnormalities and the determination of fetal lung maturity. The fluid is analyzed for the presence of surfactant, a substance manufactured by the mature fetal lung. Without sufficient surfactant, the lungs do not stay inflated and the baby will become asphyxiated.

Amniocentesis is usually done in conjunction with ultrasound. By first "viewing the works," the physician is able to insert the needle into the amniotic fluid rather than into the placenta or the baby. Risks associated with amniocentesis for diagnostic purposes are numerous. A few are placental, maternal, or fetal hemorrhage or injury, and premature labor. Read them again, slowly! The placenta is frequently damaged by the needle, which also increases the risk of Rh sensitization. Edwards and Simkin report that amniocentesis will cause one in 150 women to miscarry, and holds an overall risk rate of .5 to 1 percent.[36] A 41-page supplemental report to the *British Journal of Obstetrics and Gynaecology*, entitled "An Assessment of the Hazards of Amniocentesis," reported an increased fetal loss of 1 to 1.5 percent and a possible increase of 1 to 1.5 percent of major infant morbidity, "namely unexplained respiratory difficulties at birth and major orthopaedic postural abnormalities. These risks seem to be independent of the particular indication for the procedure."[35] According to Ettner, there have been several accounts of fetal death by bleeding because of puncture of the placenta or umbilical cord, and various fetal injuries, some permanent, caused directly by the needle. Ettner tells us that clearly, the dangers of amniocentesis demand evaluation before its use becomes common practice.[37]

Its use is already becoming common practice. Women over 35 are encouraged to have amniocentesis. They are considered "elderly" and are told that their chances of having a defective child are significantly increased. The British researchers suggest that only after 40 years of age is the indication for the procedure to detect an abnormality equal to or greater than the increased risk to the fetus.

We'd rather you were a 39-year-old, healthy, well-nourished woman who does not smoke or use alcohol than a 24-year-old smoker whose diet is poor. We'd bet our money on you and your baby any day. If women weren't supposed to have babies at age 40, the "factory" would have shut down. According to Evarts,[38] if you are under 40, it is more likely that detrimental effects from the procedure will occur than that you will produce an abnormal child. One woman in our class wrote on her records that she was 34. Actually, she was 38. "I wasn't about to have any tests, and I didn't want any hassles," she said. Her fourth daughter was fine, and she said she'll keep putting "34" on her records until she decides to stop having children.

Obviously, there are other, more involved, issues involved with amniocentesis. When the procedure is performed early in pregnancy, it is usually done with the thought of abortion if the fetus is defective. We've all heard stories of test results that are either wrong or confused. We know several women who learned the sex of their babies as "bonus" information from the amniocentesis they had undergone, and some who scheduled amniocentesis to learn the sex, only to deliver a baby of the opposite sex. We know of a situation where a healthy baby was aborted due to a "mix-up" in test results. The genetically defective baby was born to parents who had been assured (through amniocentesis) that they would give birth to a healthy baby. It is time we evaluate the many aspects of this procedure, and make a decision based on information as well as personal concerns.

Oxytocin Challenge Test

In an Oxytocin Challenge Test (OCT), the external fetal monitor, which utilizes ultrasound, is attached to the mother and synthetic oxytocin is administered intravenously. The mother is put into a bed, and the "drip" is begun, with increasing dosage every ten to twenty minutes until there are at least three uterine contractions within a ten-minute period. The monitor records the baby's heart beat and response to the contractions. If the heart tones are abnormal in any way, the mother is whisked to the operating room for a cesarean section.

In the next chapter, we will be discussing the dangers of monitors, the supine position (which decreases the oxygen flow to the baby) and Pitocin—all of which are part of OCTs. Besides these concerns, there is the strong possibility that, since mothers brought in for an OCT are often apprehensive, this in itself can alter the baby's responses.

During a contraction, the fetal heart rate slows down; it "recovers" when the contraction is over. One rationale for a cesarean is that if the baby's "recovery" isn't quick during the OCT, the placenta may already be compromised, and during labor there will not be enough oxygen for the baby. The section is done ostensibly because, according to the OCT, the baby will not be able to withstand labor. In "Obstetric Tests and Technology: A Consumer's Guide," Edwards and Simkin (1980) remark that the supine position of the mother during an OCT can result in the appearance of fetal distress when the fetus is perfectly all right. Induction, they say, is in itself a form of stress. Others believe the test elicits ominous decelerations that might otherwise never appear if labor were allowed to start spontaneously.[36]

According to Brewer, several women have reported that their doctors advised them to have an OCT on the grounds of postmaturity. Once the test was underway, the doctors tried to persuade them to have a full-fledged induction, telling them that they were already committed.[34] Ettner says that the major criterion for an OCT is calculated due date, which is notoriously unreliable but has become the mainstay of diagnoses of postmaturity.[37] If dates are inaccurate and the "postmature" baby is really a month behind, the test will be positive; the baby isn't ready to be born, so she will "fail" the test, and a premie will be delivered.

Dr. R. Freeman's study stated that OCT was disappointing as a way to predict subsequent performance of the fetus during labor. This study and others reported 25 percent false positives. If late changes in the fetal heart rate occur as a result of the OCT, then "at what point is intervention best implemented, if at all?"[39] Dr. Ettner remarks that hospital obstetricians have promoted the OCT to the point of a self-fulfilling prophecy: "The fetus is challenged and the EFM dutifully records the stressed fetal heart rate."[39]

Non-Stress Test

Another test, the non-stress test (NST), also records fetal reaction. It is based on the rationale that accelerations of the fetal heartbeat during fetal movement indicate a healthy fetus. According to Edwards and Simkin, deceleration may indicate that the fetus does not respond to differing physiologic demands.[36]

During the NST, the external monitor records the baby's spontaneous movements as well as manually stimulated responses. The test can also be performed by listening with a fetascope while the baby moves. The test is positive (or "reactive") if the baby's heart tones accelerate at least fifteen beats above the normal rate (120–160). If the test is negative, it is followed by an OCT. You hope for a positive non-stress test and a negative OCT.

The NST is considered normal (reactive) if there are at least two fetal rate accelerations of at least 30 seconds, as well as fifteen beats per minute greater amplitude during a twenty minute period. According to "More Muddy Water— Antepartum Fetal Assessment Techniques," it is well known that the wake-sleep patterns of the fetus considerably influence the fetal heart rate pattern. Thus a nonreactive NST may become reactive as the fetus wakes up. A false positive conclusion could be drawn if the test is curtailed prior to the fetus' awakening.[44] Dr. J. Patrick reports that an increasing number of stimuli, such as maternal hypoglycemia, time of day, drugs and the onset of labor, may also result in significant alterations in fetal breathing activity. He urges great caution in making suggestions based on the NST alone.[43]

Gail Brewer tells us that "placental insufficiency" is a result of reduced blood volume due to undernutrition. If a woman's diet is improved, even in the last weeks of pregnancy, her placental function improves due to the increased blood flow through it. An appropriate therapeutic intervention in cases of "placental insufficiency" is *not* to schedule the mother for more tests to see if the baby could survive delivery at this time, but to make intensive efforts to improve the quality and amount of food consumed. "The advantages of trying to improve the maternal health situation—and so the baby's environment in utero—are obvious."[34]

X-Rays

X-ray pelvimetry is often ordered to diagnose or confirm CPD. X-rays are dangerous—very dangerous—and *inaccurate* for either diagnosing *or* confirming

CPD. And remember: CPD is a wastebasket term into which obstetrics tosses its crumbled labors.

As you already know, the pelvis changes shape during active labor. It increases in size when a woman squats. So x-rays taken prior to the onset of active labor are of no value, and x-rays taken in any position besides squatting do not show the potential of the pelvis.

X-rays taken during active labor do not accurately predict the route of delivery either. A study by Campbell, entitled "X-Ray Pelvimetry: Useful Procedure or Medical Nonsense?" states that there are numerous factors that adversely affect the progress of labor, and the contracted bony pelvis is statistically among the least of these![47] The findings of a study by Kelly et al., declare the researchers, "warrant an investigation of the efficacy of pelvimetry."[54] Another study by Joyce et al. on "Role of Pelvimetry in Active Management of Labour" questioned its accuracy and stated that it should not be performed routinely.[53] Hannah, in the 1965 article "X-Ray Pelvimetry—A Critical Appraisal," says, "For some time I have been convinced that the vast majority of X-rays ordered for pelvimetry were completely unnecessary." He goes on to state that the only value in most cases is the additional time the procedure and the elevator ride give the labor.[51]

"An Evaluation of the Usefulness of X-Ray Pelvimetry," which compares x-rays with manual pelvimetry, reports that there is no significant role for x-ray pelvimetry in the diagnosis and management of CPD in vertex presentations.[49] An article by Jagani et al., entitled "The Predictability of Labor Outcome from a Comparison of Birth Weight and X-Ray Pelvimetry," concludes that pelvic measurements and birth weight do not provide a predictive tool for delivery outcome.[52] Other work supplements and supports these findings.

In most studies, x-rays' predictability rate was sorrowful. Women who were classified as unable to deliver vaginally gave birth while the cesarean room was being readied. Other women, shown by x-ray to be adequate (we are *all* adequate, remember), were expected to labor for hours; many did, without "producing." Clearly, it is more than a pelvis that gives birth. Joyce reports that antenatal pelvimetry is rarely justified,[53] and Campbell noted a lack of correlation between pelvic measurements and the course of labor. "The effects of molding of the fetal head and the expansion of the pelvis may render pelvic diameter measurements meaningless." Campbell found the incidence of truly "small" pelves in patients to be as low as one or two cases in 2500!

Why then, are x-rays still being recommended? The dangers are staggering. The U.S. Department of Health and Human Services recently published a booklet entitled, "The Selection of Patients for X-Ray Examinations: The Pelvimetry Examination." It states that in addition to an increased risk of cancer, irradiation during pregnancy may also be associated with genetic damages. There may be mutations which give rise to changes that can be transmitted from generation to generation. Such mutations are generally detrimental, it says, and may increase undesirable genetic characteristics in the population.[61]

We are the population.

In 1979, the FDA approved a statement that included the following: "Pelvimetry is not usually necessary or helpful in making the decison to perform a cesarean section." The American College of Radiology approved the statement by the FDA. The American College of Obstetricians and Gynecologists approved a comparable statement: "X-ray pelvimetry provides limited additional information to physicians involved in the management of labor and delivery. It should not be a prerequisite to clinical decisions concerning obstetrical management . . ."[61]

Christopher Norwood, author of *At Highest Risk*, tells us that 2 to 26 percent of all pregnancies in this country are x-rayed. Three-fourths of this is pelvimetry. A 1969 study noted a 7–15 percent increase in fertility in daughters of x-rayed mothers, a finding accompanied by somewhat more miscarriages and almost triple the fetal deaths.[58] By 1978, this extra fertility had markedly diminished, followed by sterility. Eighty percent more of these daughters experienced severe menstrual problems than women in the control group. The cancer that the U.S. Department of Health and Human Services reported was leukemia: almost twice as many children who died of leukemia before age ten had been prenatally exposed to radiation as had normal children.[62]

Miller reported that even small prenatal exposures to radiation may deprive the individual of some intelligence.[60] Macht reports that x-rayed children have been found to have a higher incidence of abnormalities.[56] A study in 1958 by Stewart reported that even x-rays taken preconceptually were linked with cancer in the child,[61] and one in 1965 at Johns Hopkins found that mothers of Down's Syndrome babies had had seven times the radiation exposure of the control mothers.[59]

Many reports evaluating x-ray pelvimetry question potential long-term hazards of irradiation to the fetus, and recommend a study to evaluate the impact of x-ray pelvimetry on perinatal mortality and morbidity. Do we have any volunteers to be one of the subjects?

Dr. Helen Caldicott reminds us that all radiation is dangerous. In *New Directions for Women*, she maintains that infants and children are ten to twenty times more susceptible to the carcinogenic effects of radiation because their cells are rapidly dividing.[46] If this is so, what of a *fetus*? Mendelsohn warns us about x-rays, too.[58] Even dental x-rays should be postponed during pregnancy, and Novacaine was implicated in early miscarriage by one research team. Do yourself a favor: stay away from the x-ray machine. The next time someone says you ought to be in pictures, make certain it's not your "innards" they want for their photo album.

"Don't Worry Your Pretty Little Head!"

We received this letter from a doctor in Toronto:

> My patient heard you speak on the danger of ultrasound. She has been upset that
> her baby may have been harmed because of ultrasound examinations done during
> her pregnancy . . . . I think it is prudent (and humane) to avoid raising unwar-
> ranted fears and anxieties. I think it is important when talking with pregnant
> women, who are particularly susceptible to fears and anxieties regarding their
> unborn babies, not to create unwarranted fears.

If it *is* true that women are particularly susceptible to fears and anxieties
regarding their unborn babies, perhaps it was meant to be so. Mother bears
guard their cubs with a vengeance. Are we not to do the same for our "cubs"?
Perhaps the "susceptibility" to fears that touch on our unborn is a protective
measure for our species. Let's not lose it—ever. The *truly* prudent and humane
thing to do is to alert mothers to any and all potential dangers and let them
make informed and intelligent decisions. Again, where technology and our
babies' well-being are concerned, all things must be considered guilty until
proven innocent.

We are going to have to learn the dangers of interventions and set limitations.
No one else is going to do it for us. (For example, the recommended allowable
non-ionizing radiation level in the United States is *1,000 times higher* than the
standard set in the Soviet Union. In addition, the Soviet Union has set a standard
for exposure to non-ionizing radiation for the general public. The United States
has no such standard.)

We have a responsibility to protect our babies; they can't yet say "no," so we
have to say it for them, loudly and clearly. Until interventions have been *proven*
safe, we must not allow their unwarranted invasion into our babies' bodies, or
into our own. We should make exceptions only when the information gained
from their use will clearly prevent even greater harm than the damage each
intervention may inflict.

Ignorance Is Bliss?

These tests and others like them must be reserved for the infrequent situations
in which their benefits outweigh the risks. Women with toxemia* or diabetes,
for example, may benefit from modern technology. Women who have previously

---

*For information about preventing toxemia, read *What Every Pregnant Woman Should Know*,
by Gail Brewer (New York: Random House, 1977), and *Metabolic Toxemia of Late Pregnancy: A
Disease of Malnutrition*, by Thomas H. Brewer, M.D. (New Canaan, Conn.: Keats, 1982).

had babies with genetic abnormalities may need even the "reassurance" that the procedure can provide. But to subject a whole nation of women to these tests on an almost routine basis is treating them like guinea pigs. As Lucy Evarts has remarked: "Many difficult issues must be dealt with when a couple decides what type of prenatal care they want . . . . Recognizing this complexity, the health professional should not seek to impose absolute standards on prospective parents, but should instead support their decision when it has been made."[38] Even when the decision is, "No."

Occasionally we are accused of frightening women. Interestingly, the accusation comes most often not from women but from men who perhaps want to "protect" us or keep us ignorant. Ignorance is *not* bliss; it is, quite simply, ignorance. Information, on the other hand, yields power, so birthing women need as much information as they can get their hands on to make decisions and effect change. Our intention is not to frighten but to *enlighten*, as well as to excite and to motivate.

Dianne wrote:

I've lived in four different places in ten years and it's the same everywhere. Everyone is scared. They're scared of pregnancy, of labor, and of delivery. The women are scared of the doctors and the nurses are afraid of the doctors. Doctors are scared of the midwives, of childbirth educators, of the administration, and of malpractice. Everyone's scared of the anesthesiologists, even though they themselves are shaking in their shoes. Why is everyone so scared?

We feel that there is indeed a great deal of inappropriate fear surrounding childbirth, and we want to help take some of that fear away.

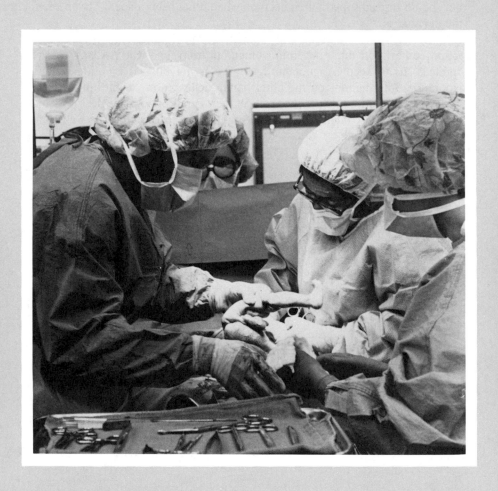

9 ❧ Birth Interventions and Their Consequences

> In a general sense, every intervention into, or
> complication of, the birth process can destroy or distort
> the delicate physiological-hormonal-psychic balance
> programmed into mammalian species through centuries
> of evolution.
>
> —Muriel Sugarman, M.D.

Elderly women in nursing homes who can hardly remember what they were served for lunch become lucid when asked about their children's births. They recall details, sensory impressions. Birth is such a powerful life experience that it lingers in memory throughout a woman's life. Its effects are immeasurable; they ripple continuously and are boundless. For this reason and countless others, birth needs to be—and can be—a time of peace, joy, and awareness.

There are many potential technical and psychological interferences and interventions that may affect labor and delivery. Each in and of itself can be a problem and one intervention almost always leads to others—a domino effect. Although medical interventions at this time, like tests during pregnancy, have occasional judicious uses, we must continually look at the possible risks, and question any procedure that might potentially cause complications. Most of the interventions can provide a direct route to unnecessary cesareans. A lyric from Linda Arnold's album "Nine Months" reads, "It's time we learned what our bodies can do all by themselves. . .it's time to celebrate what Nature can really do."[2]

When To Go to the Hospital

Most women go into the hospital too early. Cathy wrote to us:

> Since we never went into labor with our first child, we really didn't know how intense contractions get. We thought I must be well into labor. When we found out I was only a centimeter dilated, we should have gone back home. We stayed, though, and labor slowed down considerably. Labor progressed slowly, and some negative run-ins with members of the staff (nurses and residents) with regard to our "attempt at VBAC" affected me more than I would have liked. So, we ended up with a cesarean. We realize that our lack of experience coupled with negative energy generated by the staff contributed to the outcome. So, we take what we learned and help other couples in order that they may attain this goal.

Healthy, normal women don't need to be in the hospital at one or two centimeters. Many doctors are reluctant to send women home, so you'll most likely be admitted. One by one, other women enter the hospital and give birth ahead of you or are sectioned. You become impatient and discouraged. It seems as if this baby will never arrive. Early labor can last for hours. Most women who have a slow start go on to have perfectly healthy, normal labors and deliveries. There you are in a jonnie, in a room smaller than a one-car garage. Comments from well-meaning people ("You still hanging on, Mrs. J?") make it difficult to relax.

Diony Young and Charles Mahan warn us to stay at home until labor is well established. They even advise a return home if you are less than four centimeters dilated, unless labor is moving rapidly and you live a long way from the hospital.* Some women we know have rented motel rooms near the hospital or have gone to a friend's home closer to the hospital. Many go into the hospital at seven to nine centimeters rather than three or four. Many hire a private labor assistant to come to their home and help them decide the best time to "journey in." Many go in just in time to push their babies into the world. Some don't go in at all.

---

*Their 1980 pamphlet, *Unnecessary Cesareans: Ways To Avoid Them*, is available from the International Childbirth Education Association.

Upon Your Arrival . . .

"Just a Little Ride"

When you arrive at the hospital in labor, you are often greeted with a wheel-chair. You are usually told that it's "hospital policy"; all laboring women must be wheelchaired to the labor and delivery floor. In our opinion, wheelchairs are for sick people. They are of great assistance to invalids too weak to walk, or as "legs" for paraplegics. They are not for healthy women preparing to give birth.

Maybe you've never ridden in a wheelchair. Maybe you'd love a free ride up (we shouldn't assume "up" since one of the major birthing hospitals in this area set up its maternity unit *underground*). It's probably been years since someone pushed you along on wheels, and most likely it would be great fun. It might even be fun to be little again and be in a carriage and have your mommy pushing you along, without a care in the world—instead of being all grown up and in labor and, confidentially, insecure and scared. If you decide to hop a ride, it is important that you are clear about your frame of mind, since being in a wheelchair connotes passivity, obedience, weakness: qualities not generally con-ducive to self-regulated birthing.

The hospital's attitude is also important. Do they offer the wheelchair as simply an alternative way to get to your labor room, to add to your comfort? Or do they insist that you sit in it because it's "doctor's orders" or "hospital policy"? Are they truly intent on aiding you, or on establishing *rules* from the moment you enter their domain, rules that may have little to do with birthing but much to do with power and control? If you see the wheel chair as a quick and fun way of getting upstairs, enjoy it. But it's better for you, physiologically as well as psychologically, to say "No, thanks," as we shall see.

Admissions Procedures

You may be asked to stop in the admitting office on your way up (or down, as the case may be). Routine admitting procedures are appropriate for patients who are being admitted for elective surgery, not for women who are about to give birth. Many women undergo long, detailed interviews with the admitting staff while they are in active labor. They are bombarded with questions about insurance and next-of-kin. ("And in the event that you croak, my dear, to whom do you wish to leave the family jewels?") Some of the staff are kind enough to wait during contractions; others plod right through the forms to be filled out. Some apologize profusely for any inconvenience; others seem annoyed that you won't stop your contractions midstream so that they can get their work done. Some are frightened that your baby might be born in their office.

Forms can be filled out ahead of time. Some hospitals send the forms to your home several weeks prior to your EDC, or estimated date of confinement. Confinement—that old-fashioned term! Maybe you don't plan on being confined. Maybe you don't even plan to be admitted. Maybe you just plan to visit for a spell, have your baby and go home, as many women do. In some hospitals, the forms are filled out once you are "settled." In others they are even filled out after the baby is born.

The women with whom we work often go straight to labor and delivery without stopping in admission. Some have filled out forms previously, some have not. The ones who do stop are assertive enough to politely say, "While I'm having a contraction, it is important for my husband and me to concentrate on each other and our baby. We'd be glad to answer any questions between contractions."

In the Labor Room

When you get to your room, you'll probably be given a hospital jonnie, an ugly old *"shmata"* (Yiddish for "rag"), one-size-fits-all. Birth is an opening experience, and a sexual one. When you wear a jonnie, the only thing inclined to open freely is—the jonnie. It's hard to feel released, open, and sexy when you are wearing a shapeless garment whose opening keeps shifting so that one breast, your entire behind, or both, keep peeking out. Women should be wearing whatever makes them feel good. It might be a jonnie, but we rather doubt it. Why not wear your own nightgown, one that makes you feel soft and feminine, pretty and open? Or a comfortable maternity dress or jumper, or something you've made especially for the occasion? Pat Barki, head of the International Women's Council on Obstetrical Practices, has a beautiful, sexy, black negligee that she's lent to a dozen or more women, all of whom have delivered naturally (four were VBACs). "This'll do it every time," Pat laughs. "They open for ten-pounders in this!" One woman wore a jumper with bunnies and teddy bears on it "to remind me that all this work was going to produce my *baby*!"

You might not want to get blood on one of your favorite nightgowns. You might hate doing laundry and figure you are paying the hospital, so why not give their laundry the business. However, making you wear *their* clothing is another way in which hospitals subtly take control. We associate jonnies with illness, laboratory tests, and surgery. When you don one of their high-fashion creations, it is one more hospital ritual that strips away your identity. It alters your view of yourself—not a healthy normal laboring woman (client) but a hospitalized individual who requires medical attention (patient).

What you wear is one of the factors that influences where your head is at.

What if your labor slows down, *as many normal labors do?* If your clothes have been taken away, and you are in a jonnie, it will be difficult for you to go outside and take a walk, or mosey down to the gift shop to browse around, or to the coffee shop for some juice, a sandwich and a change of scenery. It will be difficult for you *to go home* to wait until labor becomes well established. If you choose to leave the hospital after your baby is born and your clothes are in the next wing, your departure may be delayed. You need to decide beforehand what you will wear, when you will wear it, and where the belongings you don't need are to be kept.

You may decide not to wear anything. Nudity enhances labor for some, inhibits it for others. Some women pull off whatever they are wearing during active labor, if the clothing feels too restrictive. "All of a sudden, I felt earthy, primitive," Jane N. said, "and primitive didn't feel like a Lanz nightgown with flowers and lace all over it." Your baby will benefit from skin-to-skin contact with you when he's born, so make sure that whatever you wear, part of your naked skin will be readily available!

Some fathers take off their shirts and their undershirts during labor and birth. Alan said, "I needed to feel closer to Elaine. It didn't feel right having layers of clothing between us." Patty agreed that feeling her husband's bare chest supporting her bare back felt wonderful.

Most hospitals discourage nudity. They seem terrified of it. Fathers are gowned from head to toe. Masks are worn. The woman is carefully, if not lavishly, draped, like some Halston creation. Only the "essential parts" are allowed viewing. Draping a woman has little to do with sterility, except in a psychological sense. Sheila Kitzinger believes that draping a woman is an act of depersonalization; it sets "the initiate" apart. The opening in the sheet, the isolated viewing area, becomes the domain of the doctor, a part he can control. In fact, draping is a ritualistic way in which the woman's genitals become separate from the rest of her. Kitzinger tells us that the ritual allows us to believe it is no longer a man looking at a woman's vagina; it is now a doctor confronting a case. She reminds us that the area is not sterile, nor does it belong to the physician! Until we accept our own sexuality and allow birth to be the sexual experience that it is, we will continue to allow the cover-up. This ritual provides a defense against sexual feelings, as well as protection from feelings of tenderness and sympathy.

Couples are rarely left alone during labor. Kissing, hugging and cuddling can help both of you relax, and it can actually stimulate labor. (Nipple stimulation, for example, releases oxytocin, which is responsible for uterine contractions.) Having your mate hold you tightly when you're feeling anxious or tense can help you feel safe, but the beds to which most women are strapped during labor (by means of a fetal monitor—we'll get to them in a little while) are too narrow for your mate to lie comfortably beside you. Pregnancy begins in a bedroom atmosphere. Perhaps the baby's birth should begin in one also.

Maternal Position during Labor

Most women are confined to the hospital bed the moment they arrive at their assigned labor room. Lisa S. said, "I had the fear of God placed in me. My physician forbade me to get out of bed. He put me on my back and told me not to move. I'm sure he would have been livid if I had dared to sneeze. I was certain that if I stood up the baby would *fall* right onto the floor. I was only four centimeters dilated when the section was done for "fetal distress." I don't imagine a baby falls through a cervix that is four centimeters dilated." Lisa's healthy baby's fetal "distress" was caused by her being forced to stay in the lithotomy position. As many of you already know, this position was popularized for us common folk after France's King Louis XIV insisted upon a better view of his many mistresses' genitals during birth. It was kinky then; it's unnecessary and dangerous now. The only advantage is the obstetrician's, not the baby's or the mother's.

You must remember that your position during labor should never be restricted! How many of you were instructed to get onto the bed, lie on your back, and stay there? This, in spite of the fact that being in bed during active labor, especially on your back, is the worst position for any laboring and birthing woman. Lying on your back reduces the blood flow (oxygen) to you and your baby, reduces the effectiveness of contractions. In addition, it positions you so that you are trying to deliver your baby *uphill*, against gravity.

Standing during labor increases the intensity of contractions, while decreasing pain. This has been reported by several researchers.[23,24,30,36] Because contractions are more effective in an upright position, the average duration of labor is significantly shortened in this position. Animals instinctively know what positions are best. We too know instinctively what position will best assist us in birthing our babies, but we aren't given the opportunity to try a few to determine this. In Caldeyro-Barcia's study of 145 women whose positions were not restricted, 95 percent chose to be vertical.[24] Efficiency in dilating the cervix is much greater when a woman is standing than when supine or in a side-lying position. Measurements of uterine activity show that contractions are far more efficient in vertical positions (standing, sitting, squatting, and kneeling) than in horizontal positions.

An ICEA review on maternal position during labor and birth reports that no other mammal adopts such a disadvantageous posture during such an important and critical event. People who live in cultures that have escaped the influence of civilization and modern obstetrics rarely assume a recumbent position. Women choose a position that feels most appropriate, according to their build and the shape of their pelvis.[29]

Women giving birth must be free to stand, sit, squat, kneel, and walk. A report by Read and others stated that initial observations indicate that in terms of progress and initial effects on uterine activity, ambulation is as effective as synthetic oxytocin for the enhancement of labor.[32] Carr declared that the recumbent and lithotomy positions for birth serve the needs of the attendant rather than the woman and baby.[25] One doctor said to Ellen B., "Oh you're another one of those bush ladies. You want to squat. American women don't know how to squat. I suppose you want me to lie on the floor while you deliver your baby?"

The advantages of an upright position and full mobility to mother and baby are extensive. When a woman is lying on her back, she risks maternal supine hypotension as the heavy uterus restricts the inferior vena cava, lowering blood pressure and uterine circulation. Women complain of dizziness, breathlessness, visual changes and numbness, all due to the circulatory deficit. A change in position will improve all symptoms. However, as the mother's oxygen supply is affected, the baby is compromised. A study by Huch found that within two minutes after the mother was rolled onto her back, the level of oxygen to the baby was dramatically reduced. Rolling the mother onto her side raised the baby's oxygen level, but it took eight minutes to bring the oxygen back to its original level.[27]

Even if the mother is "propped," damaging effects are noticed. For example, bearing down efforts are not nearly as effective as in a more upright position. Roberts states that being propped is the worst position in labor next to complete recumbency, because it closes off the pelvis.[33] Carr reports that hypotension can still occur in this position without warning to the mother, so it is particularly dangerous to the fetus.[25]

Flynn and Kelly reported that being ambulant may actually protect the umbilical cord from pressure between the fetal skeleton and the bony maternal pelvis. The mobility allows the fetus to move about and adjust to the pelvis, eliminating long periods in which the cord is compressed.[26] The cord supplies oxygen to your baby, and if it is compressed, her well-being and very life may be endangered. Carr states that, "Not only does the upright position result in a more efficient and shorter labor, but also in the virtual eradication of most common fetal distress patterns which are due to cord compression."[25]

Carr also reports that in all the studies comparing ambulation with recumbency in labor, the women preferred the upright, mobile positions and felt less pain.[25] Positions such as standing, squatting, kneeling, sitting, semi-reclining, or all-fours allow gravity to aid the mother's own bearing down efforts. Having the legs far apart narrows the introitus (vaginal opening), actually making it prone to tearing. The lithotomy position is in direct contradiction to basic principles of anatomy and physiology in labor and birth. However, it provides ready access to the perineum for forceps, episiotomy, manual maneuvers, anesthetics, and repairs.

When the mother is in a lying-down position, the newborn baby is placed on her abdomen. The baby cannot see his mother's face, nor is he close to her voice. In an upright position, the mother reaches for her infant and draws him close to her breasts, nearer her heart; her face and voice are then closer to him as well.

Why, with all the research on the importance of being upright and mobile, are women still on their backs in hospital beds? Sheila Kitzinger believes that one of the reasons so many women are put on their sides derives from the fact that in this position the woman has her back to the doctor and "he need not see her face."[41] When a woman is put in stirrups, with the doctor on his stool, he need not see her face, either. Being in bed suggests sickness, and indeed many pregnant women begin to feel weak and sick when they are placed on their backs. Here you are, a healthy woman about to give birth to your baby, being treated exactly like a gall bladder patient two floors away: you are lying in a bed, flat on your back, in a hospital jonnie, instructed not to move.

Ah, but you *can* get up once after you've had an enema. And *that* will probably be just after you have been shaved.

The "Prep"

In "Cultural Warping of Childbirth," Doris Haire informs us that research involving 7,600 mothers demonstrates that shaving of the pubic hair does not reduce the incidence of infection.[39] Since surface cells are scraped, bacteria are introduced. The infection rate is *higher* in those who are shaved! Yet, this ridiculous procedure continues.

A woman about to birth her baby shouldn't look like an 8-year-old. Brewer and Presser, in *Right from the Start*, remark that the psychological effects alone constitute basis enough to refrain from the practice.[38] The psychological effects are, indeed, important. The woman is changed from a woman into a little girl. Her concept of herself is altered and she becomes most vulnerable.

In addition, it is extremely uncomfortable when the hair begins to grow back. The physical and psychological discomforts can interfere with and affect sexual relations following the birth.

Enemas

Many physicians still insist upon giving a birthing woman an enema. Sheila Kitzinger labels this ritual just one more way the doctor and the hospital take control, of even our *inner* functionings. Enemas are pointless in terms of hygiene, she tells us; but they are not pointless in terms of fulfilling a ritualistic ceremony to "purge the initiate."[41]

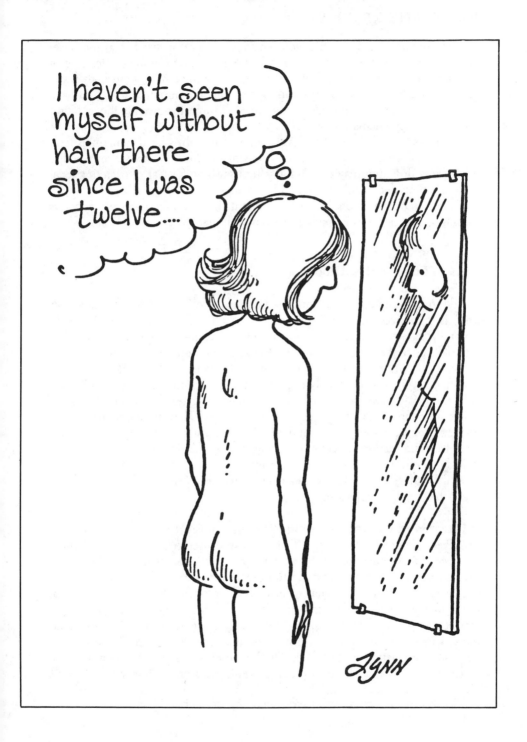

Many of you will notice that you have loose stools or diarrhea at the onset of labor. It's almost as if your body is helping you do a thorough cleaning of all your nooks and crannies. But this natural "cleaning out" is your body's way of getting ready for labor. You needn't get readied the hospital's way, and have cramps added to your contractions. You needn't subject yourself to the irritation caused by soapy enemas.

When you are pushing, the pressure from your baby's head sometimes feels as if you are going to have a bowel movement. Many of us see our body's products as dirty and may even refrain from pushing for fear of excreting fecal material. One doctor told us he orders enemas routinely because, "Frankly, I don't wish to be shat upon." Frankly, he should have chosen dentistry. If doctors cannot handle our normal body functions with grace, we're in trouble.

I.V.s vs Food during Labor

Add to the jonnie, contractions, and cramps one I.V. An I.V. (intravenous drip) is introduced into a vein in your arm so that fluids (a glucose solution, generally) can be infused right into your bloodstream—"an instant dinner," we are told. Since the fluid bypasses the stomach, you don't have to digest it. The rationale for this procedure is that it ensures that you won't become dehydrated and that a vein will be readily available if you go into shock and your veins shrivel up. We have spoken to over one hundred nurses with several thousand collective years of labor and delivery experience. They have yet to see one woman's veins collapse during childbirth. The well-nourished pregnant woman's body has extra fluid to protect it from going into shock. In the rare circumstance that shock is imminent, there are warning signs. There is plenty of time to find a vein. Besides, a procedure called a "cut down" is possible in the very *unlikely* event that a vein *is* shriveling.

Hazards of I.V.s for Birthing Women   In *Right from the Start*, Brewer and Presser note that hours of I.V. fluids can cause both serious disturbances in electrolyte balance and water intoxication. They report that needles occasionally become dislodged and the fluid seeps into surrounding tissue, causing swelling.[38] Judith Randal, science correspondent for the Washington bureau of the New York *Daily News*, urges us to remember that the first intravenous drip can be a step down the road toward cesarean.* Besides, the needle hurts. And all that fluid can cause bladder distention and impede dilation. Some women have adverse reactions to the fluid. The I.V. unit is awkward and cumbersome and restricts mobility. (It pretty much prevents you from that browse in the gift

---

*"Widely Used Technology Needs More Testing," *Washington Post* (19 Apr. 1978).

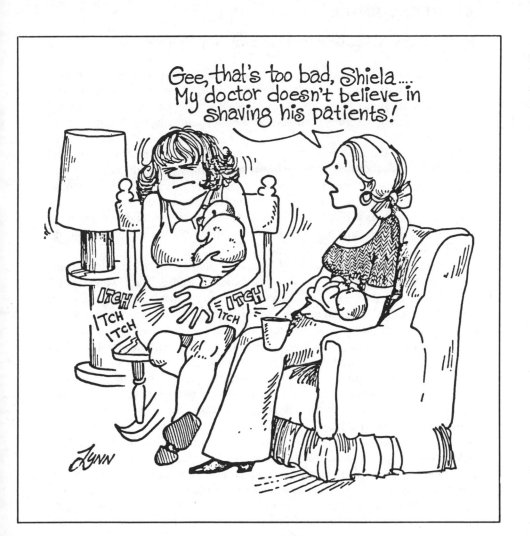

shop we suggested. Of course, you can always request the *portable* I.V. stand on wheels. . .)

In 1980, Kenepp stated that excessive maternal dextrose administration may harm the newborn, and that studies are being done to determine what amount of routine intravenous fluids are safe during labor.[40] We can only hope that the women in the studies are informed that they are, once again, being used in experiments.

If a cesarean becomes necessary, an I.V. can be inserted within minutes. But installing an I.V. routinely in every birthing woman is a blatant statement that everyone *expects* something to go wrong. It's another of the ways that the physician protects himself at your expense. Perhaps whenever you get into your car you should have an I.V. put into your arm. That way, should you be in an accident and require surgery, you'll be ready. Imagine a law requiring us all to wear I.V.s whenever we get into a car.

Another problem is that once the I.V. is in, you are a sitting duck for various chemicals or drugs that most doctors will not hesitate to use. Many women don't even know a drug has been administered until after it has been infiltrated into the I.V. solution. The main problem with using an I.V. for a birthing woman, however, is simply that it is unnecessary: you can keep *yourself* hydrated during labor. We recommend drinking soups and fruit juices. (Ironically, I.V. fluid not only does not provide adequate nourishment, it causes negative nitrogen balance, "a condition of starvation."[37]) Remember that during labor, *your body is running a marathon*! Labor requires great strength, energy, stamina, and oxygen, as your body works to peak efficiency. Can you imagine Bill Rodgers running up Heartbreak Hill with an I.V. in his arm? Or Diana Nyad swimming from Florida to Cuba with an I.V. pole? Giving birth with a needle and tube sticking out of your arm is equally ridiculous. Sick people need I.V.s, people who are not able to take in adequate nourishment—not healthy, birthing women. The fact is that most birthing emergencies that require I.V.s are predictable and the vast majority of emergencies arise because of unnecessary invasive techniques. A parody in the *National Lampoon* quotes a "Dr. Exacto" on unnecessary hospital procedures, as follows:

> I've. . .seen a number of ridiculous procedures added to our hospital routines—procedures that waste time and money, mollycoddle patients, and accomplish absolutely nothing. Take catheterization. More tubes, more trauma—all totally unnecessary! What do I do about post-op patients who had trouble passing water? I do what we used to do in med school thirty years ago. I give them beer. If they can't take it orally, I pour it in their I.V.s. And they love it. Two Buds and they're peeing like they used to in the parking lot behind the Hi-Ho Tavern. Plus, it cheers them up. I tell you, not all change is progress. There's some things tried and true, that should be left alone. . .*

---

*Nov. 1978, p. 47.

Imposed Fasting   What we've been discussing so far—restricted mobility, donning a jonnie, the prep (shaving and enema), and I.V.s—are part of *routine admission procedures* for most every woman in our country, procedures that ritualistically transform a healthy person into a patient. The woman surrenders her own gown, her identity, and then, in far too many cases, her health and well-being.

But back to Rogers and Nyad. Imagine forbidding Bill to eat for 24 hours before the marathon. Do you think he would be able to run if he'd had no nourishment at all for a full day prior to the race? Do you think Diana would be able to swim mile after mile if she'd not eaten for two days before she plunged? Yet we are expected to have our babies even if we haven't eaten for hours—sometimes days—before giving birth. Think for a minute: how do you feel if you've missed a meal? What about two? Hungry? Annoyed? A little light-headed? Weak, famished, bitchy, tired? Imagine doing a day's worth of hard exercise without being permitted to eat.

Our bodies cannot work the way they are meant to during labor without fuel. I.Vs do *not* provide adequate nourishment during labor, and we have mentioned the variety of problems associated with their use. You need to be eating! Yes, Virginia, you *can* have a sandwich during labor, or fruit, or a potato, or some cheese and crackers. You can have whatever appeals to you, as long as it's nutritious. Mendelsohn warns that even well-nourished individuals often become malnourished when they depend on hospital cuisine,[42] so we suggest you "brown bag it" to your labor.

We are the only women in the world whose nutritional requirements during labor are ignored. How sad, at a time when these requirements are paramount. Suppose a woman does not begin labor until 6:00 A.M., not having eaten since dinner the night before. In the hospital, food is prohibited. Active labor may not begin for another eight or eleven hours, in which case it will have been 24 hours since she had any nourishment. If a friend asked you to help out by moving some furniture and you hadn't eaten for many hours, you'd be sure to grab a sandwich before you went to help. You can help your baby out, too!

Without food, labor begins—and continues—in a weakened state. It's extremely difficult to feel relaxed, strong, confident, and energetic when your body is becoming hungrier and more exhausted by the moment. Psychological changes occur. You begin to feel less like a healthy, normal birthing woman, and more like a passive, sick patient. The pain of the contractions becomes more difficult to meet. You become frightened. Also, it is difficult to watch others eating when you are famished. One filet mignon for you, sir, and for you, m'dear, our delicious I.V. with house dressing, no extra charge. It's like being at a birthday party and not being offered any cake. You feel left out, angry, and deprived. One husband kept asking the nurse for juice. "While the nurse was on these refrigerator runs, I'd get Karen up and walking. When the nurse went to get more juice, I'd hand Karen the juice and she'd drink the whole thing."

Some women are able to dilate only to find they have no energy for pushing. How disappointing to get to Heartbreak Hill and not be able to make it over! These women end up with a spinal or epidural, and their babies have to be pulled out by forceps.

We are not permitted to eat during labor because, in the event that we need general anesthesia, anesthesiologists are concerned that during the intubation we could vomit and aspirate the contents of our stomachs which can cause death. They want our stomachs empty. Just as every healthy woman in our country is seen as a potential candidate for surgery, all are restricted from eating when they birth. At the 1982 ICEA Regional Conference in West Virginia, Dr. George Mahan remarked, "Lord knows that 99 percent of the women in the world eat during labor. The reason people aspirate and get chemical pneumonia is that they're put to sleep by people who don't know how to do it. It's not what they've had to eat." He explained that the problem is that women are put to sleep with a mask instead of an endotracheal tube when they are pregnant and going to have a cesarean. When this is done, they're in danger whether they've eaten or not.

Not being permitted to eat *makes* every birthing woman a candidate for surgery. Doris Haire points out that in other countries, healthy women are encouraged to eat and drink lightly during labor.[39] This practice has not been found to increase the incidence of morbidity or mortality. At the University of Amsterdam Hospital, women are allowed to eat through second stage. This practice is believed to *help* laboring women. They have not had a single incidence of vomitus in five years. It is not labor that slows digestion, Ms. Haire tells us, but *fear!* The inhalation of gastric juices alone can be dangerous, so most obstetricians require that the mother's stomach be emptied if she must have general anesthesia for delivery anyway. Nimmo remarks that drugs used for obstetric analgesia cause vomiting and influence gastrointestinal motility, and notes that the possibility "that delayed gastric emptying might be due to the administration of narcotics does not seem to have been considered"[43].

Back to our cars. Perhaps no one should be permitted to drive after having eaten. If you are in an accident and require surgery, you must have an empty stomach. So, from now on, don't drive home from a restaurant on a satisfied stomach.

Women we worked with all drank lightly during labor, and more than three-quarters of them ate. Several who did not eat either had short labors or began labor after a large meal. Many undoubtedly would have had cesareans if they hadn't eaten, since their labors were more than 36 hours. It seems unlikely that many women, no matter how well nourished they were upon going into labor, would still feel strong after 36 hours with no food.

One woman who was told not to eat in labor wrote to us. She had a large dinner and went into labor two hours later. Her doctor was angry that she'd had dinner! Two hours later her VBAC baby was born. "I was so glad I had dinner first. I'd have been famished!" Another was scheduled for a repeat cesarean and went into labor three days before the operation was to occur. She did not know VBAC was possible and immediately went to the hospital to be sectioned. She considered it a stroke of good luck that she'd eaten just prior to the surgery. "I had no problem with the anesthesia and felt strong almost immediately afterwards. I'm sure it was because I'd eaten," she said.

What of the baby that is waiting to be born? Your baby depends on you for her nourishment, and no baby should have to go twelve or eighteen hours without food. More than ten years ago, Haire said that the effect on the fetus of depriving the mother of food and drink had not been sufficiently investigated.[39] It still hasn't been. But the number of floppy, weak babies born in our country may certainly be a clue.

And what of a uterus that has been deprived of energy-giving sustenance for many hours? The percentage of women in our country who are sectioned for disfunctional labor is amazing. Failure to progress, uterine inertia, failure to dilate, dystocia—all terms for a tired, weak, hungry woman's uterus.

Some women are afraid to eat. They're worried they'll vomit everything back up. Vomiting can be caused by fear, anxiety, hormones, or even the pressure of the baby on various parts of your insides as she moves to get in position to be born. If you are going to vomit, you are going to vomit, food or not. For those of you who have had dry heaves, you know it's far less agonizing to upchuck something than nothing. So be productive in your labor and, if you are going to vomit, be productive in that as well! Listen to your body. If it tells you you need to eat, eat. At the very least, remind yourself to drink during labor.

Some women believe that the digestive system closes down during labor. Not so. Fear, excitement, and drugs cause a slowdown. Women who are relaxed during labor, who are walking, drinking, and eating lightly, continue to function normally. They urinate and defecate normally. Birth is normal. Your other systems (respiratory, circulatory, endocrine) don't shut down; why should your digestive system stop? Most obstetrical texts have few, if any, references to nutritional support in labor (although a 1962 obstetrical text stated that a potential c/section patient having a trial of labor should be encouraged to eat and drink foods such as eggs and milk).[44]

Many hospitals stock their shelves with gelatin and canned goods—not exactly dynamite for laboring women. Where are the fresh fruits and vegetables? The tofu, sprouts, and whole grains? The nuts and seeds for restoring energy and bolstering nursing mothers? One dietician, in defense, expressed sincere frustration: "Offering fresh vegetables and fresh fruits is discouraging. People want what they are used to—canned junk."

Occasionally, a woman may not feel like eating during labor. She may feel strong and need to concentrate on her body without being distracted by a menu.

Beth R. said, "I'd eaten a full dinner a few hours before my labor began. My friends were paranoid about keeping me fed. I felt like a two-year-old: 'Here comes the airplane into the hangar, Bethie! Open the door nice and wide, heeere it comes. . . .!'"

Fathers need to keep up their strength and energy, too. There should be enough food available to keep them alert and strong. Many of us have been with obstetricians who see the father munching on a sandwich and want a piece of the goods, too. Often they haven't had anything to eat all day, either. No wonder so many of them are impatient with labor: they want to get the baby out so *they* can get out—for dinner.

The physicians to whom we refer women enourage eating, walking and drinking. They do not use routine I.V.s (Norma's physician, however, was a holdout for I.V.s; he couldn't quite agree to abandon the procedure. When Norma entered the hospital and he prepared to put in an I.V., she told him that she was in such early labor it seemed unreasonable to have to "wear it" so soon. Several hours later, when labor became quite active, he again prepared to introduce that I.V. "Now? Now? When I'm just about ready to have this baby, you're going to stick me with needles?! No thanks!" she exclaimed. Norma's doctor no longer insists on I.V.s for laboring women.) Some physicians will compromise by waiving an I.V. but insisting on a heparin clip (or lock). Heparin prevents the blood from coagulating and keeps a place ready for the insertion of an I.V. needle. To us, use of a heparin lock is one more statement that birth is dangerous and requires tools, tubes and fancy gadgets. Robert Mendelsohn, M.D., tells us in his book *Mal(e) practice: How Doctors Manipulate Women*, that doctors are taught to believe that almost everyone is sick. They persuade mothers that the normal physiological process of giving birth is a life-threatening nine-month disease.[42] We don't believe that healthy women have to compromise. It's . . . er . . . compromising. And potentially dangerous. As for us, we'll say a flat "No, thanks" to the I.V., and have ourselves a delicious, refreshing, pineapple-orange juice on ice . . . or maybe a banana apricot shake . . . no, now let's see, make that a . . .

Amniotomy and Infection

You can increase your chances for having this baby naturally by refusing to allow your baby's waters to be broken. The bag of water (membranes) surrounding your baby is there for many reasons. It provides a sterile environment. The water protects your baby from the power of the contractions by acting as a cushion for the baby's head.

If your membranes rupture on their own prior to labor, you must believe that this is exactly the way your particular body needs to start this particular labor. Accept it as a sign that labor will begin sometime within the next hours or days. Appreciate that your body is giving you advance notice for the coming event. Stay close to home, relax, eat well. All women on the verge of birthing should rest every day so that they will not go into labor tired. Some midwives recommend that you shower rather than bathe, and refrain from intercourse. You needn't worry about a dry birth. Your body continues to produce amniotic fluid until your baby is born. We've worked with many women who have had PROM (premature rupture of membranes) up to a week before the birth, and they've had no problems. You can up your vitamin C, and increase your fluid intake. Before agreeing to be induced, you can try one of several *natural* induction suggestions: visualization, herbs, or castor oil (under the direction of a qualified midwife), for example. You can cuddle with your mate. Lovemaking (without sexual intercourse) and orgasm may encourage labor to begin; at the very least this will help you to feel more relaxed—and what a nice way to pass the time before your new baby arrives! You can also wait to go into labor. Remember, too, that if your water is leaking, it is possible for the membranes to reseal.

Many physicians are worried that an infection will begin now that the protection around the infant is gone. Some prescribe antibiotics prophylactically. Others ask you to take your temperature and report any rise. Some take blood tests to check your white blood cell count. Most tell you that if you haven't had the baby in 12 to 24 hours, a c/section will be performed to prevent an infection from occurring. (Fifteen years ago they used to give us 72 hours . . . we guess infections have picked up some speed since then.)

A cesarean to *prevent* infection? You already know that the risk of infection from cesarean section is very high. Most women can go *days* without an infection after their water has broken, especially if they stay out of the hospital and refuse internal exams. Mendelsohn[60] and others tell us that 5 percent of all hospital patients contract new infections they didn't have when they arrived. In a single year, 1.5 million patients were victims of hospital-acquired infections, and 15,000 of them died. He tells us that germs are transmitted from one patient to another by careless doctors and nurses who don't scrub often or well enough, and from mattresses and pillows camouflaged by "clean" white sheets. "The 'greens' worn by hospital staffs are often *filthy*," remarked one nurse. "The labor rooms wouldn't win the *Good Housekeeping* Seal of Approval, either," added another. "Make certain everyone washes their hands before they touch you," cautions a third. "You never know where those hands have been just minutes before they're touching your body." We've heard tell that the higher the staff position, the dirtier the hands,* but the *National Lampoon* medical parody calls

---

*Richard K. Albert, "Handwashing Patterns in a Medical Intensive Care Unit," *Clinical Research Abstracts*, 29 (February 1981).

this information into question: "I was an intern, wet behind the ears but cocky as all get out. As I was scrubbing up, the senior resident . . . came over to me and put his arm around my shoulder. Was I nervous? Did I think that I could handle it? Well, I just sneered at him, spit on my hands, and went to work."[*] Joan L., a nurse in labor and delivery, says, "Some of the doctors wash their hands to get them clean, but others, I feel, wash them also because they consider women's bodies unclean."

Mary Daly, author of Gyn/Ecology, tells us, "In 1861 Semmelweis published a book establishing that poor women who literally gave birth in the streets of Vienna had a lower mortality rate than those giving birth in the First Clinic (staffed entirely by physicians and medical students) of the Vienna Lying-In Hospital. For his truthful exposé, the scholar was ostracized by his profession" (p. 294). Daly adds that the response of the medical profession (to the fact that puerperal fever was carried from physician to patient to patient) was "outrage at the very idea that the hands of the physician could be unclean" (p. 257).[131] The infection rate at home births is practically nonexistent. Dr. Kloosterman from the Netherlands remarks that in America the husband is either excluded from the delivery or "recognizably disguised" in a gown, mask, and cap. "The fact is completely overlooked that he [the man with whom the woman became pregnant], her life's partner, her bedfellow, is indeed the last person who should be considered dangerous, bacteriologically and hygienically."[†]

Many doctors want to rupture your membranes as soon as you get into the hospital. You are told that rupturing your bag of waters will speed up your labor. The procedure is called amniotomy. It is quick and painless to begin with, but it results in problems for both you and your baby. Caldeyro-Barcia's studies indicate that this practice speeds labor only slightly (20–30 minutes!), and at the expense of the baby's head![50-52] When the water is broken, the baby's head loses the protection of the fluid. The fetal head suffers uneven pressure and deformation. The umbilical cord may be compressed or completely blocked. Schwarcz and his colleagues [68] concluded that early amniotomy is an artificial and disturbing interference and stated that all unnecessary interferences, maneuvers, and medication that may alter the normal evolution of the birth should be avoided. Other studies [46-48] find no significant improvement in labors augmented by artificial rupture. The authors conclude that amniotomy as a routine procedure is not of sufficient benefit to warrant its use.

During a contraction, the oxygen supply to the baby is temporarily cut off. When the contraction is over, blood flow is resumed, and oxygen is once again available. Babies have enough reserve to carry them through each contraction. When your water is broken artificially, contractions often change in character: they become stronger, longer, and more frequent. So, for longer periods of time,

*Nov. 1978, p. 45.
†Australian Newsletter on Homebirth, January 1979, p. 8.

your baby is without oxygen. We haven't enough fingers or toes to count the number of women we know whose babies have gone into distress shortly after amniotomy was performed. A cesarean is done to save the distressed baby. If the water had been left intact, allowed to break on its own, the baby would probably have been fine. The distress has been caused by an impatient physician who could not stand back and wait for a natural process to take place.

We've been told that an early obstetrical text instructs the physician how to manage labor. The doctor is instructed to go to the woman's house, break her water, and tell her the baby will come soon. He is then instructed to leave. If the baby is born before he returns, he can take credit for his intervention. If it hasn't arrived by the time he gets back, he can "do the birth" and take the credit anyhow. Medical students are *still* taught how to make themselves essential to the birthing process.

Holland stated many years ago (1922) that early amniotomy is associated with brain deformation, which is caused by undue molding of the fetal skull.[56] In his article "Adverse Perinatal Effects of Early Amniotomy during Labor," Caldeyro-Barcia reports that amniotomy is associated with changes in the fetal heart and neurological abnormalities.[50] Brotanek and Hodr's study substantiates the theory that amniotomy produces a long-lasting reduction of maternal uterine blood flow, which can cause fetal distress.[49]

Gabbe demonstrated experimentally that amniotic fluid may be critical in protecting the cord and maintaining normal umbilical cord blood flow, as well as affecting the fetal heart rate.[54] There is a danger that when the water is broken, the umbilical cord will be washed down with the fluid. This is a prolapsed cord, a serious circumstance necessitating a cesarean. If the baby's head has engaged deeply into the pelvis the umbilical cord will not be able to prolapse into the vagina; but a deeply engaged head isn't a permission slip to rupture membranes.

We were recently contacted by a woman whose water had broken at seven centimeters with her first baby. She had had a cesarean for fetal distress. For her next labor, her physician told her it would be a good idea to break her water before seven centimeters to "see if the same thing will happen." Rupturing the membranes to see if the baby will go into distress is *inviting* trouble.

Another physician insisted upon inducing a woman who had had her two previous babies in under three hours. He told Marie that she'd never make it to the hospital this time and that it would be dangerous for her to go into labor on her own, unwatched. He broke her water to induce her labor. "I had an excruciating fourteen-hour labor," she told us.

One woman was told that she'd have to spend the last week of her pregnancy in the hospital. Her two previous babies had been born in under forty minutes. Her physician told her that the moment she was "ripe," which he would determine though vaginal exams performed twice a day while she was in the hospital, he would break the water. That way, he told her, he'd be assured of being there for the birth. Our membranes are ruptured because we deliver too fast—or too slow. We keep trying to conform to *their* timetables; we'll never please them, and it's time we stopped trying.

We can only wonder how many women are truly informed when they agree to certain procedures. In one study, for example, fifty pregnant women "near term" were divided into five groups, to determine which of several methods of induction of labor was most effective. All of the women were electronically monitored, and all had their membranes ruptured. The researchers were most interested in the "role of the cervix" during an induced labor; how easy it seemed to be to forget that there was a *woman* attached to each of those cervices, and a baby who had been depending on that amniotic fluid for a while longer.

Another reason given for rupturing the membranes is to determine if there is any meconium in the fluid. Amniotic fluid is clear, odorless, and watery. Meconium is fetal waste material that is generally not excreted until after birth. It gives the fluid a green or brownish tint. It may cause the fluid to have some odor, and it may make the consistency of the water thicker. The rationale for meddling with the membranes (a good song title?) is that *if* there is meconium, many physicians are worried that the baby will aspirate it. So your water is broken to see if there is meconium. If there is, you will be wheeled off for a section presumably to "prevent aspiration" of the "soiled" fluid.

In a study done by Abramovici et al., entitled "Meconium during Delivery: A Sign of Compensated Fetal Distress,"[45] no significant difference in fetal outcome was found between babies with and without meconium—even when the meconium was thick and solid. These results support other observations that during labor, the appearance of meconium in association with normal fetal heart tones is not ominous. Meconium is thought to be a sign of "compensated fetal distress." At a previous time, when the baby's oxygen supply was compromised, the baby's anal sphincter relaxed and meconium was excreted. Miller et al. report that signs of fetal distress are not significantly different than those in the nonmeconium group. The authors state, "The presence of meconium in the amniotic fluid without signs of fetal asphyxia is not a sign of fetal distress and need not be an indication for active intervention" (p. 573).[62]

We have been present at births where the fluid was thicker than pea soup. One baby was covered from head to toe in meconium, and happy as a pig in mud about it, too. In the absence of alarming fetal heart tones, the presence of meconium need not be a ticket to the O.R. Meconium is present in a number of births—over 30 percent in some studies. We don't think that it would happen so often if it were as dangerous as we are told. We do wonder, however, if perhaps environmental causes explain the increasing frequency with which it is noted.

The doctor ruptures your membranes and tells you that you have to produce your baby in twelve to twenty-four hours. The time begins to tick away. Twenty-three hours and 59 minutes to go. "If I don't hurry and have this baby," you think, "I'll be sectioned." So you lie there, getting more and more tense by the minute, praying that your labor will pick up. At the same time, you're worried that if it does, you might not be quite ready for it. Certainly, your baby isn't ready for it.

If your husband was told that he had to get an erection and ejaculate within a certain time or he'd be castrated, do you think it would be easy? To make it easier, perhaps he could have an I.V. put into his arm, be kept in one position, have straps placed around his penis, and be told not to move? He could be checked every few minutes; the sheet could be lifted to see if any "progress" had been made. We think you'll agree that it wouldn't be the best circumstances under which to let one's body function normally!

A woman should not be made to feel pressured to have her baby a particular way within a particular time slot. Some women take five hours to have their babies. Some take five days. Both are normal. The Friedman curve, a progress guide for labor and delivery, is sometimes honored as God's word. Women do not all dilate at a similar speed! Sometimes you get to four or six or eight centimeters and your body needs to rest. Sometimes labor even stops for a time.

If you haven't dilated in a predesignated time, you are sectioned. (It is interesting to note that most physicians are eager to follow "The Curve" for dilation, but refuse to acknowledge that it allows for a two- to four-hour second stage. Most women are sectioned after only an hour or two of pushing. It's hard to have a leisurely dinner in that time, let alone push a baby into the world!)

If a cesarean is scheduled due to "prolonged rupture of the membranes," you can refuse. You can take your blood pressure and temperature; elevations in either may indicate that infection is present. Drink plenty of fluids. If you are threatened with a cesarean you can ask for a blood test and/or fetal scalp sampling to determine if infection is present. We do not consider cesarean section necessary simply because your water broke twenty-four hours previously. We urge you to keep your vagina open for the baby and closed to unnecessary, invasive, and frequent exams.

You are unique, and your baby is unique. Your water will break when it is ready to break. It should not be artificially broken. The chances of infection are slim. The outward flow of fluid, nature's design, makes it hard to introduce infection into the uterus. However, hospitals manage to introduce infections a fair amount of the time.

Vaginal Exams

One way infection is introduced is through vaginal examinations. They are invasive and generally unnecessary, even during your ninth month of pregnancy. The position of your baby can usually be determined by abdominal palpation.

The amount of dilation does not give information of value: women who are three centimeters dilated at their 39th-week checkup can still be two weeks overdue. Nancy was one centimeter dilated until two hours before her baby was born. Cathy was eight centimeters dilated six days before actual labor began. Chris dilated one centimeter every day for nine days until she "hit ten" and had her VBAC. The amount of effacement and dilation *do not* give information about when labor will begin or how long it will take to have the baby, since many factors affect labor.

Many women complain of cramping or slightly bloody discharge after a pelvic exam late in pregnancy. It's almost as if the body is complaining about the interference and asking that we leave well enough alone. Some doctors "strip the membranes" during a vaginal exam—they separate the layers of the amniotic sac in hopes of starting labor. Why should anyone start labor for you except your body and your baby? Dr. Charles Mahan tells us vaginal exams in the last four weeks of pregnancy can predispose a woman to premature labor.

Some women want to know how far dilated they are. If they are having difficulty with labor and learn that they are quite far along, it may be just the incentive they need to keep their spirits and energy high. If they are panting and blowing, and a vaginal exam gives them the information that they are only three centimeters dilated, they may reevaluate their coping techniques and find less exhausting ways to continue on. They may also have a posterior baby or a precipitous labor, which would account for additional pain or strong contractions early on. However, most women with whom we work refuse to be examined vaginally more than once or twice, and sometimes not at all. They agree only when they are convinced that the information garnered would be truly useful.

Most midwives we know do very few, if any, vaginal exams during labor. The whole process of birth is to *let out*, not to put something in. Most attendants can tell how far dilated a woman is by watching her during labor. By placing their hands on the woman's abdomen, they can gauge the intensity of the contractions. *You* can *tell* your attendants how your contractions feel. The vagina is a private sexual part of a woman; just because you are in labor, and just because someone is garbed in a green uniform, that doesn't automatically mean that you are "open for business" or must give "carte blanche." The fact is, people don't need to be constantly putting their fingers up your vagina.

Some women have eight or ten vaginal exams during the course of a "normal" labor. Some have more! The doctor tells you where you are. He's in the driver's seat. It doesn't make any difference if you are five or six centimeters dilated. Your cervix *will* open and your baby *will* be born. One woman felt certain that her baby was going to be born at any moment. Her doctor told her it was impossible; he'd just checked her and she was only four to five centimeters. Five minutes later her baby was born. Ellen's doctor told her that at the rate she was dilating, she'd have her baby before lunch. At 10 P.M. that night her baby was born. No uterus wants to punch a clock, and every baby should be allowed to punch its own.

Another thought about vaginal exams: each one should be done with your permission, to ascertain only essential information, and only by the fingers of your choice. You do not have to permit three different nurses and/or residents to examine you. This also prevents discriminatory evaluation. One resident says, "You are five centimeters." The other examines you and says, "She's three." Is it the size of their hands, or their inexperience that gives them different perceptions? It may be that a woman's body can actually begin to close if she feels unprotected or invaded. Jay Hathaway, director of the American Academy of Husband-Coached Childbirth and author—with Marjie Hathaway—of *Children at Birth*,* tells us that if Mother Nature wanted the cervix inspected, the cervix would be on our outsides.

Columnist Erma Bombeck once wrote a telling tale called "Giving Birth to Immodesty." She tells us, "I lost my modesty when I gave birth to my first child. . . . The skimpy gown—I've had blemishes bigger than that . . ." As Ms. Bombeck was laboring, "two hundred or so people moved in and out of the room," and once when someone walked in, she just "threw back the covers and waited for the probing fingers." It was the custodian, who had come to clean under the bed. "Few people check out of the hospital the same as when they went in," Ms. Bombeck astutely observes.†

A Breath of Fresh Alternatives

Strictly speaking, this little section doesn't belong here, but we thought that by about now—since you've been reading about one harmful and unnecessary routine after another—you might be getting awfully discouraged. The power of the medical establishment can look pretty overwhelming even when you're sober and not in labor. So on these few pages, we're pointing out very firmly that *labor really doesn't have to be managed the medical establishment's way*, and we're suggesting very specifically how *you* can vary the routines. This is a sort of preview of the suggestions we offer in more detail in "Labor Support" (Chapter 11).

You have already learned that an upright position increases the effectiveness of your contractions. If your labor seems to be going slowly, change positions. Take a walk. Mosey on down to the bathroom and urinate frequently during labor. Emptying the bladder, giving the cervix more room, can turn a previous

---

*Sherman Oaks, Cal.: Academy, 1978.
†*Boston Globe*, Feb. 28, 1978

diagnosis of failure to progress or CPD into a healthy newborn. Have something to eat. Get a massage. Give one. Get a change of scenery. Use their water: take a shower! Leave your own water alone! It'll break whenever it's ready. Thirty percent break during dilation, twenty-five percent during pushing, and ten percent at birth. If your water has broken on its own before labor, you're in good company, and it's just the way your particular body needs to begin this particular labor.

Showers are wonderful during labor. Dr. Pachiornik from Brazil recommends twenty-minute showers to increase relaxation. His cesarean rate is only 5 percent. There is nothing more soothing than warm water trickling all over your body to stimulate you and relax you at the same time. Many women with whom we work spend hours in a shower! Some take five or six during the course of labor. Some stay in until the baby's almost ready to be born. Noreen said her baby had the cleanest mother in all of history. Make certain the hospital you choose has showers or tubs. One hospital in the area has two showers, both in the doctor's lounge, but they clean out the lounge for any laboring woman who wants to shower. We applaud them. We suggest that husbands and L.A.s bring bathing suits to the hospital. They will then be able to assist the woman if she wants or needs companionship during the shower, and if they'd prefer not to be nude in that setting. At the Birthing Center in Pethivier, France, women birth in wading pools filled with warm water! The warm water relaxes the mother and helps stretch the perineum. Maybe they even use the built-in slides occasionally!! (So don't give away that little kiddy pool with the turtle pattern on it: some day you may want to lend it to a pregnant friend!) A group based in California believes that birth should take place under water and is currently working with pregnant women who wish to birth this way.

Water is very soothing. Some women like warm compresses placed on their backs or abdomens. Others like to feel water being dribbled over their bodies. Warm compresses on the perineum during pushing feel wonderful. Most of the women we work with bring a crock pot to the hospital and heat the water to the desired temperature. It saves running to and from a sink. Cold compresses on the forehead often feel wonderful too: just make sure the *cold* ones go on the *forehead*!!

. . . Back to the Labor Room

Induction of Labor

The number of women in this country whose labors are artificially begun is staggering. Amniotomy is one method of induction. Stripping membranes is another. Anything that encourages or initiates labor at a time when labor would not have begun on its own is a form of induction.

Pitocin is a synthetic hormone created in the laboratory to stimulate uterine activity and duplicate oxytocin, the body's *normal* labor stimulant. It is a potent chemical that is difficult to control. It causes unusually powerful uterine contractions, which can compromise the baby's oxygen supply, and it is associated with uterine rupture in completely intact uteri. Pitocin often makes it difficult for a woman to work with her body. The contractions become overwhelming, the woman fretful. She is likely to ask for medication, no matter how much she had planned not to use any. Contractions last minutes. Often there is no end to one contraction before another begins. There doesn't seem to be any time to catch your breath. *Nor for the baby to catch hers.*

In one British study, 50 percent of noninduced women birthed normally.[41] Only 8 percent of the induced mothers did. Women who are dosed with Pitocin ("pitted") become frightened, unable to cope. They begin to lose confidence in themselves and in their ability to birth. Normal labor is also difficult and painful, but we believe that women can be strong enough to work with their body's own labor. However, they may not always be able to cope with an artificially induced labor.

No one knows exactly how labor begins. Many theories abound. (We all watch for a full moon!) However, it is generally agreed that a certain balance in hormones in combination with a certain balance in other body chemicals and a certain state of the baby and uterus all contribute to the onset of labor. When a labor is artificially begun, or a labor in progress is artificially augmented, the balances necessary for normal labor may be thrown off. Your cervix may not be *ready* to dilate. Your uterus may not be ready to contract powerfully. Your baby may not be ready to drop down into the pelvis. Your pelvic ligaments and the pelvis itself may not be as giving and flexible as they will be when your natural laboring time begins. The team, necessary for a normal labor, isn't warmed up yet. No matter how hard you work, the team isn't ready. It can't win the game until everyone is in position and ready to play.

Dr. Mendelsohn reports still more hazards of induced labors: malpositioning of the fetus, which makes delivery more difficult; cranial hemorrhage in the baby; maternal hemorrhage after delivery; and, of course, c/sections because of fetal distress caused by the induction. He says that the doctor's primary motivation is his own convenience; but that, rather than admit to it, the doctor will say that the mother wasn't strong enough to cope with the ordeal of labor.[60] Even the FDA cautions the use of drugs to induce labor, since they have not been sufficiently tested to guarantee the safety of the baby. G. Peterson says that oxytocin, used to stimulate labor, increases neonatal shock and metabolic disorders. She reports that an infant is more likely to have fetal distress, to require help in breathing, and to need intensive care when the mother's labor is chemically stimulated or when the baby is delivered by forceps.[64] Dr. Mehl tells us, "Nurses should give of themselves instead of medication." "In my clinical experience, each warm, supporting, loving person in the delivery room is worth about 75 milligrams of Demerol."*

Many women are induced because their doctor is going away for the weekend and they only want *him* to deliver them. By the way, doctors do not deliver babies; women deliver babies. Many women see their doctor as the person who is going to get the baby out. *You* are the person who will birth your baby! While your own particular doctor's presence may be important to you, you need to begin seeing his presence as secondary. If you were in the backwoods of New Hampshire, or the wilderness of Colorado, or anywhere else, and you couldn't get your car started, and you went into labor, you'd have your baby, doctor or not.

Mehl and Peterson talk about "locus of control."[64] A woman must believe that the location of strength to have this baby lies within herself. Women whose locus, or focus, of control rests totally with the doctor usually have forceps deliveries or c/sections. They depend on "The Doctor" to get the baby out and leave their own sense of strength, confidence, trust, and power behind.

Labors are often induced when women are "overdue." Sheila Kitzinger reports that seven out of ten babies arrive after the due date.[41] Nine out of ten of those "late" babies put in an appearance within ten days of the due date. More than 60 percent of the VBAC women with whom we have worked were "overdue."

If you made the same exact cake batter, using the same exact recipe as Lois and Nancy, and you put yours in your own oven, Lois put hers in her oven, and Nancy put hers in her oven, at the same temperature, would they take the exact same time to bake? One cake would be ready in 58 minutes, perhaps, another in 60, and another in 62. Our ovens work basically the same way, but there are always individual variations! We think it's important to have a general time in mind, not a *particular due date*, since few women have their babies on the "due date" anyway. You need to know that your baby will be born when it is ready, when all systems are go. You can use the "overdue" time to reflect on your pregnancy, appreciate your body's ability to grow a baby so well, and rest for the upcoming birth. (One childbirth instructor suggests to her "very overdue" couples that they make love—not exclusively through intercourse but not necessarily excluding that, either—every day, and not to stop until the woman has had several orgasms per session. "What a homework assignment!" they tell me. But labor almost always begins within hours of the first evening.†

*From a lecture on the psychophysiology of childbirth given in Boston in 1975.

†According to *Our Bodies, Ourselves*, women in some cultures who are ready to go into labor make love to help bring on the labor. We are told that abstention from intercourse prior to and following childbirth in our country may stem from doctor's discomfort "with the idea that we can

When the lovemaking comes from the heart, it helps everyone, and everything, be more open for the baby.) Besides, we all know that the worst thing about being overdue is having to wash your hair and shave your legs every day so you can go into labor "well groomed," right?

We've already talked about speeding up labor. Why must it be speedy? To fit into Friedman's curve? We know few women whose normal healthy labors have fitted onto the curve and we would like its use tempered or abandoned.

Dr. Mahan from the University of Florida states that adherence to the curve is one of the biggest problems in the increase in the cesarean rate. "We weren't made all alike," he reminds us. He says that he and his colleagues don't use the curve at all. They keep it in the back of their minds. "As long as some progress is being made, that's fine. If not, we figure out how we can help the woman out."

Perhaps your doctor wants to get back to his office or home to dinner? We've already mentioned that more cesareans are performed at particular times of day and particular days of the week. Be smart. Let your baby decide when it is to enter the world. An obstetrician's life can be frustrating and unpredictable. He may never be able to schedule anything definite or arrive at a meeting on time, but your baby need not accommodate him.

Let's look at some studies on the dangers of chemical uterine stimulation. Saldana says that oxytocin is of little value. In his study, it led to instrumental delivery in all circumstances.[65] Those babies were clearly not ready to be born! They had to be pulled out. Granat reports that oxytocic drugs are frequently implicated in excessive uterine activity and are associated with uterine rupture even in the absence of a scar.[55] Caldeyro-Barcia found that contractions stimulated with Pitocin can cause dangerous pressure on the fetal head.[50,51] In his excellent article "Hospital Technology Breeds Pathology" (1977), Dr. F. Ettner wrote that when Pitocin is used, the baby is stressed before its very first breath.[53] Mendelsohn notes cranial hemorrhage in "pitted" babies.[60] Pitocin is associated with jaundice in the newborn. It has also been shown that the mother's bearing-down urge may not be in effect in an induced labor.

The literature reporting the dangers of oxytocic drugs is abundant; despite it, their use continues. And if these drugs aren't dangerous enough on their own, there's more. Can you stand it?

Since Pitocin is so dangerous, there needs to be a "safeguard" while it is being used. A monitoring system, if you will. We hope that you won't.

---

be sexually active and potential mothers at the same time (don't mix sex with motherhood). These unscientific cautious beliefs can deny us our sexuality and prevent us from maintaining a closeness to the man we're involved with when that closeness is much needed." New York: Simon & Schuster, 1976 (2d ed., rev.).

Electronic Monitoring Devices

There are two kinds of devices that are used to monitor labor, the Internal Fetal Monitor (IFM) and the External Fetal Monitor (EFM). In most labors, neither one is safe or necessary.

First, the IFM. According to an article from the Feminist Health Works, this machine was originally designed as a diagnostic tool for the exceptionally high-risk labor;[73] but it is now considered standard procedure for normal healthy labors.

The mother must lie flat on her back. We know by now that that position in itself contributes to fetal distress; and that "except for hanging by the feet," it is the worst conceivable position for labor and delivery.[36] It also requires artificial rupture of the bag of waters, another problematic procedure. Rupturing the membranes is necessary so that two electronic catheters can be inserted into the vagina. One punctures the fetal scalp to monitor fetal well-being and the other lies between the fetus and the wall of the uterus to measure the pressure of the contraction.

The IFM can cause minor vaginal and cervical lacerations. Often the catheters become dislodged and have to be reinserted. The most consistent fetal complications to the baby are scalp bleeding, abscesses, and other bodily injuries. Sometimes the scalp electrode is misplaced and put into other places, such as an eyelid or a fontanel (soft spot). Ettner points out that this indwelling equipment provides a route for entry of bacteria from the vagina into the fluid with the results of infection and inflammation. It also can puncture the umbilical cord. It has been reported that cerebral spinal fluid has been caused to leak when the electrodes were incorrectly placed.[53] It has been suggested by many researchers[53,76,77] that the monitor causes the attendant to do more vaginal exams, which further increases the infection rate. Gassner and Ledger report a 40 percent infection incidence associated with cesarean section in monitored women compared to 20 percent in unmonitored women.[76]

Several studies comparing the effectiveness of IFMs to auscultation (listening to the baby's heart with a stethoscope or fetascope) showed no difference between the groups.[70,72,77,80] Striking, though, is the increase in cesareans performed for fetal distress in the monitored group. No one is watching the woman: everyone is more interested in the machine. The woman begins to feel abandoned and fearful, too. The *mother* goes into distress, followed by her little one.

It is well known that monitoring is associated with increased c/section rates, with no apparent improvement in infant outcome. Haverkamp's study shows a threefold increase in section with no difference in infant outcome.[78] Thompson and Cohen also show a tripling of the cesarean rate that occurred with the popularization of IFM. Until the uncertainties of IFM are resolved, they say, routine monitoring of low-risk births might itself be viewed as risky strategy.[96]

Drs. R. H. Paul and E. H. Hon tell us that the potential benefits of IFM are questionable.[90] Its questionable accuracy is an important consideration, not to mention countless problems with misinterpretations of results.

The EFM, in contrast, consists of two straps placed around the mother's abdomen. One belt is a pressure gauge that monitors the pressure of the contractions. The other belt contains a device that measures the fetal heart rate. The machine translates information onto a sheet of paper that is excreted from a noisy machine next to the woman's bed. The woman is asked *not to move* from the bed, for her movements can alter the readout. Sharon said, "When the monitor was attached to me, I was made to be flat and told not to move. I was told that the monitor wouldn't work if I didn't keep still. I was *yelled at* several times because I tried to change position. I felt like a caged animal."

Perhaps one of the most important considerations is that the external monitor utilizes ultrasound, the dangers of which were discussed earlier in this chapter.

The use of fetal heart monitors during labor is widespread and thoughtless. Originally designed as an aid in monitoring high-risk women, the EFM is often required by hospitals for all laboring women. We've accepted these potentially harmful devices because no one warned us of their dangers and we never thought to ask; or, if we asked, no one knew the answers.

Ettner concludes that such monitors show an entirely false sense of precision and that the information is inadequate as much as two-thirds of the time.[72] Dr. John Patrick, of St. Joseph's Hospital, London, Ontario, remarks that fetal monitors were in widespread use in hospitals before a study of their value was even begun. He believes that no one should have installed the machines until it was known whether or not they were of value, since there are risks involved. He also believes that doctors still don't know what the measurements on the machines mean, and there are 30 to 50 percent false positive results.* Some hospitals now have technicians who are specifically trained to interpret EFM readouts, since there is a wide variation in what is normal. There may not be room for a friend to be with you in labor, but of course, there is room for an EFM reader, since *his* role is important. . . .Patrick reports that one of the reasons the monitors are inaccurate is that the fetus moves and affects the measurements. There are those who would have us anesthetize the baby. Or yell at it not to move. Or slap its hand.

Banta and Thacker's article, "Electronic Fetal Monitoring: Is It of Benefit?" reports that careful review of the literature indicates little, if any, increased benefit from EFM compared to auscultation.[70] The risks, they say, are substantial. The National Institutes of Health task force on cesarean childbirth concluded that auscultation is an acceptable method of monitoring normal

---

*Is Fetal Heart Rate Monitoring Worthwhile?" Paper presented to the American Association for Advancement in Science, Toronto, Canada, January, 1981.

labor.* Jarzembski does not feel that physicians are qualified to choose between different brands of monitors, much less to use them reliably.[80] Ettner tells us that the benefits of electronic fetal monitoring do not outweigh the risks.[72] Despite all this evidence, the trend toward universal EFM continues unabated.

The issues of control and ignorance are ever-present. There are political and monetary overtones. Banta and Thacker estimate that EFM involves an annual cost to our society of $411 million, if the costs of cesarean sections and complications are included.[70] Hospitals buy the monitors, we pay for them . . . in more ways than one.

About three months ago, a woman in Massachusetts was sectioned for fetal distress without benefit (we use the term loosely) of anesthesia. The fetal heart monitor signaled distress and was unable to locate any fetal heart beat. The woman was told the baby had to be born immediately. The anesthetic hadn't taken, but the surgery was begun. A perfectly healthy, pink baby was born to a mother who was screaming too loudly to care. Later, she was grateful to the doctor for "saving her baby's life." We spoke to a nurse who was present. She told us that no one had taken the time to listen for the baby with their ears. "If they had, they would have known the baby was fine. It wasn't fetal distress— it was physician distress. And now *I'm* distressed from working at this hospital!" Evidently, situations like this one occur fairly often, although they are hushed up. Mendelsohn,[86] Ettner[72] and others emphatically alert us to the fact that monitoring *causes* the distress it professes to detect. Murphy remarks that values from monitors are no better than "simply tossing a fair coin."[87]

That was true in our own "study." Out of 50 mothers we surveyed who were sectioned for "fetal distress," 48 had babies with Apgar scores of eight to ten.† We are certain that when they were rolled over onto another table for the section, their baby's oxygen supply was reinstituted. We are certain that when the electrode was finally taken from the baby's scalp, the baby breathed a sigh of relief (wouldn't you?). And, given the facts of c/section procedure, we are certain that the distress of the other 2 infants was caused by the anesthesia administered to their mothers.

Of 173 VBAC women, less than 6 percent had monitors. Most were women who lived far from Boston and could not find doctors who would agree to labor without a monitor. The others had the monitor hooked up periodically during labor: the doctor's "protective" measure, and an unnecessary and dangerous practice for women and their babies. All of the other women, including many with more than one previous cesarean, had their baby's heartbeats lovingly auscultated with fetascopes by human attendants.

The psychological implications of machine monitoring are incredible. Here

---

*NIH Cesarean Childbirth Consensus Development Conference Summary, vol. 3 (1980), no. 6.

†The Apgar score is a numerical assessment of the baby's well-being during the first minutes of independent life.

you are, about to give birth, wanting to feel open and relaxed. Instead you have tubes hanging out of your arms and your vagina, or belts strapped around your belly. The machine is making noise and drawing lines over papers that fall on the floor. This is not birth. This is a scene from an outer-space movie.

Often when a woman asks for a stethoscope or fetascope, the staff thinks she's crazy. "You want tuna fish when you can have caviar?" they ask. On most tours of a local maternity unit, the virtues of EFM are routinely extolled to prospective parents. "And of course, here is our all-new deluxe fetal monitor. We have one in every room." Lucky you. When asked about some of the risks involved with EFMs, many nurses don't know. Many nurses and doctors have little experience *listening* to the baby's heartbeat.

One couple wrote, "They make you feel guilty for refusing an electronic device; or they listen and don't tell you how terrific your baby's heart rate is and you wonder and worry. . ."

Another couple had the same experience:

> *We asked that the monitor not be used. We were told that they were far too busy to have to take the time to look for the heartbeat with a fetascope. It was most evident that they felt terribly inconvenienced and even threatened by our request. We told them that we weren't trying to be difficult but had legitimate concerns about ultrasound. They looked at us in total disbelief. They reluctantly listened to the baby's heartbeat with a fetascope and walked out of the room without any reassuring words. When we asked about the heartbeat, we got a noncommittal "Yes, it's all right."*

Yet, it's so hard to refuse! women say. It is even more difficult *to move* with a monitor (although they are now coming out with a newer, more versatile model, a mobile unit. . .) It's even harder to be hugged and "loved up" a lot when there are straps around your belly—or in your vagina—leading to a noisy grey machine. It's even harder to think of yourself as normal, healthy, strong, and capable. It's even harder to shower. (Several women we have been with have avoided a monitor by remaining in the shower. Whenever a monitor was suggested, they hopped into a shower. When they turned into prunes and couldn't look at another drop of water, they came out. If a monitor was still being pushed, they said they had forgotten their soap and went back into the shower.)

And when you stay in bed and on your back, there's a good chance you'll end up with a cesarean, and a good chance it will be for failure to progress (FTP) or CPD.

Drugs

There is no drug that has been proven safe for a pregnant or laboring woman or her baby, yet the vast majority of women in our country take drugs during these times. It may be of interest that the FDA does not guarantee the safety of any drug, even those it has officially approved.[112]

Drugs cause problems. To name a few, they cause nausea, confusion, raised or lowered blood pressure, and blurred vision—and all these conditions will also affect your baby. Brewer and Presser add that on drugs, the "patient" even experiences hallucinations, muscle spasms, a loss of urinary retention, headaches, tremors, and convulsions from toxic reactions.[103] Drugs affect the uterus's ability to contract. We've lost count of the number of women who were sectioned for failure to progress after a drug was administered.

Most of the effects of a particular drug are not known until it is too late. For example, Bendectin, a drug commonly prescribed for women with nausea during pregnancy, is now linked to *severe* birth defects. According to Dowie and Marshall, authors of "The Bendectin Cover Up," the effects of the drug have been known for a long while, but have been ignored by the FDA.[105] Bendectin might very well be a teratogen (a drug or chemical that causes congenital malformation and defects in human and animal fetuses), like Thalidomide, the authors state, and their article is well researched and well documented.

Pain medication given to a laboring woman carrying a 7½ pound baby may be more harmful when given to a woman of the same size carrying a 7 pound baby: the smaller baby receives more drugs per unit of body weight. It is impossible to assess a drug's effects on a baby, since many factors affect the efficiency of the placenta. Nutrition, before and during labor, the stage of the labor, the size of the baby are only a few of many factors to be considered.

Brain disfunctions are now being linked to drugs given during labor. Fetal distress is a common reaction to these drugs. Maternal distress is equally common, since the drugs can cause irritability, depression, and "spacing out" in a woman as well as in her baby. Brewer and Presser say that the most damaging aspect of drug use during labor is that almost all drugs, when taken in amounts large enough to be effective in the mother, constitute an overdose for the baby.[5] Most drugs work by depressing the central nervous system, and they can cause your baby to be limp, pallid, and unable to breathe on her own at birth. Drugged babies sometimes choke on their own mucus.

One laboratory has developed a drug to counteract in the fetus the narcotic effects of drugs given to the mother. "Our drug," they boast, "rapidly reverses narcotic effects to help insure a more responsive beginning." The onset of action, they tell us, is within two minutes following I.V. administration. Twin I.V.s. One for mom, one for baby: like mother-daughter dresses. And, folks, you can repeat the dose at two- to three-minute intervals if the initial dose doesn't give the desired degree of narcotic counteraction and improvement in respiratory function. "When you suspect that depression in the newborn is due to narcotic analgesis in labor . . . Xxxx is the name." Soon we'll have a third agent to counteract the first two: *if* our babies are still alive to test it out, that is. In "Cultural Warping of Childbirth,"[39] Doris Haire says:

Many professionals contend that a "good experience" for the mother is of paramount importance in childbirth. They tend to forget that, for the vast majority of mothers, a healthy, undamaged baby is the far more important objective of childbirth . . . to expose a mother to the possibility of a lifetime of heartache or anguish in order to insure her a few hours of relative comfort is misguided kindness [p.19].[111]

Drugs, rather than skillful emotional support, are employed to relieve the mother's apprehension and discomfort. Elkins wonders why "verbal anesthesia" isn't employed over chemical analgesia.[106] Brackbill, a leading authority on the use of drugs in pregnancy, concurs: mothers do not receive adequate information on the adverse drug reactions, or on alternatives to drugs for relief of pain.[100] In "How the FDA Determines the Safety of Drugs—Just How Safe Is 'Safe'?"[11] we learn that just because a drug is FDA-approved does not mean that the drug has been subjected to properly controlled scientific evaluation and follow-up studies.[112]

In an extensive report entitled "Research in Drugs Used in Pregnancy and Obstetrics,"* presented in July 1981 to the Subcommittee on Investigation and Oversight of the House Committee on Science and Technology, we read, "In addition to a drug's direct action on the mother and fetus, there is the risk of the drug acting synergistically with other drugs and obstetric stresses, increasing the drug's adverse effects on the fetus and newborn." The following factors were set forth to demonstrate the complexity of determining how a drug will affect each individual mother and child: they include the size of the pregnant or parturient woman; the condition of the pregnant or parturient woman; the condition of the fetus; the time the drug is taken or administered relative to conception, fetal development, labor, or birth; the quantity of the drug ingested or administered and whether it is given in single or repeated doses; the route of administration of the drug; the absorption characteristics of the drug; the rate of placental diffusion of the drug; the rate and ability of metabolism and excretion of the drug by the mother and fetus; the concentration of the drug or its metabolites left within the circulation and tissues of the infant when she is detached from her mother's circulatory system at birth; the rate and ability of metabolism and excretion of the drug by the newborn infant as affected by environmental factors such as temperature, nursery procedures, or drugs administered postnatally; and others.

When one considers the difficulty of predicting the effects of a single drug, it is easy to see that it is almost impossible to predict the effects of combination drugs on the child exposed to drugs in utero.

Yet many drugged babies are given generous Apgar scores. "Some doctors have never seen a ten baby," remarks a local midwife. "They see only drugged babies, so their criteria are low. It's rare for them to see a really healthy baby."

---

*By Doris Haire.

Giving high scores is also a way of "proving" that, even with all of their interventions, they still deliver "perfectly fine" babies.

With Pitocin, I.V.s, ruptured membranes, vaginal exams, and fetal monitors, it's hard *not* to need drugs. It's hard to relax and feel normal. No one tells you the many risks that accompany drug usage. "Why not just take a little something, Mrs. S.?" Don't forget, Mrs. S., that little something could permanently harm your baby.

Doris Haire makes the point that it is the mother who must ultimately bear the major burdens of a damaged or impaired child. It would seem prudent, she says, to make every effort to prepare the mother physically and mentally to cope with the sensations and discomforts of birth in order to avoid possible hazards from drugs and anesthetics. [112]

Ronald Glasser, in *The Greatest Battle*, says:

> We are now aware that drugs used during pregnancy can and do cause gross physical congenital defects. Yet the deeper concern is not with gross defects caused by chemicals, but the subtler and more difficult-to-evaluate effects of drugs on a developing child's personality, his intelligence and mental abilities as well as his motor coordination and psychological growth. If drugs can cause arms not to grow and faces to be left open, then they can certainly get into fetal brain cells leading to poor electrical transmissions or storage-ability, interfering or coupling with subcellular structures, not enough to kill the cells but to affect their functioning, leading to seizures, hyperactivity and decreased intelligence [p.73]. [109]

Suzanne Arms, author of *Immaculate Deception*, writes:

> How many times must it be said? Drugs get to the baby. Drugs adversely affect the baby. Drugs may permanently damage the baby. Any doctor who tells his patient that any drug used for any reason—including tranquilizers, sedatives, caudals, epidurals, saddle blocks, paracervical blocks, spinals, generals, or whatever—will not affect the baby is telling her an untruth: no drug has been proven *not* to affect the baby . . .[p.58]. [98]

Abraham Lowbin, writing in the *Journal of the American Medical Association*, reports:

> Gestation and birth thus form an inexorable leveling mechanism; with the brain marred at birth, the potential of performance may be reduced from that of a genius to that of a plain child, or less. The damage may be slight, imperceptible clinically, or it may spell the difference between brothers, one a dextrous athlete and the other an "awkward child" [p.1214]. [116]

Janet Leigh, R.N., midwife and lecturer on the art of labor support, reminds us that there is a process of learning to labor. Drugs prevent us from learning about our normal labor and finding ways to be with it effectively. When a doctor prescribes a drug, he may be embarrassed about the sounds you are making. He might be anxious to "quiet you down." Noise-making is normal, appropriate, and healthy. Many of the sounds are similar to those made during lovemaking, although one woman said, "The sounds that came out of me did not resemble those in lovemaking. It was more like a seriously constipated cow." When someone eagerly offers you a drug, he or she may be dealing with *his or her own* fears about pain in labor. If those around you are nervous, suggest that *they* take something! Drugs undermine a woman's confidence. Offering a drug often suggests to the woman that she isn't doing well enough, or that things are going to get worse ("Here, honey, you ain't seen nothin' yet").

A study by Alan Gintzler at Downstate Medical Center in New York[9] suggests that a woman's pain tolerance may be increased before birth. Beta-endorphin, the brain's own morphine-like substance, is present in the human placenta as a natural antidote for the pain of childbirth. The endorphin system is responsible for this effect, and drugs can alter endorphin production. A preliminary study by Akil et al. at the University of Michigan[1] showed that endorphin levels are six to seven times the normal level in pregnant women and jump even higher during birth. A study by Kimball[12] suggests that elevated maternal endorphin levels may evoke prolactin secretion (prolactin is a mothering hormone: if it is given to roosters they run around looking for little chicks to care for) and thus be related to maternal-infant bonding. According to Dr. Kimball, prenatal understanding and reassurance about the powerful anesthetic effects of endorphins (which can be obtained by active participation in labor) provide much incentive and confidence for expectant mothers. Goodlin[110] reports that drugs may interfere with the production of endorphins in the fetus, thus causing birth to be more stressful to the baby than need be, and possibly contributing to fetal distress.

Second Stage

Some women do manage to dilate to ten centimeters in spite of interferences in the birth process. At this point, the second phase of labor—the pushing phase—is said to begin.

Occasionally a "lip" of the cervix remains. Pushing at this time may cause the cervix to swell or tear. Heather, a home birth VBAC mother, patiently waited several hours for a persistent lip to "disappear" finally. "Those were the most difficult hours of my life, but worth every minute. Of course, had I been in the hospital, I would have been sectioned, since I'd had two previous cesareans." Patience is necessary until the lip pulls back. Occasionally a persistent lip can be held back for a moment to allow the head to descend; it then acts as a wedge and assists in holding back the lip. Upright positions usually encourage the cervix to dilate symmetrically.

One woman wrote that she had had no urge to push immediately after dilating. Ten minutes later she was told that something was wrong with her uterus. As she was being moved to the operating table for a cesarean, she felt the urge to push (no surprise to us, since changing positions often activates this stage). It was "too late," she was told, the operating staff was ready to proceed with the surgery.

Another woman was fully dilated but her baby was not engaged in the pelvis. Some babies "drop" before labor begins. Others don't begin to descend until pushing is *well established*.

Many women are instructed to inhale deeply, hold their breath as long as possible, and push as hard as they can. In a lecture entitled "Management of Second Stage Labor: A Physiological Approach," Frahm and Smith* remark that this kind of pushing gets some babies out, "but at what unnecessary expense to them and their Moms?" Migraine headaches (from increased intracranial pressure), possible burst blood vessels in the eyes, and angina or heart pain from lack of sufficient blood and oxygen flow are but a few of the consequences of this kind of pushing to the mother. According to Frahm and Smith pushing in this manner is very dangerous to the unborn child. Fetal distress is common due to the lack of oxygen that occurs when this method is employed. Not infrequently, a mother trustingly follows these instructions and is then rushed into the O.R. for a cesarean section to "save" her baby.

Some women find pushing painful, others find it wonderful, exciting, and extremely satisfying. Some women push for two or three contractions and out comes their baby, while others push for five or six hours. We are in a fast society: quick hamburgers, ten-minute car washes, quick-stop cleaners. We are expected to birth our babies quickly, as well. It took time to grow your baby. Allow time for him to be born, too! Cohen reminds us in "Influence of the Duration of Second Stage Labor on Perinatal Outcome and Puerperal Morbidity" that terminating labor simply because an arbitrary period of time has elapsed in the pushing phase is clearly not warranted. He tells us that the practice of subjecting patients to potentially traumatic operative procedures merely because they have not delivered within two hours after the second stage has begun "should be decried."[130]

Generally, women do not need special instructions to push. Each woman must listen to her body and push with her own rhythm, with as much force as her body dictates. Time and time again, we have seen that this works. We do not believe that your body dilates to ten centimeters without knowing how to complete its task.

Often, during the pushing stage, women are moved from one room to another.

---

*Marion Myers, "1982 ICEA Convention Notes," *Pacesetter Newsletter*, September–October 1982.

For most, this policy is disorienting and unnecessary. It is another tactic employed by too many hospitals; it confuses women and disrupts labor. One father wrote:

> A nurse came in to check Karen and panicked after seeing the top of the baby's head. "Oh my! We're having a delivery! Don't push now! We have to get you to delivery!" She half led, half carried Karen to a labor bed and flew her down the hall to the delivery room. Meanwhile, I had to put on a mask and hair cover, and hop on one foot while I got my shoe covers on. The nurse was trying to wake the doctor and push Karen through the delivery room door. The doctor tried to squeeze in the delivery room but the nurse, our midwife, the bed, and I had the door blocked. It took us all about three tries, but we were finally all "in place" for the birth.

In the Delivery Room

Anesthesia

Several types of anesthesia are given to women in labor. Many of the dangers of anesthesia have already been discussed. Local anesthetics not only can cause problems in the newborn but can interfere with the mother's natural bearing-down capacity as well. When an anesthetic is given at the end of labor, the woman's experience of her child's birth is damaged, not enhanced.

Erickson remarks that it is indeed a paradox that the drugs most toxic to the fetus and newborn are precisely those which produce the most desirable effects from the obstetrician's point of view, and are most widely used.[133] Caudals and saddle blocks necessitate the use of forceps and cause a drop in the mother's blood pressure, which affects the baby. Paracervical blocks promoted as a minor regional anesthesia that will merely "take the edge off" may not relieve back labor and may cause severe changes in the baby's heart rate. If given too early, they can slow labor. Some babies have died from paracervicals! (Did you watch the program "20–20" on the dangers of anesthesia? We can only venture a guess as to the hundreds of surgical operations that were canceled the next day!)

Dr. Kloosterman, head of the department of obstetrics and gynecology at the University of Amsterdam, remarks that the move toward "daylight obstetrics" creates unphysiological conditions, "as natural activity of the uterus is highest during the night hours, lowest during the daylight."[11] He tells us that 70 percent of all births start spontaneously between 8 P.M. and 8 A.M. "Daylight obstetrics thus lowers the pain threshold again and creates more demand for analgesics and anesthetics. The result: more epidurals . . . [which lead to] more forceps and more cesareans."

Forceps

If you are flat on your back, trying to push your baby against gravity—remember, an upright position assists gravity and increases the capacity of your pelvis—your efforts may go unrewarded.

If you don't push quickly enough, or are "ineffective" in your pushing efforts, your baby is likely to be born with the "aid" of forceps. These steel blades, which resemble salad tongs and would be better wrapped around a green pepper than your baby's head, can cause a multitude of damage. However, they are used frequently in this country to shorten the second stage of labor.

Fundal pressure is also used by some physicians to hurry the birth. This is dangerous! Fundal pressure can cause the baby's oxygen supply to be severely compromised. It can cause premature separation of the placenta. Some doctors are known to use fundal pressure *and* forceps simultaneously. (OUCH!)

Infants delivered by forceps may sustain skull fracture, intercranial hemorrhage, cord compression, brain damage, damage to the facial nerve, facial paralysis.[10] Damage to the central nervous system is common. Brewer and Presser report that the delicate spinal and neck vertebrae are easily pulled out of alignment by excessive and forceful extension of the infant's head with forceps.[127] It takes *seven years* (!) to assess the neurological results of forceps delivery.[10,13,101,102] Death from forceps is noted in the literature.[137] In many countries, the incidence of delivery by forceps is 5 percent. In some American hospitals it is well over 65 percent.[10]*

Harriet's doctor told her he could turn on some "Pit." "I can deliver the baby with forceps—the head is right there anyway—and have the placenta birthed within minutes." Harriet wrote, "It felt like he was trying to get this thing 'cleaned up' and I thought, 'Now I really understand the meaning of killing two birds with one stone.' I couldn't believe the pain."

Lacerations of the cervix and of the pelvic floor tissue and muscle, rupture of the uterus, injury to bladder and rectum, fracture of tailbone, and urinary tract infection are but a few of the complications a woman can expect from a forceps delivery. Brewer and Presser caution us that everything possible should be done to avoid the need for forceps. When they are legitimately required, they should be used with minimal traction. They report that the addition of a pressure gauge to the handles of forceps has been advocated so safety limits are not exceeded.[127] We wonder how long it will take for this suggestion to be considered.

Some women have been told that all VBACs require forceps. Some are frightened to push because they fear that too much pressure at this point will rupture a previous cesarean incision—although no research substantiates this.

---

*NAPSAC News, 4 (Summer 1979):3.

RECIPE

Preheat operating room to 68°F.

Ingredients:

> 1 hungry laboring woman
> 1 tired, apprehensive, expectant father
> 1 hospital jonnie
> 1 resident, assigned to the "case"
> 1 EFM
> 1 I.V.
> assorted drugs (optional)
> 1 amnio hook
> 1 pair forceps
> 1 typical American obstetrician

Directions:

Place woman in jonnie. Add other ingredients, except obstetrician. Mix. Spread onto one narrow hospital bed. Simmer for twelve hours or until baby's heartbeat begins to drop. Place all ingredients in preheated operating room, on operating table. Roll them over. Do not allow to rise. Make well in center and add one package of anesthesia and the obstetrician. When ready, slice evenly.

Jennifer wrote:

I had a short labor—only four and a half hours. The doctor feared strain on the scar and insisted on forceps, even though the baby was moving rapidly down the canal. It was done without any anesthetic although I asked for it. I was told I'd feel as bad with it. I begged for time to catch my breath during the probing, but the doctor would not stop. He ignored me. Incidentally, the mid forceps was begun by the resident under my doctor's supervision. My baby suffered a huge hematoma.

*The doctor's treatment was callous. His poor treatment and unnecessary interven-
tion endangered my life and my baby's. There was no warning to me or my husband
as he introduced the forceps—my first knowledge of them was the excruciating and
sickening feeling of their introduction. All this took away the benefits of a natural
birth. I was unable to hold or observe the baby because of the pain and trying to
remain still during suturing. I feel worse after this birth than after the cesarean
as I feel a* perfect *birth was snatched away by an interfering doctor. My Christmas
presents to all my pregnant friends will be* Confessions of a Medical Heretic *and*
Mal(e) Practice.

Contrast Jennifer's and Harriet's experiences with those of a VBAC woman
from Nebraska. Bobbi wrote:

*Somewhere after the fourth hour of pushing I started to leak meconium. My labor
attendant was listening to the baby and the fetal heart tones remained good at all
times. I pushed for another two and a half hours, at which time we discussed with
our doctor the possibility of low forceps (mostly because of the meconium). I will
never forget his calm manner and gentleness. He reminded us to bring my warm
compresses and oil to the delivery room! He gave me the choice of a pudendal block
and I elected not to have one. He used the forceps for only a short time and helped
to bring the baby's head down (meanwhile, the hot compresses above and below felt
wonderful). He then said, "You do the rest, Bobbi," and I pushed my baby into
the world." During the crowning he reminded me to reach down and touch her
head. Our daughter is strong and healthy and beautiful, and I had no I.V., no
monitor, and no drugs. It was actually fun!*

Unfortunately, Jennifer's experience is far more apt to occur than Bobbi's.
She is only one of dozens of women who have written to us who are bitter
because of a "thoughtless and barbaric butcher who masquerades as a physician."
She is only one of hundreds of women who endure painful and unnecessary
techniques performed without knowledge or consent. As one midwife in Massachusetts has put it, "What goes on in delivery rooms without words is a
progression in incompetence and insensitivity." Another woman wrote, "Insurance companies and golf games must run doctors' practices, because good, caring
judgement certainly does not." Still another wrote, "Lambs, all of us, lined up
for slaughter."

NAPSAC's *Safe Alternatives in Childbirth*[149] reports that Dr. Delee, who
introduced forceps and episiotomy around the turn of the century, stated just
before he died that if he had his whole life to live over, he would do home
births and nothing else, realizing that the majority of his work was probably
going to do bad instead of good.

Episiotomy

When a forceps delivery is done, episiotomies are performed as well. An
episiotomy is a cut made into a woman's perineum to enlarge the vaginal

opening. This "innocent" slice of the knife turns every birth into a surgical procedure.

Our vaginal openings don't need enlarging! The vagina is made up of pleats of elastic tissue, ready to open and stretch. Episiotomy is a painful, unnecessary procedure. Doctors tell us that they will cut us in order that we won't tear. It has never been shown that cutting is preferable to tearing. As a matter of fact, the opposite has been shown. When an episiotomy is done, the doctor makes a cut through a thickened perineum. Tears, on the other hand, occur at a place where the perineum has stretched out to its fullest. In Janet Leigh's lecture on the art of labor support, she says, "How do you avoid an episiotomy? You don't allow one!"

Scandinavian countries have less than a 6 percent rate of episiotomy. The United States is well over 90 percent! Our perineums are no different than those of our Scandinavian sisters. There are very few situations that warrant an episiotomy. But we lie on our backs as our doctors make an incision into our genitals. "I'm just going to cut you a little," we're told. Yet if we told a doctor we were just going to cut his penis a little bit, he'd be halfway to China before we picked up the knife.

Banta and Thacker, in "Benefits and Risks of Episiotomy: A Review of the Literature 1860–1980," tell us that there are "significant risks associated with episiotomy that have not been adequately studied."[124] They believe that the episiotomy rate in the United States could be reduced by more than half. Since episiotomy is "essentially unstudied," they recommend carefully designed studies to determine the circumstances in which the procedure is clearly indicated. Unfortunately, most doctors believe it is clearly indicated all the time, and not one of their clients escapes "a little snip." Most endure a super snip.

Kitzinger[137] believes that episiotomy is an act of ritual mutilation that we accept as necessary. It is an operation performed on the body of a healthy woman without enough information or her consent, she says. She believes that childbirth education prepares women to adjust to, rather than avoid, this unnecessary assault. She believes there is a punitive element: if I don't push quickly enough, he'll cut me.

Women are usually draped for the birth of the baby. In *Vaginal Politics*, Ellen Frankfort alerts us to the fact that drapery not only depersonalizes the woman by making her faceless and bodiless *except* for her vagina, it also prevents her from seeing what the doctor is doing. He is usually doing an episiotomy. She advises women to discard the drapes by throwing them on the floor. If the doctor replaces them when he enters the room, throw them on the floor again. If he questions your behavior, tell him doctors in California are no longer draping. And if you're in California, tell him doctors in New York have stopped this strange custom (p. 266).[134] If you are upright, the "sterile" drapes will fall away.

Kitzinger's study concludes that women with episiotomy have far more pain than those with lacerations, and that the pain of an episiotomy lasts longer and is more severe.[137] It affects lovemaking for months. Although episiotomy is done to avoid tearing, third-degree tears occur with episiotomy rather than in its absence.[41]

Kitzinger supports the accusation that physicians cut much too soon. "'Let's get this baby out,' doctors say, even when there is no medical reason to do so. They chop through an unstretched perineum . . . Excessive bleeding is common."[41] In *Spiritual Midwifery*, one woman remarked that she could have gotten two babies out of the cut simultaneously.[8] Many physicians do not support the perineum after the episiotomy and allow the woman to tear clear back to her rectum. Evelyn from New York writes:

> I had a beautiful VBAC and cries of "We did it!" and "She's beautiful" still ring in my ears. But I did not escape the knife. My own doctor was away. The doctor who attended the birth had made up his mind about an episiotomy from the time he entered the delivery room. I yelled "No episiotomy!" but he wasn't too keen on VBACs and was very keen on episiotomies. I would have liked to have that last push. As with the cesarean, I have learned another important lesson. Hundreds of dollars worth of surgery to repair the botched episiotomy and a rather difficult sex life have taught me never again to let an obstetrician with a knife near my body.

A doctor in Boston tells women, "I am a male chauvinist. I do episiotomies because sex isn't any good unless you've had one." In Andrea Dworken's book *Our Blood*,* Dr. Herbert Ratner tells us that some doctors do cesarean sections and episiotomies as a contribution to lovemaking. Deep down, he says, the American physician thinks he is preserving the woman's vagina for sex. Dworken generalizes that the epidemic of cesarean sections in this country is a sexual, not medical, phenomenon. The vagina is saved to serve the husband.

Many VBAC women say they'd gladly exchange a cesarean incision for an episiotomy. VBAC mother Sharon felt like her "guts were falling out" for a month after her episiotomy, although her cesarean incision hadn't been much more than "itchy." Her doctor assured her the pain was completely normal! The mentality that we must suffer and be cut at some point on our bodies frustrates us. Women think they must make an exchange, a sacrificial offering of at least one part of their body in order to birth vaginally. You needn't be cut *anywhere!* And you needn't tear.

One way to condition your perineum is by doing Kegel exercises. These should be done frequently before and during pregnancy. Your Kegel muscle, also called the pubococcygeus muscle, is the one you use when you deliberately want to stop urinating. Strengthening your Kegel, by alternately contracting and releasing it, will aid you before, during, and after birth. A healthy Kegel equals

*New York: Perigree (1981).

a healthy pelvic floor. A healthy pelvic floor keeps a woman's "innards" from prolapsing. (Many physicians perform surgery on women who are incontinent. They don't suggest Kegel exercises, which could improve the situation to the point where surgery would be unnecessary. If surgery has already been done, Kegel exercise can prevent it from becoming necessary in the future.) An excellent description of the pelvic musculature and the importance of Kegel exercises is found in Elizabeth Noble's *Essential Exercises for the Childbearing Years.** Being able to release your pelvic floor during pushing will aid your baby's descent into the world. You can Kegel when you are stopped at a traffic light. You can Kegel when you are making love. You can Kegel to music. Ready? And-a one, and-a two, and-a three. . .

Some women do perineal massage during pregnancy. Some couples include it as part of their lovemaking. Good nutrition contributes to good muscle tone and elasticity of the skin. Upright positioning during pushing will help. Let your body *ease* the baby out, slowly and gently. Allow your perineum to stretch. Warm compresses and pure vitamin E oil applied during pushing can help. In "On Avoiding Episiotomies," Carol Harris reports that first-time mothers do not need episiotomies, but much depends on the delivery position and the skill and the patience of the birth attendant.[136] Ina May[135] tells us that scar tissue is stretchy. Even if you have had an episiotomy, you can give birth without one.

Caldeyro-Barcia[128] reminds us to bear down with our bottoms: many women are instructed to hold their breath and push with their brains. Doctors—telling women how to push! You need only push for as long as your body tells you to push. This will prevent oxygen deprivation to the baby. It will also slow the birth somewhat, giving your perineum time to stretch and reducing the need for a knife. Herbert Ratner tells us ironically, "Apparently God, who could make a tree, knew not how to make a perineum."

Just in case you are not convinced about the problems associated with episiotomy, Dr. Robert Mendelsohn gives us the following information: often a local injection is given for the episiotomy. Occasionally, a needle is jammed into the baby's brain when the anesthetic is administered, causing its death; often the knife goes too deep and slashes the anal sphincter; when a doctor performs an episiotomy, he cuts through muscles and nerves, producing a numbness that sometimes persists for years; repairing an episiotomy usually takes longer than the delivery itself; the operation increases the risk of infection and is responsible for about 20 percent of maternal deaths.[144]

Don Creevy, an obstetrician, tells us that there is no value to routine episiotomy except "cost effectiveness": by shortening the second stage episiotomies make room for other women in the delivery room. He tells us that the doctor gets to cut and suture and "act like a surgeon."

---

*Boston: Houghton Mifflin (1976).

Stirrups

To put it briefly, stirrups are for horses. Doris Haire dreams of the day when putting a woman in stirrups for no medical reason will be considered malpractice. If you are in stirrups, you'll most likely end up with an episiotomy and a forceps delivery. Leave the stirrups to equestrians!

Birthing the Placenta

Often, after the episiotomy is done and the baby's head is born, women are given another shot of Pitocin. "You need this in order to contract your uterus and so the placenta will birth," we are told. However, women in other cultures who do not have the benefit of synthetic contracting agents are not walking around with their placentas still attached to their uteri. Placentas separate all by themselves! Unless, of course, the woman is lying flat on her back, weak from lack of nourishment and so drugged that her uterus and placenta are *unable* to function as they're supposed to . . .

In "Cultural Patterning and Perinatal Behavior," Margaret Mead and Niles Newton tell us that sight and sound together facilitate the delivery of the placenta. They believe that seeing the baby and hearing him may trigger a biological releasing mechanism.[143] Kitzinger tells us that in a *really natural* birth (what we call "purebirth"), the first physical contact with the baby produces a rush of emotion; this is accompanied by oxytocin, which keeps the uterus firm and causes further contractions.[41] In our group of 173 VBAC women, there has been only one placenta that needed assistance; it separated only partially and was helped along by the physician 25 minutes after the birth. There were no additional problems. No one jumped on these women's bellies or yelled at their placentas to hurry and get out. Most placentas arrived within minutes of the baby; a few took up to 60 minutes. Mead and Newton's article tells us that in some cultures a fire is built to speed the delivery of the placenta, but the woman is never touched. They let gravity help.

Cord Clamping

Kitzinger[41] tells us that clamping the cord immediately at delivery may make a retained placenta more likely. If the cord is not clamped until after it has stopped pulsing, there is less chance of retained placenta and postpartum hemorrhage. (Alcohol can predispose a woman to hemorrhage, so you may want to save the champagne until your baby is several hours old.) Rahima Baldwin, author of *Special Delivery*, tells us it is a shock to the baby to have the cord cut too early. It forces him to depend on his lungs as the sole source of oxygen sooner than nature intended.[123] In an article entitled "Brain Damage by Asphyxia at Birth,"[125] we are told that immediate cord clamping is equivalent to subjecting the infant to a massive hemorrhage, because almost a fourth of the fetal blood is in the placental circuit at birth. Depriving the infant of that blood can be a factor "in exacerbating an incipient hypoxemia and can thus contribute to the danger of asphyxial brain damage"(p.78). Ina May Gaskin[135] suggests that the cord be allowed to finish pulsating—it takes about five minutes—before it is clamped. Speir states that the cord should be neither tied nor cut, and believes that to do so is "a violent act that disturbs the natural birth process (p.1)".[173] She tells us that the cord will dry up and fall off naturally.

Women often hear that it was a good thing a cesarean was performed—the cord was wrapped around the baby's neck. *Lots* of babies have wrapped cords! By the way, the cord should never be pulled, as it can break away from the placenta. Treat it lovingly; it too, was a comrade to your baby. When the time is right, you (or your mate) can cut the cord. It seems only fitting that you bring your baby into the world and then free her from your body.

Another word about your placenta and your umbilical cord. Just that: they are *yours*. Take a look at them—they provided *life* for your baby! It's amazing, when you think about it. The whole process is amazing!

In Jordan, the placenta is considered the sister, or comrade, of the baby. It is treated with respect. United States hospitals use some placentas for tests, and some for skin-grafting procedures. Most are discarded. "We couldn't let them throw my placenta away," said one woman. "So we brought it home and planted it in our yard with a little apple tree. It enriched the soil, and every spring, when that tree blossoms, we are reminded of the life that it brought to us as well."
Judith Dickson Luce, a midwife in Boston, tells us that childbirth in our country is fast becoming childbirth without mother. She says that it is possible to have a "natural childbirth" with an epidural, fetal monitor, and the "drug of your choice." The baby's welcome and the labor and delivery are all engineered and controlled by the doctors. She believes that we are being robbed of the experience of actively shaping and creating our birth experiences. She believes that we are also robbed of our right to pursue our own instincts of tender loving care to our newborn during the first moments, hours, and days of life.

We agree, for after your baby is born, the interventions *continue*.

"Welcome to the World, Dear Child":* Baby's Own Interventions

The birth of your baby is not, by any means, a grande finale. As a matter of fact, it's just the beginning; the beginning of a precious new life, a new family, and, unfortunately, more interventions. Because the health and well-being of the baby is one of the primary motivations for a VBAC, we cannot leave this chapter without information—and cautions—about what is done to most babies after the actual birth is over.

In an article entitled "The First Day of Life," Charles Spezzano and Jill Waterman comment, "If first impressions count, as we are convinced they do, perhaps we should be more attentive to the kind of welcome we give our children." They tell us that the first minutes and the first hours of the baby's life may be just as crucial as the first year.[174] Yet, the number of mothers and babies unnecessarily separated during the first hours—and days—is outrageous. Before you even have time to hold him, love him, let alone count the fingers and toes, he is whisked away for a variety of hospital procedures. Even when the baby is "allowed" to be with you after birth, many hospitals still view the baby as their possession. The time *will* come when hospitals will ask your permission whenever they touch your baby. They should be doing it *now*. They are holding *your* precious treasure, and should certainly have your consent before "handling the goods."

Babies, feeling safe enough to be born, optimistically greet the world. Before they are minutes old, they are suctioned, tagged, scrubbed, weighed and footprinted, and occasionally cultured. That's the best part. Silver nitrate is dropped into their eyes, and vitamin K is injected into their bodies. If they are little boys, they may have the tip of their penis cut off before they are hours old. Is it any wonder that no one trusts anyone in this world anymore? They trusted us all enough to be born, and look what happened! (Claudia Panuthos asks: "Is it any wonder that most of us have difficulty in front of groups? Our first group experience was in the delivery room, folks.")

The room is often cold, a shock to baby's system. And babies are still being held by the feet like prize fish! Vernix, baby's own soothing skin cream, is washed away. He gets a bulb syringe in his mouth, lights in his eyes, a slap on the bottom, and perhaps a tube down his throat for good measure. In spite of prepared childbirth classes and natural childbirth movements, most babies in our country are subjected to one or more of the above. Those that have been drugged are subjected to their own set of procedures. In *Changing Childbirth*, Young remarks that included in the disturbing trends among childbearing women in our country is the relinquishing of responsibility and care for our babies to the nursing staff and hospital.[201] Dr. Charles Mahan warns that nurseries often

---

*We recommend that you listen to "Welcome to the World," by Robbie Gass. Available at Spring Hill Music, Ashby, Mass.

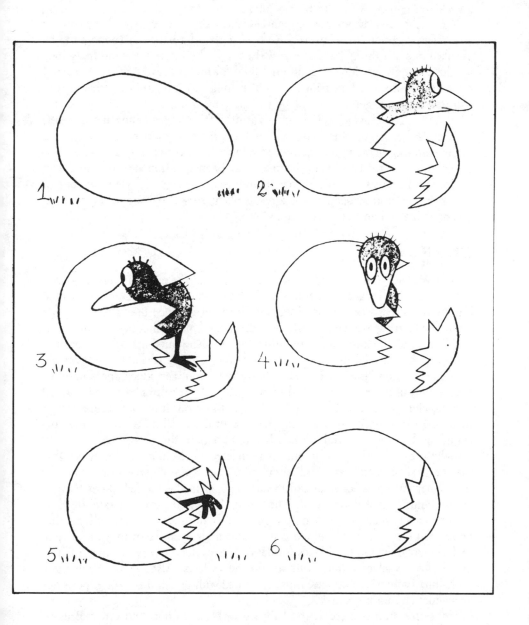

look like "production lines at the Ford Company" and tells us that the best place for a sleeping baby is next to his sleeping mother.*

We credit Leboyer for raising consciousness about a newborn baby's plight at a medical childbirth. However, we believe that if a baby was supposed to be plunked into a bath right after delivery (Leboyer's "solution"), the mother's body would somehow provide the additional fluid for this endeavor. Since it doesn't, we can only assume that baby does not belong in a tub, rubber duckies notwithstanding, but gently greeted by his mother's arms, her touch, her voice. The warmest, safest place is in mother's arms, skin to skin, nursing at her breast, with a blanket around the baby and mother. Instead, most babies are placed under warming lights in a container that looks like oversized Tupperware. (Indeed, even the *safety* of baby warmers has been questioned. The American Academy of Pediatrics[185] states that neurological damage, dehydration, burns, and even death have occurred as a result of their use.) No sooner do they get "comfortable" when the "fun" begins.

Silver Nitrate

In most states, it is required by law that silver nitrate be placed in the newborn's eyes within moments after birth. This is done ostensibly to prevent congenital blindness caused by gonorrhea infection in the eyes, since the baby's eyes can be infected during passage through the birth canal if the mother has the infection.

Silver nitrate is caustic and inflammatory. A classic nursing textbook reminds nurses to take special precautions against dropping any silver solution on the face and to allow time for the baby "to recover from the shock and smarting" before putting the drops in the other eye (p. 344).[168] It causes pain, redness and swelling, temporary blindness, and prolonged irritation. It is not always effective in killing the gonococcus bacteria. Because of the swelling of the tissues surrounding the eyes as a result of the silver nitrate itself, the gonorrhea that might initially cause the same symptom goes undetected. Mendelsohn believes that the use of silver nitrate is a "ridiculous rite." He says it may be responsible for the higher incidence of astigmatism and myopia in the United States than in other countries that don't use it. There is no basis to believe it is safe, he says. Its side effects include blocked tear ducts and conjunctivitis. He tells us that babies can see until silver nitrate is placed in their eyes. Then they are unable to focus on their mothers' faces for days. Tetracyclene or erythromycin is just as effective as silver nitrate, without the side effects. Also, they do not mask opthalmia, which, by the way, must be treated with penicillin or other powerful antibiotics should it occur.[165]

If the infection is present, the baby's eyes begin to ooze. In Great Britain, baby's eyes are watched for the first weeks of life. If no "prevalent discharge" is noticed, the baby's eyes are left alone.

---

*From a lecture given in Wheeling, W. Va., 1 Aug. 1982.

A baby can't pick up gonorrhea if the mother doesn't have it. Putting silver nitrate into all babies' eyes presumes that all women have the veneral disease. Doctors proceed on the assumption that all women have gonorrhea, are all infectious, and have all infected their babies. This is an insult to women who do not have gonorrhea. Mendelsohn tells us that he teaches his students to comply with the law, but to do it by squirting the chemical in the general direction of the baby from ten feet away.[165]

Most of the couples with whom we work refuse silver nitrate. Because some laws require the physician to administer it, the physician who neglects to do so runs the risk of being fined by the state. After several "offenses," he may lose his license. Fortunately, there are doctors who are willing to take the risk and do not insist upon its use. Some, like the professor just mentioned, put the material on the babies' cheeks and say, "Oops, I missed." Some tell couples they must do it, but give the couples clear water to rinse the baby's eyes immediately afterwards. Others hand it to the nurse and tell her to do it.

We think it is offensive to have to put something ineffective and inflammatory into a newborn baby's eyes. However, if you decide to go along with the law, we suggest that you wait at least until your baby is several hours old. Let her adjust to the world a bit. Let her hear your voice, drink your milk, feel your touch and your love. Let her see your face and your smile before she is temporarily blinded from them.

According to Nancy Whittaker and Judy Strasser, researchers have developed accurate means to detect gonorrhea in the pregnant woman. This affects the reasonableness of the concern underlying the silver nitrate laws, that gonococcus bacteria can lie dormant for several years within the mother's body and nonetheless infect her infant. "A mother who has had good prenatal care, including a routine gonorrhea culture which has indicated the absence of the bacteria, presents virtually no risk to her unborn child. Her infant should not have to be subjected to silver nitrate or any other routine preventative measure" (p. 27). The law ignores that there are safe and effective alternatives to silver nitrate and also effective antibiotics to treat the infection. Some hospitals have release forms that read:

> I release the hospital, its physicians, and its employees of any or all liability should any untoward effects result, due to failure to permit the administration of the prophylactic eye medication silver nitrate drops, one into each eye and/or the prophylactic intramuscular injection of Vitamin K (aqua-mephyton) routinely administered to all newborns.

If we were you, we'd sign on the dotted line.

Laws that are inappropriate and insulting need to be challenged and changed. Fortunately, many couples have laid the groundwork. Several states have revised their laws on silver nitrate. In the meantime, newborn after newborn makes his way into the world only to be greeted by an unnecessary inflammatory and painful agent. It certainly doesn't seem *lawful*. As a matter of fact it seems criminal.

Vitamin K, Circumcision, and Jaundice

Most babies in our country are routinely given vitamin K—without our permission! Vitamin K, which influences blood clotting, is manufactured by the body. The baby does not begin to manufacture her own until after birth; but there is no reason to believe that she is vitamin-deficient at birth. Brewer and Presser tell us that the baby's liver should have sufficient vitamin K to meet her needs until she can start synthesizing her own. They add that, given what babies have to endure in standard hospital nurseries, vitamin K may be the least of their problems.[155] Mendelsohn tells us that administration of vitamin K to newborns may produce jaundice—which gives the doctors an excuse to treat them with bilirubin lights. These lights expose the babies to a dozen documented hazards that may require still further treatment and possibly affect the children for the rest of their lives.[165]

One reason for administering vitamin K immediately after birth might be that your baby required surgery. Another reason might be circumcision.
We suggest that *if* you are going to have your son circumcised, you wait until he is at least a week old. Give him time to be with you, to adjust to life, to feel good about the world, and to manufacture his own vitamin K before subjecting him to a painful operative procedure! Let him learn your voice and your smile and your face so you can soothe him after the surgery.

In the Jewish religion, circumcision is part of a covenant with God. It is part of the religious heritage, although, for the first 2000 years, the practice merely involved nicking the top of the foreskin.[179] Males are circumcised on the eighth day by a trained *"mohel."* We're certain God took into consideration that babies needed time to synthesize vitamin K. Joan, whose father is a mohel, writes:

> *Ritual circumcision performed by a* Mohel *merely involves loosening and lifting the foreskin from the glans, the emplacement of a protective shield, and the actual cut with a surgical scalpel. From the beginning to end, the procedure often takes less than a minute. As the* Mohel *is a specialist in this procedure and has performed thousands throughout his career, his experience and adroitness are generally assured. Medical practitioners, on the other hand, usually employ complicated surgical clamps or other specialized equipment, which are supposed to minimize bleeding. However, the proper positioning of the apparatus is often a lengthy and delicate procedure, sometimes lasting many minutes. A prior incision may be required, all of which increases the potential for pain and discomfort. When it is recalled that under medical auspices, the circumcision may be performed by someone with little experience in the procedure, often by a hospital intern, the possibilities for problems become obvious.*

The true contrast becomes apparent by noting that as observed by religious communities, the procedure is generally performed in full public view: parents, family and friends are typically present. In contrast, physicians are typically most reluctant to have any nonprofessional audience of onlookers when they perform their procedures; even parents are usually ushered into another room, out of eyesight and earshot.

Circumcision provides no established medical benefit. The American Academy of Pediatrics does not consider it an essential component of good health care, and remarks that there is no absolute medical indication for its routine practice.*

The Painful Dilemma, a book about circumcision, tells us that babies do not always cry during the surgery: sometimes they lapse into semiconsciousness because of the trauma. Mendelsohn says that next to the needless episiotomy, circumcision is the most frequently performed surgical procedure. "Doctors enriched themselves by lopping the foreskins from nearly a million-and-a-half penises in 1979." Occasionally, he says, the knife slips . . .[165]

Some argue that a son must look like the father. Why? We don't look much like our mothers, or our sisters, or our friends. Some of us have large breasts, some small. Some of us have flabby thighs and tight tushies, others have tight tummies and flabby fannies. Some of us have stretch marks and others look like Suzanne Somers. Sexual identity and positive feelings about male sexuality do not come from having—or not having—a foreskin.

If you do decide to circumcise your son, we suggest you wait until after the first week of life. Brewer and Presser suggest that a small dose of local anesthetic seems to be the humane thing to do. They agree with Mendelsohn that circumcision is "big business."[155] We recommend that you hold or touch your baby in some way while it is being done. If you've had some wine or alcohol an hour or two before the surgery, it may calm your baby (through the milk). For information about circumcision, send a SASE to INTACT, 6294 Mission Road, Everson, Wash. 98247; or the Newborn Rights Society, Box 48, St. Peters, Pa. 19470.

Many a mother is told that her baby has jaundice (a yellow discoloration of the skin and eyes caused by an accumulation of "bilirubin" in the blood, which happens because the baby's liver is immature and slow to metabolize and excrete bilirubin). All newborns have some degree of jaundice; almost 60 percent of healthy, full-term babies show signs. Something that common must be normal and harmless; in fact, it seems to be a natural part of the newborn's adjustment to life. In most of these babies, the jaundice is "physiologic"—normal and benign. It occurs around the second or third day of life, and disappears after the first week or so, as the baby's system gradually begins to decompose the bilirubin.

---

*A two-page summary report on circumcision may be requested from the American Academy of Pediatrics, P.O. Box 1034, Evanston, Ill. 60204.

Rarely (in about .5 percent of cases), jaundice is caused by a substance in the mother's milk, and the baby may remain jaundiced for several weeks. Breast milk jaundice usually does not appear until late in the first week after birth, or during the second week. If this occurs, contact doctor and La Leche League leader. The major concern with jaundice is Kernicterus, a damaging staining of the brain cells by bilirubin. Kernicterus is *extremely* rare (it is noted more often in babies with Rh negative problems and in premature infants) and has not been reported to occur at levels of bilirubin below twenty.

Physiological or benign jaundice is vastly different from pathologic jaundice, which results from abnormality or disease. Any jaundice present at birth or evident during the first 24 hours is not likely to be physiological. "The best, perhaps only rational, management of the physiological jaundice is encouragement of frequent, unsupplemented breastfeeding, beginning immediately after birth," reports Betty Ann Countryman, R.N., in her 1978 report on jundice.[158] Water or supplements given to the newborn to "flush out" the jaundice are harmful in that they interfere with breastfeeding. Gartner[159] states that there is no cause for concern and no evidence that physiologic jaundice of the type seen in the average healthy full-term infant causes any damage.

In spite of literature on physiologic jaundice, babies are whisked away from their mothers and subjected to repeated heel pricks (to test the bilirubin level in their blood) and phototherapy; "bililights," which have been said to mask rather than assist the condition. Phototherapy causes diarrhea, interferes with parent-infant attachment, and eliminates visual stimulation (the baby's eyes must be shielded). It is associated with vitamin deficiency, skin rashes, a change in the baby's temperature, anxiety, lethargy, and a variety of other consequences. One local physician remarks that physiologic jaundice can be "admired and ignored."

PKU (Phenylketonuria) screening is done in all maternity hospitals in the United States. PKU is an abnormality of the metabolism in which the baby is unable to process the essential amino acid phenylalanine because of an enzyme missing in his liver. According to the American Academy of Pediatrics committee on genetics, "early diagnosis and treatment [via a controlled diet] largely prevent the mental retardation associated with untreated PKU."* Babies that are home from the hospital before 24 hours of age should be rescreened before the third week of life, since test results prior to this are unreliable. We recommend that you nurse your baby or cradle her during the heel prick.

As for the other routine procedures and interventions, we'd just as soon cram them into a barrel and send them down the River Lethe.

One father who would agree with us wrote:

Our son was suctioned and then given silver nitrate. He was shipped down to the

---

Pediatrics, 69 (1982), p. 104.

nursery. *Pat was wheeled into recovery. I spent the next several hours trying to get them together. I ran back and forth between the two of them. The nurse said he was cold and put him under lamps. She lanced his right heel to take a blood sample. She said he needed sugar water. I told her Pat was going to nurse and questioned whether sugar water was a good idea. She became defensive but didn't persist. On a subsequent visit, I noticed that two ounces of the glorious stuff was missing. The nurse also shot Andy's leg with vitamin K, adding, "All the babies get this now." Finally, he was returned to his mother.*

Childbirth educator Debra Evans writes: "Women are injured without being aware of the assault. Their babies are removed from their bodies, often surgically, and returned only at a suitable time. How this suitability is determined has little to do with how a mother feels and much to do with the efficiency of routinized institutional care. Why does it alarm us when mothers frequently feel detached from rather than attached to their offspring?"

Going Home ("Hate To Eat and Run . . .")

We recommend that you leave the hospital as soon as possible after your baby's birth (don't forget that baby needs to be in an approved car seat). It will help insure the least amount of trauma to your newborn. The less separation from your older children, as well, the more reassured and secure they will feel. If you remain in the hospital, we hope you have found one that encourages siblings and grandparents to visit. If not, you are in the wrong place. If you continue to give the institution your money, the policy will never change.

A Note about Breastfeeding

Being long-standing and staunch supporters of La Leche League, we cannot leave this chapter without mentioning to you that there are virtually hundreds of reasons to nurse your baby—and very few, if any, not to. All the values of breastfeeding have only begun to surface. Most of them we'll never even know, but they're there, in every drop.

Formula, cow's milk, is for *calves*! The most significant of the many differences between cow's milk and mother's milk appears to be the "abundant supply of nutrients most needed for the rapid growth and development of the central nervous system, including the brain," and its effectiveness in protecting the infant against infection. Yet, so many women in our culture refuse to nurse their infants.

The excuses women give ("My breasts are too big," "My breasts are too small,"

"My husband wants them for his own," "I didn't nurse my first and I don't want to play favorites," "I don't have the time") are supported by physicians, mostly male, who are often uncomfortable with the functional and nurturing aspects of breasts, and who prefer formula because they can control it. Mendelsohn points out that when babies are breastfed, doctors have nothing to treat. The nursing relationship is so intimate that many husbands, doctors, and women themselves feel puzzled or threatened by its intensity and move away from it. We must claim it, not reject it.

Let us not allow ourselves to schedule feedings or limit nursings the way our labors are scheduled and limited. Let's not permit artificial supplements into our babies' bodies the way artificial labor stimulants are pumped into our own. Let us allow our natural mothering hormones to flow as breastfeeding is established. Let's not leave our babies to cry, as many women are left during labor. Let's give our babies the very best we have to give. The very best does *not* come in bottles from an animal that has three stomachs, chews its cud, and says, "Moo."

Judicious Use of Medical Interventions

Normal, healthy women, with tubes coming out of their arms, belts wrapped around their bellies, catheters and electrodes hanging out of their vaginas—this must be a parody. Unfortunately, we have yet to find the humor.

This is not a book about necessary interventions. Any obstetrical text and many childbirth books will give you all the "reasons" to intervene. However, there are a few circumstances when intervention can be useful. For example, if a woman is at eight or nine centimeters for several hours, rupturing the membranes may help. Sometimes a catheter is beneficial. Once in a blue moon a fetal monitor is useful. (Once you've got the information you need, take the thing off!) If labor has been going on for hours and hours, and the woman is unable to sleep, a narcotic may be considered. Pitocin is occasionally helpful; in certain situations it prevents cesareans by aiding uterine contractility or prevents hemorrhage postpartum. Maltau and Anderson[141] report that an epidural block tends to restore uterine contractility in prolonged exhaustive labor. (We are reminded of a situation involving a woman in our area. Upon examination at her 40th week checkup, it was determined that her baby's arm was resting over his head: a "compound presentation." The doctor told her it would be dangerous to go into labor. She went to the hospital and was anesthetized for a cesarean. The doctor did a vaginal exam in the operating room just before the cesarean and remarked that the baby's arm had slid down into position: only the head was presenting. He said, "You are here, you might as well have your baby."

The woman, a nurse, agreed. She called us two weeks later. "I could kill myself," she said. "I could have waited until the anesthesia wore off, gone home, and had my VBAC. It was hard to think clearly strapped to a table in the hospital!" If you do have an epidural or spinal, make certain your doctor checks to see if "things" have changed. You might be able to have a safe vaginal birth.) In Maltau and Anderson's study, nine women considered for cesarean section delivered vaginally after pain relief and oxytocin infusion.

Sometimes a baby needs to be born quickly. Forceps or an episiotomy may be necessary. (We are told that vacuum extractors, rather than forceps, are the latest rage in birthing. Babies can now be sucked out, as well as pulled out.) Once in a while the cord needs to be cut quickly; for example, if it is too short or is too tightly wrapped around the baby's neck. These interventions exist for the infrequent situations when nature needs an assist. Occasionally, once in a while, infrequently—not routinely—each medical or obstetrical procedure has a place at a birth.

For the most part, however, we depend on trusted, knowledgeable individuals rather than technology at birth. A human ear to check the fetal heart. Human hands and minds to assess health, in conjunction with feelings and sensory judgments reported by each mother. Human hearts to trust in all of us, and in pregnancy as a state of *well*ness. When normal, healthy women say "no" to the purveyors of technology, the believers in machines, they say a confident and loving "yes" to themselves and their babies.

One physician remarks, "Everyone has their favorite interventions. Dr. A. insists upon I.V.s, but could care less about monitors. Dr. B. demands the use of monitors, but has a nonchalant attitude about I.V.s." Perhaps the dissension within the field will ultimately provide women with the fuel they need to refuse all but the most necessary interventions.

Why Reinvent the Wheel?

> Let it be, let it be
> Let it be, let it be
> Whispered words of wisdom:
> Let it be.
>
> —J. Lennon and P. McCartney

Many years ago, Oliver Wendell Holmes, Sr., speaking of the woman in childbirth, said, "God forbid that any member of the profession to which she trusts her life, doubly precious at that eventful period, should hazard it negligently, unadvisedly, or selfishly." Before him Dr. Delee remarked that the first stage of labor is one of "watchful expectancy." The duty of the attendant, he said, is "to observe the efforts of Nature, not to aid. There is nothing so reprehensible as meddlesome midwifery." How unfortunate that their wise words have reached mostly closed ears in our culture.

We received the following letter from a man in Canada:

> Despite my objections, the doctor performed all of the following on my wife: I.V., rupture of membranes, internal fetal monitor, catheter, oxytocin, stirrups, and episiotomy. However, thank goodness, there was no pubic shaving and no enema, so we avoided some interventions! We were told our babies can easily die if they are not electronically monitored. We were told that the membranes have to be ruptured in order for any progress to be made and to stop being stubborn.

Later in his letter, this husband went on to say, "A c/sec is one of the worst mutilations that can be perpetrated on a woman, as well as a denial of a fundamental right of a woman to experience childbirth." Although his wife managed to have a VBAC, we assert that the management of her labor was dangerous and disgraceful; like many women in our culture, she was denied the right to experience childbirth. How sad that their obstetrician was unable to appreciate and observe natural processes.

On her recent trip to the Orient, Doris Haire visited many maternity facilities. "I was heartened to find that by minimizing obstetrical intervention, the Japanese Red Cross Medical Center in Tokyo have reduced their cesarean rate from 15 percent to 6 percent," she said. WHEN ARE WE GOING TO MINIMIZE OBSTETRICAL INTERVENTION? In the name of our precious unborn: WHEN? When are we going to "dispel the massive ignorance and crippling fear concerning the human experience of birth"?*

In his book *Mal(e) Practice*, Robert Mendelsohn tells us that doctors know they can't afford to allow women to perceive childbirth as the normal, typically uncomplicated process that it is. "If they did, women wouldn't need obstetricians."[165] Professor G. J. Kloosterman, chairman of the department of obstetrics of the University of Amsterdam, has said, "The spontaneous labor in a healthy woman is an event marked by a number of processes so complex and so perfectly attuned to each other, that any interference will only distract from their optimal character. The attendant must comply with the first rule of medicine, that of 'nil nocere': injure nothing" (p. 203).[1] Most doctors, always on the lookout for pathology and eager to interfere, too often change true physiologic aspects of human reproduction into pathology, says Kloosterman. Is anyone within the medical establishment listening to these people?

In *A Woman in Residence*,† Dr. Michelle Harrison writes that the sacred act of birthing has been turned into an ugly ritual because of the attitudes with which birth is viewed. "It's like considering the beauty of those moments when

---

*Marilyn Moran, in *New Nativity Newsletter*, no. 21, 1982, p. 1.
†New York: Random House, 1982.

sexuality takes on a spiritual quality and comparing that with . . . pornography" (p. 111).

In *Safe Alternatives in Childbirth*,[149] we are told that natural delivery has had the longest clinical test of any procedure in obstetrics. (Why re-invent the wheel?" asks CPM director Esther Zorn.) Most doctors don't want to hear that, though; they are too busy rupturing membranes, prescribing drugs, and using their instruments. It is our responsibility as women to hear it, to believe it, to know it. It is our challenge to open others' ears.

Childbirth educator Debra Evans tells us that we now have many men who study birth from a variety of perspectives, but who all lack the principal vantage point, the ability to give birth themselves. They attempt to eliminate the hazards of birth and to minimize the risks. They are given fantastic sums of money for doing so. "These men dictate the terms of birth and control the passage of women through territory that is uniquely feminine. It is sheer folly! *How did we ever allow this to happen?*"†

In *Of Woman Born* Adrienne Rich warns us that as long as birth remains an experience of passively handing over our minds and our bodies to male authority and technology, other kinds of social change can only minimally change our relationships to ourselves, to power, and to the world outside our babies.[209] As long as we continue to internalize the physicians' view of birth as unclean and unsafe, and women and babies as unfit, our relationship to the birth process will be sorely affected. More significantly, our babies' health and well-being will continue to be severely affected.

In "The Hazards of Hospital Childbirth," Robbi Pfeuffer reminds us that one routine after another is established because more often than not they rely on each other to be effective.[208] *Let us not start a chain of events that we cannot stop.* Lester Hazell, author of *Commonsense Childbirth*, tells us that it is the mother who will live with the results of her choices about birth, whether they are ethical, spiritual or produce a nightmare. This is so, she says, whether the mother is conscious of it or not.[205] It is also *the child* who will live with the results. *So let us be conscious. Let us not produce nightmares.* Let us resort to assistances only when their uses are truly warranted. The quality of the life we create and bear depends on it.

---

†*ICEA Sharing*, 8 (Jan. 1981).

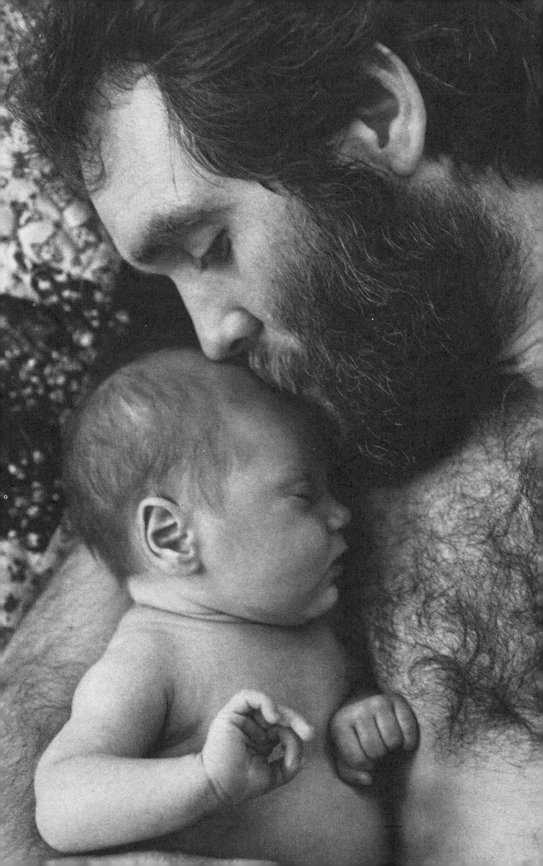

10 ❧ Paternal Perspectives

Since it is not within the scope of our book to analyze or report in any great detail the reaction of many numbers of cesarean fathers to cesarean section or VBAC, we will offer you instead two individual birth stories through the eyes of two cesarean/VBAC men—our husbands.

Paul's Story

On June 17, 1972, *several men were caught breaking into the Democratic National Headquarters at Watergate, while our son was being born by cesarean section. In their own ways, both of these events would shake this country. The fallout from Watergate has settled, but the effect our son's birth had on obstetrics as practiced in America has only just begun.*

It wasn't supposed to happen this way. We were supposed to be together. We had gone to our classes and had practiced our breathing. Nancy was healthy and her pregnancy was fine. So why was she upstairs on an operating table alone? Why was I downstairs pacing in the father's waiting room? I was totally unprepared for this unexpected separation.

I felt frustrated, angry, and betrayed. As a dental student, I had performed oral surgery, been present in operating rooms, and been taught by the medical school faculty. I knew the language. I was almost a member of "the club." Why was I being excluded now?

I felt like a failure. I had let Nancy down. Nancy had depended upon me emotionally. She had wanted me to be with her as our baby was born. She needed my physical presence as well as my emotional support. She wanted me to hold her hand and tell her everything would be okay. But I felt I had no choice but to leave.

211

So there I was pacing in the father's waiting room. I was trembling and scared. I was even crying (secretly so no one would notice). I felt very lonely. I had been suddenly and forcefully banished from my child's birth. No one was there to reassure me, console me, or explain to me what was happening upstairs. The hour I spent seemed like ten.

I felt guilty being downstairs while my wife was on the operating table. It should have been me, I thought. I was better suited psychologically to accept the surgery.

When I did get the call from the doctor, the emotional roller coaster started. In an instant, the stressful exhaustion of the previous hour was replaced by joyous anticipation and relief. My adrenalin was pumping as I raced upstairs to see Nancy. I found her outside of the operating room on the way to recovery. I was so relieved to see her, and to see that she was healthy. Now I could calm down.

Nancy told me we had a son. A SON!!! I had a son!!! I was delirious with happiness. My tears of fear and concern were replaced by tears of joy.

I vaguely remember Nancy saying something else before she was wheeled to recovery. She said that the cesarean was unnecessary . . .

I raced to special-care nursery. Why was my son in the special-care nursery? Was something wrong? The nurses assured me that it was routine procedure for all cesarean deliveries, and that my son was fine. I stared at him for the longest time. He was more than fine, he was perfect. As I gazed in amazement, I was in awe of this whole miraculous process of procreation. Nine months ago, my sperm and Nancy's egg met. Like magic. The product of that conception was now a perfectly formed newborn. I was so high, I had never felt like this before.

My wife and son were doing fine. Well, my son was doing fine (as fine as a baby can be without anyone to hold him, I think in retrospect). For some reason, Nancy was not nearly as excited as I was. Maybe this was the postpartum depression they talked about in class.

As time passed it was evident, even to a first-time parent, that Eric's birth had caused a scar in Nancy that would take longer to heal than the incisions in her uterus and abdominal wall. For reasons I did not understand at the time, Nancy could not be totally happy about the birth. I felt scared for her emotional well-being, and frustrated that I could not make it all better for her. I vascillated between wanting to support her concerns and questions about the birth, and being impatient with her prolonged depression.

When it was clear that Nancy was serious about questioning her obstetrician's management of her labor, I became very upset. How could she embarrass me by daring to disagree with THE DOCTOR? I was one year away from becoming one myself. Some of my basic courses were taught by the medical school faculty. The respect and prestige accorded to that title were part of what I was working so hard for. Indirectly I felt sabotaged when Nancy questioned the doctor. At this point in my life, I was a mere dental student looking up. I did not question authority or "make waves." Why couldn't my wife do the same and just accept her fate? It would make things easier on everyone else. (If she had, there would be no book to write.) I could not understand what was behind Nancy's obsession with this birth. Why could she not be satisfied to have a healthy son?

The next months were difficult for us sexually as well as emotionally. At first

Nancy was sore and weak from the surgery and tired from her new mothering responsibilities. She hated the scar. She was embarrassed at the sight of it, especially since she had been extensively shaved. I was afraid to touch her or approach her. But the more significant issues were not physical. After the scar healed and the pubic hair grew back we were still apart, as if a cloud hung over our relationship. Try as hard as we could, we could not reach the closeness we had shared in all the years before the birth. I felt confused, blamed, or in some way held responsible for Eric's birth because I had left Nancy alone. This question of physical and emotional support during labor became a crucial one at our next two births.

Nancy recognized that there was a limit to the depth of my understanding and patience with the issues surrounding Eric's birth. She sensed a frailty or weakness in my overall support for her. The level of trust between us was shaken somewhat. What pains me most was my passivity at this time. I was scared about what was happening to my wife and to us, but I did not do much to improve it. I tried to deny the problem rather than accepting it and working to solve it.

During the postpartum months, Nancy found solace and support from other cesarean mothers. Being involved with C/SEC helped both of us with our difficulties adjusting to the consequences of Eric's birth. With both mothers and fathers sharing, we gained support for our own postpartum problems and began to realize that our respective mate's reactions were not uncommon. I was very thankful that the organization gave to Nancy what I could not. It wasn't that I didn't love her or didn't care. But, for me, Eric's birth was separation, fear, relief, and then exhilaration. I had great difficulty understanding why what went on in the operating room was so upsetting to Nancy. Eric's birth was not something we shared together, but rather something we experienced separately, and perceived differently.

Our second pregnancy was clouded by the shadow of the cesarean and all its ramifications. Much of the time and effort was spent on arrangements for this birth, to make it as positive an experience as possible. We felt deprived of leisure time to enjoy the pregnancy. I felt irritated about the amount of time and money Nancy's commitment to helping other cesarean couples was taking away from us. We screened doctors, wrote letters, and had numerous discussions until the early hours of the morning. I was terrified at the severe depths of depression that would accompany another horrible birth experience. It was crucial to Nancy's mental health for her to be given every reasonable chance to birth this baby vaginally. Her self-esteem as a woman had been sorely challenged by the cesarean. Her obsession with having a VBAC was born out of self-preservation.

Part of what gave me some reassurance was the obstetrician's willingness (albeit reluctant) to allow Nancy a "trial" of labor. He stood to risk ridicule, as I did, if things did not go well.

I did a lot of soul searching. What finally convinced me to support VBAC was the strength of Nancy's obsession to avoid surgery. If it meant so much to her that she might be risking her life for it, I could not deny her my support—tentative as it was at first.

Distance became a problem for us. Support for a VBAC was nonexistent in Portsmouth, N.H. The closest acceptable doctor and hospital were 75 miles away in Boston, and I feared driving that distance while Nancy was in labor and having to deal with some complication I could not handle. As it happened, we were visiting in Boston when labor started. I was anxious and excited. All the efforts to make the best arrangements and to negotiate the most natural birth possible were behind us. The starter had fired the gun, and the "contest" had begun. No time outs. Ready or not, this was it!

Nancy called the doctor to tell him her labor had begun. He asked us to come into the hospital. When we got there he examined her and told her she was one to two centimeters dilated. He picked up the phone to call Admitting and tell them we needed a room. Nancy objected. She said we would go back to our friend's house for a while. In the car she told me "Last time we came in I was only one to two centimeters dilated. He got impatient, broke my water, and the whole zoo began." I wouldn't have suggested we go back to our friends', but I was glad that Nancy had the presence of mind to do so.

Several hours later the doctor called us. "Get in here," he said, "on the double!" Later we learned that he had received many negative comments from his peers. "What? She's had a previous cesarean and she's in labor at home?"

Entering the hospital produced a level of tension not present when Nancy was laboring in the comfort of our friends' home. The difference was support. There, Nancy and I had positive, loving support, and Eric was with us the whole day. At the hospital, we faced the pressure of having to show constant progress. One false move and Nancy would be in the O.R. again. We went from a loving and supportive atmosphere to one of doubt and fear. Would the doctor waver in his support and start to put limits on us? And if so, to what point could I resist him? How strong was his commitment to us now that we were in labor in the hospital rather than just talking in his office?

God was with us. In spite of all that was against us, Nancy finished transition with a healthy uterus and a healthy baby. At this point I didn't care how the baby was birthed, as long as the birth was nonsurgical and the baby was healthy.

I felt like celebrating. I sensed a sigh of relief and a lessening in the level of tension in the room. The obstetrician indicated that we had reached the point where the birth would be vaginal either with or without forceps. We had done it! Now the baby just slides out after a few pushes, right? Wrong! Nancy was told to push. She pushed for a few contractions. The doctor became impatient and I got nervous. He suggested a spinal and forceps. Anything was acceptable to me as long as it was nonsurgical. When we had reached the point where it was obvious this would be a VBAC, my expectations for this labor were realized. I had no motivation to question the doctor. We had been victorious. We had fought for something and we had won. I felt magnanimous in victory. As a result it made no difference to me if Nancy pushed the baby out or the doctor "did his thing." Unfortunately for Nancy and Elissa, I didn't protest. With the proper support from me and the nurses, Nancy could have avoided the anethesia and forceps.

Nancy was exhausted. She was told by a nurse (one chosen by the doctor) that she wasn't pushing well. She was flat on her back with the monitor wrapped around her and an I.V. sticking out of her arm. She hadn't eaten for 24 hours, since early labor had been ten hours, off and on. She had no energy or support to "fight to *the finish." As she was lifted onto another table to wait for the spinal to be administered, she got her first urge to push. I was in another room, dressing in my "greens." Nancy later told me that she became very excited and happy. She yelled, "I finally have the urge to push!!" The anesthesiologist and obstetrician disregarded her enthusiasm and within seconds she was totally anesthetized from her waist down.*

I entered the delivery room for the first time as an expectant father. I felt excited almost to the point of being giddy. I was going to witness the birth of my child. I did my homework. We passed all the tests. I deserved to be here. As I watched, a beautiful baby girl, Elissa Rachel, was born. A GIRL. A beautiful baby girl. I could not believe I could be so happy. Not only did we have a healthy baby, but she was a girl. There she was, the miracle of birth, and we were all together this time.

I experienced so many different emotions during this labor and delivery. Aside from the usual spectrum of feelings triggered by a successful birth, I had to deal with additional situations peculiar to this birth and its special circumstances. I had felt the pressure to "perform" perfectly. I questioned the amount of support our obstetrician would lend to us, if our labor did not progress properly or if it deviated from the norm. I felt pressure to succeed from those who knew we were trying. I felt pressure to succeed because trying to explain any complications or compromises to mother or baby, considering what we were trying, would have been humiliating. I could not bear to face the accusations of irresponsibility and foolishness I would be the target of if we failed. But we didn't fail, as far as I was concerned. We succeeded. We succeeded in a scope I could not fully appreciate at the time. I felt button-popping proud. I believed we had accomplished what we had set out to. We took a risk in that there were no footsteps to follow. We had to blaze the trail. We had to set the precedent. In this respect I felt like a pioneer. Also, I felt happy for those couples who would follow in our paths and be able to have a VBAC.

As revolutionary as this birth was, it was less than perfect. Although Nancy and I were physically together, we were not as close as we would have liked during labor. As a labor coach, I was a great disappointment. I felt very ineffective. I spent most of the time watching the fetal monitor, so I could warn Nancy when the next contraction was coming. Although I was holding her hand, I was focusing on the foolish machine, and not on my wife. I hadn't considered the problems the monitor might present. Not only did it immobilize Nancy, but it was also physically between us, making it difficult for me to be close to Nancy and look into her eyes. As a result, Nancy labored at arm's length, somewhat alone. We were both physically present for this birth, but we still were not emotionally together.

Nancy was fairly happy about the birth—for about two days. Then her anger and frustration began. She felt she had been abandoned at the very end. She had needed a little extra support to get the boat safely into port and no one was there to guide it. She had been grateful to the obstetrician for "allowing" us this experience, but became furious that, once again she "was delivered" of her infant. She hated the remarks the doctor made about tying her up "nice and tight" for a better sex life, after he had done a large episiotomy. She began to read about forceps and was appalled at how dangerous they were. She was furious that without our knowledge or informed consent, our daughter had been x-rayed after birth. Once again, my support vascillated between understanding and impatience.

Three and a-half years later, we experienced a Marriage Encounter weekend. We had had a very strong marriage, but M.E. helped to make it better. I learned not only to recognize, accept, and share my feelings, but also to accept Nancy's feelings without judging them. Although I may not have understood her feelings, I did respect Nancy's right to have them. The M.E. weekend and the time and effort we have put into our relationship since then have had a profound and long lasting effect.

It was only during the months after our M.E. weekend that I began to understand why Eric's birth had been—and was still—so devastating for Nancy. Working through what went wrong between us at the first two births was crucial for the success of the third birth.

At this time, I needed surgery for a hernia. I had never been operated on before. I wasn't the least bit nervous about it—until the night before the surgery. I began to worry that the anesthetic would never wear off and I'd be paralyzed. This fear seemed irrational but nevertheless, it existed. When the operation was over I tried desperately to move my legs. For a while I thought my worst fears had come true.

This experience gave me some insight into the helplessness and lack of control Nancy had felt during the births. It gave me some understanding for her feelings of fear about going under the knife and being anesthetized. I also had a sense for the physical pain encountered after a surgery—and I didn't have a baby to care for after my surgery, either.

Nancy's efforts in the area of childbirth had also benefitted me. I refused to go into the hospital the night before the surgery. I was at home in my own bed. We held each other. I also left the hospital within 24 hours of the surgery. The doctor was amazed. I questioned everything.

Our next pregnancy ended in miscarriage in the third month. The closeness we had maintained since our M.E. weekend helped us to deal with the frustration, helplessness, and pain. However, it took a while for Nancy to understand my reaction. I was more upset for her than for the lost pregnancy. During the first two pregnancies, I didn't begin to "feel pregnant" on a psychological level until the last trimester. Since the third pregnancy ended in the third month, I wasn't at the point where I felt a strong bond yet. It's not that I wasn't excited about the pregnancy; I was, and very much so. But I wasn't experiencing pregnancy on a physical level. As a result I had difficulty grieving.

The fourth pregnancy began with some apprehension. The fear of miscarriage seemed to follow us like a shadow those first few months. Fortunately, it never became more tangible than that—a fear, not a reality.

Nancy and I were concerned. The hospital policies in our area were less than acceptable. This would perhaps be our last pregnancy. We wanted no interventions, and we wanted our children present at the birth. There was difficulty finding a combination of doctor and hospital that suited our needs. I began to wonder if Nancy's reputation as a pioneer in childbirth had intimidated some people, making them less cooperative than they might be with someone else.

Not surprisingly, the question of a home birth appealed to Nancy. Most midwives at the time would not attend a woman with a previous cesarean. I did not take the idea of a home birth seriously until Nancy found a midwife who would support her at home. What kind of foolishness was this!? How irresponsible this was to our baby! Only two midwives in the whole area would agree to attend Nancy at home. How could Nancy think they were right and the others were wrong?

I was looking forward to meeting the midwife. I wanted to make her look foolish. There was no way she could answer my questions to my satisfaction . . . or so I thought. To my surprise, the midwife was very knowledgeable and professional. She calmly answered all my questions. Although I wasn't sold on a home birth after our first meeting, I agreed to consider it. We took home birth classes. I felt that the information would assist us in the hospital.

Two factors greatly influenced my feelings about a home birth: understanding Nancy's feelings about this birth and reading Immaculate Deception, by Suzanne Arms, and Spiritual Midwifery, by Ina May Gaskin. The communication skills we learned from M.E. helped me understand Nancy's fear about entering a hospital and thus losing control of the birth. Reading Immaculate Deception impressed upon me the remarkable difference between verbal and physical support, on the one hand, and medical intervention, on the other.

I came to believe that with loving support and a sense of confidence, Nancy would be better off birthing this baby at home. I was surprised that I had come to the point where I could consider having a baby without a doctor present. These feelings grew inside of me until I was more afraid of the hospital than of being at home. In fact, I became enthusiastic and excited about a home birth.

I was not surprised when the due date passed uneventfully. A week later, after two days of off-and-on contractions, my enthusiasm was being overshadowed by impatience. (Thank goodness Nancy knew she could eat—she'd have starved herself and the baby if she had listened to a doctor's orders and stopped eating at the first sign of labor.) Late Saturday night when the water broke, labor began and then shifted into high gear. It happened so quickly, so smoothly, it was incredible. 1-2-3, a baby! What a baby! What a birth! Here in the very bed in which she was conceived, and in the presence of her brother and sister, Andrea Jill was born.

I felt so close to Nancy. We shared this together. I felt so good that during the labor I held her and she held me. I felt so proud and happy that we birthed Andrea with no medications or intervention whatsoever and that we were all present to greet her. It was the best birthday gift we could give her. I felt proud that we had worked for this and achieved it, in spite of the general lack of support we encountered (but we were used to that already). I felt proud of the beautiful and positive experience we had shared with Eric and Elissa.

I was impressed by our midwife's calm and support. I knew that if we needed any assistance, she had the necessary skills and expertise. She supported Nancy and me, and let Nancy's body do the work.

I felt close to Nancy because this was the first birth during which I did not let her down. I supported her during the whole labor. We had shared what each of us needed from this labor beforehand. Together, we birthed our daughter in the love and security of our home, with our other children and our friends close by. I felt *proud of the step we had taken for all VBAC couples. Before labor, my thoughts were not about this larger issue at all. As the significance of Andrea's birth struck me, I realized how monumental an event this was: to think that a woman with a previous cesarean not only delivered vaginally, but at home.*

I feel a great sense of pride and accomplishment for the positive steps we took. We worked hard to improve our postcesarean births, and we succeeded. But I can't take any credit as an innovator. If we had had to depend on my assertiveness and initiative to affect change, we would have had three cesareans. Nancy was the motivator. Her indominable will, perseverance, and unwillingness to let her scar condemn her to a lifetime of surgical births fueled our efforts.

I am very fortunate to have three wonderful children who entered this world their own unique ways. I love them very much and will always remember each of their births as very special times in my life. As a result of all that I have experienced in the past ten years, I have some observations about childbirth that I would like to share.

I have gained enormous respect for birth as a natural and miraculous process, not to be tampered with lightly. I have come to more fully appreciate the female anatomy which is ingeniously designed to nourish, support, and then deliver the baby without fancy machines or equipment. I have come to believe that babies benefit most from a pure, unaltered birth. I have come to recognize that the husband's role during labor is to love and support his wife. This can be effectively done only when the man trusts in the natural process of labor and lets go of any fear he may have of it. I believe that men have a right to be at their children's births. I have come to know that they, as well as women, need support during labor. I have learned that it is important to set a goal but to recognize that there may be many different paths that lead to it. Finally I have come to question why is it that in America skilled surgeons manage the births of healthy women.

In the wake of Watergate, the American people saw how power corrupts and destroys the integrity of once respectable men. Watergate caused our country to reevaluate the questionable morality that fostered such a shameful scandal. Certainly birthing couples will soon begin to question the dramatic number of cesarean sections that are being performed on healthy women. They will begin to reevaluate the attitudes and procedures that foster this other shameful scandal.

Martin's Story

Until the time of our second pregnancy, I never would have considered myself to be a good prospect for VBAC fatherhood.

When our first daughter was born by cesarean section, the method of delivery did not upset me. Instead, my overall feeling was a high-level excitement. It was a peak experience. Holding my beautiful ten-minute-old baby girl in my arms while we stared into each other's eyes remains one of the greatest moments of my life. I never knew I could love so much or so freely. I was in another world.

It is hard for me to believe that only seconds earlier I had been infuriated. The *operation had not gone well. We had gone to the hospital much too early, and Lois had been subjected to all the usual interventions—I.V., external fetal monitor, hospital jonnie, hospital bed, no food, no water, countless internal exams, countless nurses, interns, residents; plus, after nine hours of "uneventful" labor, Pitocin; and, after three more hours, anesthesia—an epidural.*

Throughout all of these interventions, I remained very accepting, reasonably calm, and respectfully cooperative. I did become very concerned and worried during the three hours between the commencement of Pitocin and the administering of the epidural. I am convinced that it is a rare woman who can tolerate Pitocin without anesthesia. Once the "pit" was on, we kissed our childbirth education course goodbye.

But Jordana was breech, and thus there was some cause for concern. I knew that the delivery could be complicated. Even more problematic was the fact that Jordana had not dropped into the birth canal. So at about 1:00 A.M., after we had been at the hospital for almost fifteen hours, it was decided that it was time for the final intervention—cesarean section. It is interesting to note that the reason for the cesarean is officially listed in our medical records as "uterine inertia" rather than "breech."

I suspect that the epidural had left a "window." Lois had great pain during the operation. In the operating room, I was the only one who noticed. Finally, I advised the anesthesiologist, who was looking intensely at all his dials and screens and other paraphernalia. He had never noticed that Lois was in pain. I was enraged. Perhaps he had forgotten that all those mechanical marvels were connected to a human being. My fury found my tongue. My punishment was to be summarily evicted. Lois was given a dose of something that knocked her out, and she never knew that I had left.

It was then that I was given Jordana to hold.

The emotional flip-flop from anger to adoration was so intense and so lasting that the events in the operating room suddenly became unreal. It was as if I had been watching a movie of someone else's cesarean. I suddenly became detached from the whole procedure and still am. Since then, I have never again been angry about anything that had to do with Jordana's birth.

Lois was not upset either. Like me, she pretty much forgot about the birth as soon as she got her hands on Jordana. The important thing was that we had a beautiful, healthy baby. I still believe that.

But I did feel just a bit disappointed. I had failed as a "coach." Maybe if I hadn't been so compliant, I thought, it would have been different. Yet I didn't really believe that. It felt as though we had really practiced and trained for the big game only to find that the other team was just too good. We were beaten. In fact, they whupped us pretty good. Before the birth, we had defined failure as merely needing anesthesia. Having a cesarean made for a very lop-sided score.

I really did not carry my disappointment around with me very long. I was thrilled to be a father. I have never in my life been more obnoxiously boring, telling everyone about my baby as if in the course of human history this were the first time a man and a woman had produced offspring.

I gave the whole matter of the delivery very little further thought until Lois became pregnant again and mentioned to me that she was thinking about not having a second cesarean. "What?! Are you mad? You want to die? That's great, leave me here with Jordana and maybe even another child, and you'll be quite dead. No, thank you, dear. Forget it."

I was not open to it. Actually, I was frightened. But it was a fear born of ignorance. All I had heard was, "Once a cesarean, always a cesarean." I was afraid that labor would cause the uterine scar to rupture. I had a picture of Lois's insides exploding. I pictured her blood and guts flying around in a twenty-foot radius like something out of a Grade B war movie.

In fact, like most cesarean fathers, I did not know the first thing about uterine rupture or VBAC. But I have always been willing to learn. After some preliminary research and much discussion, Lois suggested that we take Nancy's course on VBAC. I agreed, and it proved to be an amazing education.

Nancy had done her homework. She had the facts and figures—she'd read every available bit of research. She debunked the myths, and she assuaged my concerns.

I did some studying on my own, and my mind was changed. We were going VBAC. Now I was excited. I knew that we were in the vanguard of VBAC, and that the doctors and hospitals were not necessarily going to be all that supportive.

We prepared. We had already changed doctors; now we engaged a labor assistant. After a while, the rightness of VBAC gave me so much confidence that I was really looking forward to the birth.

On Hillary's own chosen birthdate, at 5:00 A.M., I awoke to find that Lois had been up for a while with mild contractions. Neither of us was ready to accept that she was laboring. First, she was eleven days early (according to the prediction); second, our labor assistant was on vacation; third, we knew that our doctor's brand-new associate, rather than our chosen physician himself, would be the one on call at the hospital that day. Because of our prior experience (26 hours of labor culminating in a cesarean section), we were reluctant to leave home too soon. By 9:00 A.M., however, it was clear that Hillary was soon to introduce herself to us. A quick call to the doctor and a less than placid ride to the hospital put us in the delivery room by 10:00 A.M. From that point forward, it was easy. Lois was ready.She pushed once, and we discovered that even though the baby's head was crowning, Lois's waters had not broken. Our doctor broke the waters (Intervention #1). A couple more pushes, and there was significant crowning. The doctor prepared to anesthetize Lois for an episiotomy. I questioned this, as we had specifically stated that there was to be no routine episiotomy. He reacted as if I had insulted his honor. "I'm not going to argue with you," was his tone. I remembered how I had been ejected from the delivery room last time, and I was intimidated into compliance. The doctor's argument was that there was meconium in the amniotic fluid and that this posed a risk of blockage of the breathing passages. I have since learned that this is a low-risk concern. My opinion is that this doctor may not have known how to allow a baby to be born vaginally without an episiotomy. What little I know of evolutionary theory proscribes a reasonable belief that within the last 25 years, women's vaginas have become so small that they are now unable to expel an eight- or nine-pound baby without being cut wide open. Obviously, it can be done.

Nevertheless, the episiotomy was performed (Intervention #2). Quite expectedly, Hillary popped right out, and the average Little League shortstop could have caught her. Her cord was cut, and she was immediately given to the pediatricians (Intervention #3) to suction the meconium, if any, from her breathing passages. She could at least have been shown to Lois and me for a second. Ultimately, we got our Hillary about ten minutes (it seemed an eternity) after her birth.

I suppose we did win this time. We got knocked around a little bit. There were interventions, despite our vigilance and the fact that we were well prepared and well informed. It is no wonder that the cesarean rate is so high. The uninformed are like so many cattle being herded through the O.R. rooms. At least, Hillary was born vaginally—our VBAC baby.

I was left with extremely mixed feelings. I was happy that we had avoided the cesarean. But I was sad, and still am, that so much of my emotional energy had to be expended trying to guard against medical interventions. Parents in the process of giving birth should be allowed to focus on the glory of the miracle that is birth. Instead, we must be alert and vigilant lest the birth be taken from us.This is wrong. The obstetrical profession has, in large part, forgotten that its purpose is to serve people. Physicians often seem more interested in medical high technology and as-sembly-line productivity than in the people who are in their care. They have created a monopoly of control over the birthing process. This must stop, and a duty of utmost good faith to birthing couples must be imposed on the obstetricians, so that they are required to be not only competent but honest. We must stop letting other people "deliver" our babies. Parents must reclaim what is a fundamental right: the right to give birth.

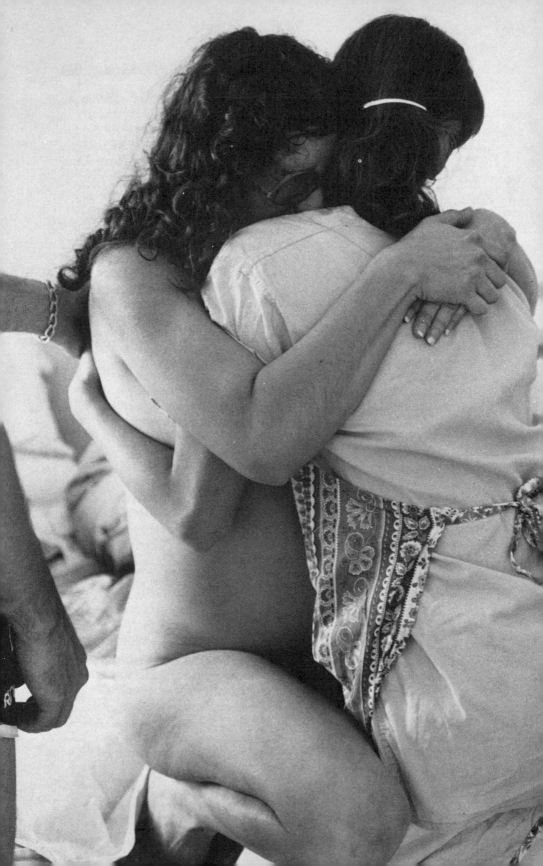

11 ❧ Labor Support

From writer Ellen Goodman's column in the *Boston Globe*, September 16, 1980:

> It seems that no less than five medical doctors, all specialists, working with grants from two foundations and the Public Health Service, have startled the medical world with the following information: It's better for women not to go though labor alone.
>
> **STOP THE PRESSES.**
>
> To arrive at this blockbuster of a notion, the men traveled to a hospital in Guatemala. . . .[and found that] women assigned a companion got through labor and delivery more easily than women alone and had a better attitude toward their babies. . . . So, in a truly risky conclusion, the obstetrical quintet said, "The findings of this study SUGGEST the importance of human companionship during labor and delivery . . ."

Ms. Goodman went on to say that although she does not doubt the sincerity of the doctors, their findings aren't exactly fresh information. "It seems to me," she said, "that these men could have gone onto the streets of Cleveland, whence they cometh, walked up to the first two dozen women they met and asked them, 'Would you feel better going into labor alone or with someone holding your hand?' "

"The Climb"

In previous chapters we have likened giving birth to running a marathon and swimming an Olympic race. Now, we'd like you to take a little analogous mountain climb with us . . .

223

The sky is a deep, cloudless blue. The sun is shining brightly. It's a *perfect* day for mountain climbing! You and your mate pack up your backpacks. You arrive at the foot of the mountain. "We'll get to the top in a jiffy," you tell each other, "and then we'll have a marvelous picnic lunch."

Hey! This is terrific. Nothing to it. A nice trail, the clean fresh scent of woods and pine, a few little babbling brooks. Neato! "Should have done this much sooner. Can't fathom why we've put it off," you tell your spouse.

An hour later the trail becomes a little less defined and you notice that you are definitely *ascending*. "I'm tough," you think. "I can handle this." You look at your spouse climbing with vim and vigor. "The rat. Well, I can keep up with him," you think. "What a show-off!"

Later, you decide to stop and rest for a bit. As you rest, you begin to think what a sissy you are. Two hours, and already you're wishing you could turn back. Where's your sense of adventure and excitement?

With renewed enthusiasm, you start up again. It's getting a little chilly. The beautiful blue—well, blue-gray—sky is still overhead. "Hey, where's the sun?" you groan. No problem, it can't be behind that cloud for more than a minute. The climb is getting steeper. This isn't as easy as you imagined it would be. Your legs are *killing* you. There are aches in muscles you never knew you had. The trees are thick, and you can hardly see the sky. "This is stupid, let's turn back," you think. "No, he'll never let me live it down! To the top!"

Rain comes pouring down. It's become so steep that you begin to lose your footing. You'll have to find cover, but where? At this point, both of you are not only wet and tired, but scared. The thunder and lightning are terrifying. The wind is awesomely powerful.

You are scared. How could a simple holiday turn into such a nightmare? It was silly to begin a mountain this steep. This one isn't for amateurs. People have killed themselves climbing mountains, you recall.

Grasping each other tightly, you resume your climb. If you thought it was steep before, you hadn't seen anything. Step by step you ascend. You are tired, scared, hungry. You are also determined. Your hearts are beating rapidly, and you have some difficulty breathing. You can't speak, so you communicate with your eyes. Every muscle in your bodies is working. You are past the point of pain. You tread on a patch of earth that doesn't hold, and you lose your balance. But step by step, you climb toward the top. Finally? Yes! There it is! The clearing that marks the summit. You run the last 50 yards straight to the top and then fall down from exhaustion.

You lie there for a moment, gasping. You take a deep breath and open your eyes. You *can't believe* what you see. The sun is shining in all her warmth and glory. You are above the clouds, and the sky is blue. Not blue, azure. Sparkling. You can see for miles and miles and miles. The view is *breathtaking*! Magnificent! Incredible! Powerful! Overwhelming! The colors, oh, the colors! Vibrant!

Clear! There isn't a picture postcard or a poster in all the world that comes close to portraying this view. You look at each other. There are no words. They aren't needed.

You know that in this experience you have grown. You are grateful, proud, exhilarated. You have an incredible sense of wonder and pride, and you feel at one with nature and God and all of the universe! You did it! You feel closer to each other than ever before. You climbed the mountain!

*   *   *

If giving birth is like climbing a mountain, being sectioned is like being dropped off on the top of the mountain by helicopter. The view is the same, but for most women it *feels* different. It's still beautiful, but not the beautiful that puts goose bumps on your skin. The exhilaration is there, but its edges are fuzzy. The colors are lovely but a bit pale. The sun is bright but not nearly as warm as you had imagined . . .

What is different about the view is *the participation in the climb*. The sense of accomplishment and pride that accompanies a difficult task is missing. The "We did it, we really did it!" feeling. The wanting to shout to the world, "Go climb that mountain! It's *incredible* up there!"

Unfortunately, many couples birthing in hospitals do not make it to the top of the mountain on their own. They run into too many misplaced streams, thunderclouds, high winds, rocky terrains, fallen limbs, and grizzly bears. They often end up hitching a ride on the helicopter.

The Climb—with Help

We know that inviting a labor assistant or labor advocate (L.A.) of your own choosing to your birth can help you get to the top of the mountain. In other cultures, when a woman gives birth, she is surrounded by familiar, trusted, loving faces. Other women, schooled in birthing, hold her, talk to her, and guide her through delivery. Studies have shown that the incidence of natural birth increases with loving, caring, confident support. Yet, in our culture, we are often left alone, or surrounded by people we don't know.

Having with you someone who has climbed the mountain before, or someone who can tell you which path to take in order to see the best possible view, greatly enhances the experience. You need someone who is familiar enough with the climb to inspire your trust so that you can forge on ahead; someone to check weather conditions while you rest, or talk, or cuddle together. You need someone who can tell you where to put your foot so that you won't lose your footing; someone to guide you as you climb. You need someone who will say, "Shhh. . .look *quietly* over there; see, there's a mother deer and her fawn!" And, "Behind those bushes there's a beautiful spot for resting." Most people are so intent on the climbing that they lose sight of their goal and miss much of the intriguing scenery along the way.

The couple in our story grew, but their growth was the result of fear and tension. We prefer that *you* grow out of *love* and harmony. It's hard to maintain support when you are cold, tired, hungry, unsure, and scared. During labor, both man and woman need support. Often, they cannot offer support, each to the other, because their own wells are dry.

"No Drugs—Just Hugs!"

Labor is a time of great strength, but also great vulnerability. The strongest woman can lose just enough of her "centeredness" if she is led to believe that her baby is in jeopardy. If she is told her labor isn't working well, it is difficult to remain in a positive mindset and to continue flowing with contractions. Without support and encouragement, it's easy to lose confidence in your body.

When a woman is begging for medication during labor, we believe she is really asking for support. She wants information that what is happening to her is okay. She wants reassurance that the pain she's feeling is normal and that she's not alone. She wants a loving touch from someone, and eye contact. She wants someone to remind her that she's strong and healthy and there's a baby coming! She wants suggestions to make her labor more relaxed. She needs, perhaps, a change of scenery or a change in position. She needs to know how much she's loved. She needs to know at what point she is on her mountain climb: if she's asking for medication, chances are she's getting near the top. Remind her of the view that awaits her! She needs to be reminded that every wave comes to shore and that this contraction has an end as well. She needs to be reminded to take each contraction one by one. That's all she needs to do. Thinking about the next five contractions can be overwhelming and defeating.

Perhaps she needs to be reminded that every contraction brings her one step closer to her baby. Perhaps she needs to laugh a bit—this is a BIRTHDAY PARTY! Perhaps she needs gentle reminding to keep her mouth and throat loose—this will help her vagina open.

A woman needs to be in an environment where she (and her mate) can feel uninhibited and where everyone present respects birth and feels comfortable with it as an intimate expression of human sexuality. (Interesting to see how quickly the room clears when a laboring woman is really "loved up" by her man. Jerry said, "All I had to do was start licking her ear or rubbing her thighs suggestively, and we were all-of-a-sudden completely alone!")

She needs to be in an environment that appreciates the beauty and strength and power in her body and flows with it. She needs an environment that says "yes" to her labor. She needs to know that there is someone who will help insure the best environment for her particular birth.

Some couples feel threatened by having an L.A. They disdain intruders in their private experience. They want to do it themselves. They think it won't be the same if someone has to help. One cesarean father said, "I didn't help her enough last time. This time I'm going to fight tooth and nail. We're going to do it by ourselves this time."

Birth should not have to be a time of war. It is, or should be, a time of energy and peace. Anger and hostility produce tension in a women and make it difficult for her body to work effectively. The father should not have to be "on guard." His energies should be directed toward loving and supporting the mother, not patroling the whole mountain. It's difficult to be peaceful and totally supportive if you are waiting for someone to knife you in the—um—belly.

A good L.A. is like a rainbow: illuminating and beautifying nature—from a distance. Oftentimes, you hardly know she's there. Her roles vary. Sometimes she is very active; other times, she is not. She can be an advocate for the couple, a protector, or a caring *"significant* other." Her presence alone can minimize the probability of unnecessary outside technological and psychological interferences or stresses. She is no stranger or intruder into the birth experience, but someone who is known to you long before labor begins, chosen by you, and welcomed by you.

Although there are exceptions, an L.A. is generally not a friend. She is not a relative, and certainly not male. She is someone who is knowledgeable about birth, is objective, and is *not* associated with the hospital or physician. She is someone who is a staunch advocate of cesarean prevention and VBAC.

Remember, she is not a "coach" who is criticizing your performance. An L.A. may very well stand at the sideline, but only to give the "team" plenty of love, and occasional drink, and oodles of moral support.

An L.A. does not "coach." A coach sits on the sidelines and yells at the team. He tells the players what they are doing wrong. Women in labor don't do anything wrong. They do the best they can. They give it their all. An L.A. assesses the labor and accepts what a woman and her mate are doing. If it helps them, she supports it. If something else might assist them, she suggests it. She helps the woman find *her own* strength and coping abilities. If that strength and coping are already *present*, she gracefully fades into the background.*

An L.A. is usually someone who has had a baby naturally, although this isn't absolutely necessary. Some of the most sensitive L.A.s have not had a purebirth experience. They remark, "It feels good to help others do what I didn't." Linda,

---

*From a lecture on labor support given by Elizabeth Shearer in Boston in May 1981.

an L.A. from New York and cesarean mother of three, says, "I can help women by pointing out *my* mistakes!" L.A.s are committed to safe, personal, joyous, purebirths for as many families as possible.

Why Not the Hospital Staff?

There is no guarantee that the nurse assigned to you in the hospital will share your deep commitment to noninterventive birthing. On the contrary, there is a good chance that she will not. You can always ask for another nurse, but if it's a busy night on the floor and everyone else is occupied, no one else may be available. You may have absolutely no "reason" to want a particular individual to leave; you just do! You need no reason. This is *your* child's birthday party and *you* make out the guest list. Maybe the nurse reminds you of your Aunt Winifred, and Aunt Winifred hates kids. Maybe you just don't like her touch or her voice.

You may find yourself surrounded by supportive, loving nurses. However, at 11:00, when the shifts change, a whole new crew arrives. If you are well established in labor, those first-shift nurses might choose to stay by your side, but if it looks as if it's an hour or more to delivery, most will elect to leave. Their job will be waiting the next day; their commitment to you is temporary.

An L.A., on the other hand, will be there for you no matter how long your labor may be. When someone whom you have begun to trust ups and leaves while you're in active labor, it can be very disconcerting. No laboring woman should have to be introduced to new faces during her labor and birth. Energy in the room changes as new individuals come and go; you should not have to be concerned with negative energies, no matter how fleeting.

You are not even guaranteed that your physician will be at your birth. Nancy's back-up physician was called out of town only days before her due date: his father had died. Lois's physician took on a new associate just before she was due, and it was his "turn" when the big day arrived. Your physician's back-up may not share your concern about interferences. He may not be as comfortable with VBAC as your own doctor. At the very least, he won't be as emotionally invested in your birth. It could be that he's a terrific guy, but maybe he's clean-shaven and you only trust men with beards!

Hospitals that don't "permit" an L.A. obviously don't understand or care about the laboring woman. To deprive her of an L.A. of her own choosing, someone she has met prior to the labor and with whom she feels trusting, confident, and released, is a clear statement by the hospital: We are in control here, thank you, and we shall manage your birth on *our* terms! It also suggests a total lack of understanding about birth as a time of nurturing, of strength drawn from established relationships. It speaks of the hospital's power and control over the woman. By preventing that one person, or those several people, whose presence could do more than any drug ever marketed to maintain the woman's sense of security and well-being, they strip her of her rights, her strengths, her adulthood. Once again, hospital rules such as this are actually rites of initiation: the woman becomes a pliant patient, doing what she is told by *hospital* personnel.

By causing the woman tension, hospital policies also hurt the baby. They contribute to the number of labors that require drugs. Of course, the more chemicals, drugs, and equipment you use, the longer your hospital stay, and the easier it is for the hospital to pay its bills. Hospitals have an interest in *not* supporting natural birthing.

We repeat: An L.A. is not associated with the hospital or the doctor. If she is associated with a particular doctor and hospital and then contradicts them, she might lose her job. For example, if the doctor restricts mobility and orders a fetal monitor and she's depending on him for her paycheck, she'll have to support his orders. As one nurse said, "I live in a small town. There's only one hospital. If I lose my job, my children will go shoeless. But every time I hook up an I.V. to a healthy laboring woman, I cringe. The I.V. is just the first of a whole series of procedures I'm *ordered* to do." Fortunately, more and more nurses are confronting their fears of antagonizing doctors, and reversing their loyalties: what is *safest* for birthing women and their infants is taking precedence over blind submission to *doctor's orders*. From one enlightened nursing staff: "No more routine enemas, preps, and I.V.s. Next, we pull the monitors!" There is strength in numbers.

Another important consideration: a nurse affiliated with a particular doctor or hospital is rarely free to be with you at your home. An L.A. will come to your home when you are ready for her support, to wait with you until your labor becomes strong and active and you are ready to be in the hospital. Together, as a team, you go to the hospital. She bears no allegiance to a particular doctor or hospital. She is *for you*.

Mates as Labor Assistants?

A woman looks around during labor, sees her husband—occasionally exhausted and often pale green—and hears, "It's okay, honey. You're fine. Everything is just fine." Then she sees her doctor—usually male—and hears: "You're about seven centimeters dilated, Mrs. H. Everything looks all right up to this point."

She wants to believe them; after all, she loves her husband and she trusts her doctor. But something deep inside her says, "Wait! How do *they* know this is all right? This kind of pain couldn't possibly be fine! Neither one of them has ever had a baby!" She begins to feel mistrusting, frightened, and very alone.

When another woman, whom she has chosen, and whom she trusts, who knows about and has personally experienced birth, wraps her arms around her, puts her nose up to her face, looks into her eyes, and says softly, "I *know* what you are feeling. I *know* it's overwhelming and that it hurts so much you feel swept away by it. But it really *is* fine. Your body is working exactly as it is supposed to," there is a sense of trust and relief. She's been there. She *knows*.

In "Studying Childbirth: The Experience and Methods of a Woman Anthropologist," Brigette Jordan remarks that women bring their female bodies and experience as childbearers to birth. She states that regardless of the number of births observed or technical expertise acquired, regardless of any amount of empathy men may feel with women in the throes of labor, "in fundamental ways they cannot know what the experience is like." She believes that women experience a "physiological synchrony," a "collaborative co-laboring." She concludes by remarking that there very well may be biological as well as cultural reasons why women are uniquely suited not only to the participation of birth, but to the supporting of other women during the process as well.[10] L.A.s rely not only on their specific knowledge about birth, but also on their intuitive understanding of a particular woman's needs. In French, the word for an L.A. is *"sage-femme"*: "wise woman."

We believe that a woman can birth alone or with her husband or with friends—without an L.A.—if she is at home. But given the situations, attitudes, and machines just standing around our hospitals waiting to be activated, we recommend that every couple consider bringing its own L.A. to the hospital birth. Asking your mate to be your sole "coach" is like asking an accountant to be a carpenter or a dentist to be a belly dancer. Labor support is an art that requires experience, sensitivity, knowledge, and objectivity. While your mate might be knowledgeable and sensitive, his experience with labor is limited at best, and his objectivity during labor and delivery may be obscured by his own intense personal involvement. His sensitivity to you and his inexperience may cause him to make or support decisions that are *not* in your best interest. For example, there are many situations in which a woman asks for pain medication. Her mate, totally out of fresh suggestions to help her deal with the pain, agrees that medication is the best thing. Asking him to be the *only* L.A. puts a great deal of pressure on him to remember all he has learned: it delegates to him a tremendous amount of responsibility for making decisions he may not be qualified to make.

Some fathers are resistant to the idea of an L.A. They don't want any "outsiders." (It is interesting that neither doctors nor hospital staff are considered outsiders by most people in our country.) Why a "coach?" men ask. "Why isn't the doctor enough? Why isn't *my* presence enough? What will be left for me to do? Why do we need another expense?

David was unapproachable about an L.A. Midway through a 40-hour labor he changed his mind. Fortunately, someone was available. "She was terrific. From the moment she arrived, we both relaxed."

Once fathers understand the L.A.'s role, most feel relieved to have her at the birth. Sam wrote:

> The midwife became part of our plan to have every bridge covered. Our first experience had convinced us that Sean should be our only child. Neither of us could handle another birth like the first. As the desire to have another child grew, so did my fears. My wife said she also needed to prove she could deliver normally. That scared me, but we decided to make this birth the birth we were robbed of. It was my wife's determination that enabled us to go the whole way, but knowing someone was around if we got fouled up again helped us both. If we'd had a cesarean, we would have known it was a necessary one this time.

Jim said, "Touching doesn't come easy to me. Having Judith with us was like an insurance policy. When I felt uneasy, she was there willing to help."

Situations arise when an L.A.'s presence might have been useful. "When the doctor said Anne needed a cesarean last time, what could I say? He put his arm around me and said, 'Of course you understand.' I understood *nothing* at that point. I nodded and told him to do whatever was 'best.' I wish there had been someone else there for me to confer with."

In reviewing their births, many women remark that the husband and doctor seemed like cohorts ("two men conferring in the corner, deciding my fate"). We remind you that men must accept feelings of helplessness during labor: fathers, because there will come a time when there isn't very much they can do to change the pain, and doctors, because unless they are comfortable with feelings of helplessness, they are going to want to *do something*.

In "Taking Care of the Little Woman: Father-Physician Relationships during Pregnancy and Birth,"[21] Coleman Romalis remarks that the physician may try to establish a "male bond"—"a political strategy for building a male coalition to 'handle' the woman during this 'difficult' and 'sensitive' period." He remarks too that not only does the obstetrician have rare intimate access to the wife, but technical understanding of her inner workings "which even the husband does not possess," as well as the position to inquire into, regulate, and even prohibit certain types of their most private sexual activity. "The relationship between the two males in this triad is highly asymmetrical." Romalis believes that the father must struggle with and overcome feelings of inadequacy and immaturity with feelings of self-assurance and potency, for the physician is plainly King of the Castle.

One father called and said:

> I had to play the heavy. The doctor walked away when I asked questions. I had to grab his shoulder and say, "Look, I'm asking you rational questions." He said, "This isn't a sporting event. In two minutes I'm washing my hands of this whole

case. I am concerned about the baby." AS IF I WASN'T! The baby's heartbeat
went down to 90 during some of the contractions but went right back to 140
afterwards and stabilized. When I pointed this out to the doctor (who said the baby
was going into distress), he seemed angry that I knew anything about anything.
I really helped, but after several hours, no encouragement, or suggestions, or support,
and more and more scare tactics, I gave up.

Men are trained to be "chips off the old block." They are trained to imitate
their fathers and to seek approval. Advancement in the business world depends
on these adaptations to male authority. Male physicians represent powerful male
authority figures, symbols of fathers to be pleased, approved by, and even feared.
During birth it often happens that men feel a need to confront male physicians.
They must be demanding in a way that goes counter to cultural father-son
programing. With female obstetricians, men are faced with the fears that "talking
back to mother" invite. Men can be confronted with a lifetime of inner fear and
disapproval during childbirth unless this approval programing is managed, and
adult self-acceptance and self-approval are experienced within.

Another aspect of cultural conditioning may prove even more intimidating
and, indeed, may paralyze a man who attempts to confront an obstetrician
during his woman's labor and delivery. This is the man's concern that in any
male-to-male confrontation, the vulnerable laboring woman might be made to
function as a hostage or pawn. Thus, if the man refuses an intervention favored
by the obstetrician—or if he merely questions the physician's authority or knowledge—the woman and infant may be made to suffer as the doctor re-establishes
his authority over his turf.

Some men don't want to be at birth, and in a relationship in which the man's
presence causes anxiety, pressure, or problems for the mother, his presence may
need to be evaluated. In *Spiritual Midwifery*, Ina May Gaskin suggests that
some people are "passengers" at birth. She says the birth can be slowed down
by hours or even halted until some change takes place in the energy. Anyone
whose presence is not an actual help, she says, is siphoning off the emotional
support that should be flowing to the birthing women. Remember, a woman's
feeling safe is one of the prerequisites for letting the baby be born. If there is
tension stemming from the father's presence, *the most loving decision* that couple
could make for the baby's sake—and each other's—would be to have the father
leave.

However, many articles substantiate one in the *American Journal of Orthopsychiatry* on father-infant attachment, which stated that the father's presence
at birth establishes nurturing patterns that continue throughout infancy and
beyond.[19] One man wrote:

There are a few days in a man's life that he'll always remember. Most of those days
are important because they represent the accomplishment of what the man considers
to be a major goal. A very few are significant because they signal a change in

direction: *the beginning of a new experience that is so significant it will continue to shape his life from the moment the experience begins until the end of his life.*

The day of my daughter's birth was one of those latter days. The experience was so intense that I felt that I was experiencing the most joy a man could attain. That joy was so powerful that, at the moment of her birth, it was almost painful. It will be, I think, one of the last things I remember when I die. A man who has not been with his wife at the moment of their child's birth has missed something no one will ever be able to describe or explain to him.

Supporting the Laboring Woman

Although we will offer suggestions for supporting the laboring woman, there are many different ways to show that support. Support does not necessarily imply agreement, nor does it always mean physical assistance. The way we support, touch, and care for others stems from aspects of our own personalities, including how we ourselves have been supported. Each individual relationship manifests its own nurturing behavior. We'd like to give you some illustrations.

Ed told us, "A few years ago I wanted to take a portion of our hard-earned savings and invest it in a friend's new business. Anne wasn't nearly as enthusiastic as I was, but she told me that she respected me and loved me and would support my decision and stick by me whatever the outcome. Now the tides have turned. I don't understand or share her enthusiasm for a vaginal birth, but if it's what she wants, I'll do whatever I can to help."

One midwife related a story about a couple during labor who had no contact whatsoever. As a matter of fact, the husband sat in a chair four feet away during the entire birth. He rarely offered anything in the way of verbal support. She continued:

Frankly, I thought he was a loser. He sat like a king on a throne. Even when the baby was born, he remained in his chair, leaning over only slightly. However, as the mother gently took the baby from her body and into her arms, she immediately turned to her husband and blew him a kiss. With tears and love in her eyes, she said softly, "Thank you, I couldn't have done it without you." Meanwhile, I had been contemplating taking him into a dark alley and punching him in the nose. All this mother needed was his presence, not his words or his touch. She felt his caring, and the fact that no one else did was superfluous.

A second story related by the same midwife presents a much different scene. During this birth, the father was working as hard as the mother. He rubbed her back, ran for cold compresses, and breathed along with her. Halfway into the labor, his shirt was hanging out of his pants, his hair was disheveled and his eyes were red and swollen. He looked as if he'd just run from a pack of wolves. As the pushing stage progressed, he pushed and grunted right along with each contraction. By the time the baby was born, he was wiped out. As soon as the baby was born, his wife jumped up, thanked her obstetrician, and hugged him. Meanwhile, the husband, tears streaming down his face, stood by. "By the way, her OB was more than willing to accept all the credit," said the midwife. "I wanted to cry."

If you ever have an opportunity to hear Janet Leigh speak on "The Art of Labor Support" as she lectures around the country, don't miss it. If you don't have an opportunity, make one. Janet's respect for birthing women, her insights into birth, and her suggestions for supporting laboring women are inspirational for anyone attending birth. We are grateful to her for her work and for helping to raise consciousness about the value of support during labor and birth.

Midwife Peggy Spindel offers further thoughts for those who attend a woman in labor. "It is not a man's role," she says:

> Nor the job of an obstetrician. This person does not assist a doctor and is not a medical worker. If she is a nurse, she must forget she is a nurse . . . She is not a wielder of technology. She does not define life, risk, death, happiness. She does not do the decision-making. She does not control childbirth. She does not manage labor. She does not deliver babies. What she does is attend. She puts her knowledge and experience at the disposal of the childbearing family. She knows birth, and she loves women.

In "The Theft of Childbirth,"[20] we are told that every woman must "*buscar la forma*"—find her own way—during labor. Each woman must manage her labor in the way that is best for her. In *Creative Visualization*, Shakti Gawain tells us, "You don't have to 'effort' to get where you want to go; you simply put it out clearly to the universe where you would like to go and then patiently and harmoniously follow the flow of the river of life until it takes you there" (P. 59).[8] The river may take a winding course toward your goal. It may even temporarily seem to be going in a different direction; yet, in the long run, it is easier to get there effortlessly than through struggling and striving. You just "go with the flow."

In an article on labor support in *Childbirth Educator*,[22] Beth shares the following:

> My job is to help the woman find her own ways of coping, of using the built-in strength every woman has for giving birth. Although I can offer ideas I've learned from other laboring women, each woman has to find what best helps her. . . .My role does not conflict with the father's. I support him as well . . . relieving his anxieties and freeing him to be as supportive as he can.

During the birth Beth explains that she gives explanations, offers suggestions, interprets sights and sounds, and gives emotional support. Beth makes it clear that she has no authority over doctors and hospitals; "only the couple does."

Let's face it. The hours of employment for labor support aren't terrific. Babies often pick the wee hours of the night to make their appearances. Hour for hour, the money is rarely "equal" to what is given. Women who attend births do so out of a deep and abiding commitment to women and birth. They put their hearts and souls into safe and joyous birthing.

An L.A. can be the anchor that moors your family to security and peace. Your labor might want to sweep you along with the strength of a powerful gale; but the "anchor" you have chosen keeps you linked to your beliefs and wishes. She will help you to sail and to weather the gale safely, triumphantly.

Ellen Goodman concludes her article on labor support with:

> Under the advice of their doctors, women have been going through labor alone. Now we have more experts telling us what our grandmothers knew in the first place. . . .Even in an overly 'experted' society like ours, doctors don't need a report by their peers to believe that labor support is essential. All they have to do is listen.

All they have to do is listen.
Amen.

Choosing a Labor Assistant

In choosing an L.A., perhaps the most important criterion is: does it feel as if she is the right person for you? Does her presence provide you with a sense of peace and trust in yourself? Is she compatible with your life-style? Is she someone who is not affiliated with a particular doctor or hospital? What is her training? What are her attitudes about birth? Is she consumer-oriented? How often will you see her prenatally? What are her preferred affiliations and why? Has she attended births with your physician or at the hospital you have chosen? What are her fees? Is she supportive of the father's role and the needs of the family? Does she have any personal limits? What are the services she offers? Is she readily available? When does she vacation? How can she be reached? Who is her back-up? Does she have any other clients due near your due date? How many clients does she accept per month? What are her own birth experiences? Does her manner help you feel confident? Is she enthusiastic, confident, responsive? What does she expect from you? Do you share common goals about the birth? Will her presence be an asset?

Labor Support: "Where Can I Find It?!"

There are several places to check in your search for an L.A. Every community has midwives, and many of them will agree to provide support if their time permits. They may also be able to put you in touch with women who are qualified to be your L.A. You can also talk with the local childbirth educators; some double as L.A.s. Often nurses who have had their fill of hospital obstetrics leave that scene and offer their services as an L.A. Often a group of women who are committed to supported birth come together, learn from one another, and are available to assist the laboring women in their community. Occasionally one has to be extremely resourceful: Liz couldn't find anyone who was willing or able to provide assistance, so she flew an L.A. across the state to be with her. Hopefully, the time will come when the demand for L.A.s will increase the supply and finding a good L.A. will be a snap.

If you can't find one, and you can't afford to fly someone hither (or thither), find someone who's interested in helping you. She can read, take any one of a number of basic courses, and put her knowledge together with her intuition about birth and her desire to help. Even if she isn't able to take a course, she can talk to other L.A.s, or learn by attending births and watching other support people. Every L.A. has to start somewhere, and maybe the novice that you choose will someday be the woman who helps to teach other women in your area about labor support by sharing her knowledge and experience.

Additional Support

You must be the one to decide whose presence would be most beneficial and whose is not necessary. Your decisions may change, depending on your mood or on your labor. At any time, right up to the moment of the birth and beyond, it is *your right* to be surrounded by those who can best love you, respect you, and support you. If you want your children at the birth, or your mother, that is your decision. If you want friends at the birth, or an aunt, or your grannie, that, too, should be your decision. If you choose to birth alone, or alone with your partner, that is your right as well. A woman who wrote to us had lost her sister six years before her VBAC. She invited and allowed her sister to be with her in spirit by keeping thoughts of her sister's love and caring present all during the labor and delivery. Certainly God will be with you, but it's also nice to have someone who can put hot compresses on your bottom!

Labor Assistants Are Not Magicians!

Although we know that an L.A. can make quite a bit of difference at a birth. We also know that she cannot work magic. As one L.A. has written to us:

I am absolutely convinced that without my presence, many of my clients would have cesareans. I feel happy & satisfied each time my belief in a woman's body—and her own belief in herself—is realized. I think, "Perhaps this birth will give the staff a new thought that a natural birth is possible even with a narrow pelvis, or a "prolonged" labor—if the mother is determined and if calm, gentle, confident, loving support is provided."

However, I have a great sense of sadness and frustration, and this is shared by other L.A.s with whom I work. Often, our very presence is resented. I want to emphasize that is the role symbolically that seems to disturb some staffs. We are always as polite as we can be, not arrogant or demanding. We try to accommodate the couple's wishes without offending the staff in any way. Still, we are often seen as intruders or trespassers. We must all love the laboring woman enough to accept that an L.A. might be what's best for her; when egos get involved, we are all in trouble.

The issue of control is ever-present—and so useless! It is the staff's "territory" and they have a certain amount of authority and "control" that can't be argued. Their familiarity with the facility and the other staff members give them an advantage "over us." We don't want to be "over" them—we want to work with them, & on the occasions when we all work together, it is wonderful for everyone.

Often times, doctors are patronizing. If I ask that an episiotomy not be done, or the cord be allowed to stop pulsing, they look at me—no, through me—and do what they please. After all, what could I know? More than once I have seen a doctor do an episiotomy, cut the cord, or stitch so fast it seemed as if he had left a red-hot lover anxiously awaiting him back in a private lounge. Many seem resistant to learning anything from those of us who do labor support.

I cannot have my eyes everywhere all at once, although I try, and sometimes I am seconds too late to help. The couple is so vulnerable—and often oblivious—at these times. Once I asked a doctor not to do an episiotomy just then. The mother, anxious to get the baby out, said, "Oh, it's all right," even though we had agreed to avoid one. More than once a doctor or nurse has done something totally invasive and unnecessary (given a shot of Pit to contract the uterus or done an episiotomy, for example) while I'm holding the mother or breathing with her. Why must we be on guard every single second? Why do many doctors and hospitals take advantage of the couple's vulnerability? When I am with a laboring woman, I am so involved with her, that in my love for her, I too am vulnerable. How sad I feel that I must learn to put the vulnerability aside and put up an impenetrable fortress with which to "protect" them. Even as I am an assertive and protective advocate for these parents, there is an element of impotency. With it comes the element fear—fear that something will be done to the woman, couple, or baby, that will take away part of the joy and safety from their birth.

I could choose to attend only home births and come home happy and peaceful. Instead, I often come home from hospital births tense, frustrated, and sad, for no matter how joyously the parents perceive their births (which is ultimately what is most important), in so many subtle ways, the wool is pulled over their eyes. Yet, if I stop attending hospital births, the important things that I can do—and do—will be lost.

You must recognize the values of an L.A., and also the limits placed on her by your own vulnerability during labor, as well as by the environment in which you birth.

Consumer Power

What if the hospital doesn't allow an L.A.? Go elsewhere! Write a letter explaining that you will not use their facility until they begin to support positive birthing. Hospitals need your business to survive.

Many years ago, a maternity hospital in Boston boasted a program called LIFT—Love Is the Family Together. However, they did not permit siblings at birth. Are other children, the baby's brothers or sisters, not members of the family? What about grandparents? One letter of complaint didn't make a difference. But 5, 10, 15 . . . and the policy was changed. When most hospitals in the Boston area did not permit fathers in for cesareans, C/SEC suggested that couples use only the two hospitals that did. When the restrictive hospitals heard from two or three couples that they would not use their facility for that reason, it did not make a difference. But when 10, 12, and ultimately 18 couples wrote, it did. (As far as we know, there isn't a hospital in all Massachusetts that still prohibits father from cesareans.) Letters to hospitals and doctors either praising them or admonishing them are extremely important.

A couple from Michigan who could not persuade the local hospital to support their wishes for an L.A. flew to Boston. They got media coverage: a TV interview and the front page of their newspaper. When a second couple threatened to fly to Boston, the hospital changed its policy. Those of you who continue to use hospitals not supportive of normal birthing concepts are giving tacit approval to their nonsupportive policies. Your business thus helps to maintain the status quo. Hospitals will never change unless consumer pressure, with its threat of lost dollars, forces that change.

If you can't travel, change physicians, or, as some couples have done, stay at home until labor is extremely active; then go to the hospital, have your baby, and leave. Others have brought their L.A. to the lobby, or the gift shop, or the cafeteria, or to a nearby motel room, and have labored with them *there*. One couple borrowed a van. With two midwives, they drove to the hospital and parked outside. They had their daughter in the van and drove home! They did not feel comfortable with a homebirth but were told if they came to the hospital their L.A. would be denied entrance, and that a fetal monitor and I.V. were absolute requirements for a VBAC. "We were unwilling to birth with unfamiliar attendants or to accept the risks of such interventions at our baby's birth." Many couples have shown great creativity and uncovered a wealth of resources at times when it seemed their birthing plans were being sabotaged.

Siblings at the Birth

In Cathy Romeo's words, "Birth is a time for families to grow together, to nurture and support each other, to strengthen infinitely the commitment they share." Sharing this belief that birth is indeed a unique vehicle for strengthening family ties, growing numbers of birthing couples are including their older children in the new baby's birth. Some siblings have been present at births in the hospital; others, at home. Having your children present is an option that should be open to you. There is available a burgeoning collection of current literature for those of you who are considering having your children present and for those of you who would like suggestions for preparing your children for the coming event.

Having the newborn's siblings present can be a positive experience for the whole family. The older children won't have to deal with separation at a time of highly charged energy and excitement. Child psychologists are increasingly urging the inclusion of children in *all* major life events: books have been written recommending that children actively share in family experiences whether they be painful ones, such as death; traumatic, such as separation from family or home; or joyous, such as birth. Even the painful or upsetting surprises that life deals out seem better handled by children when they are included, along with adults, in a response; children's imaginations can create far more fearful or damaging visions than the reality ever was.

Some women find that their children's presence calms them, centers them, and helps them to birth more easily. One woman said, "I never could have relaxed if Michael had been with my in-laws. He was in and out of the room, but not in a distracting way. Rather, I could focus better *knowing* he was fine." Another said, "I had a thought that I could help my girls (ages 8 and 5) feel better about birth than I ever did. It was very special having them with us. I know it was a wonderful experience, and I hope they'll bring the warm feelings of joy and family to their own births." A third said, "My son saw his cat birth her kittens—he just *assumed* he'd get to see his brother be born, too!"

For those of you who are planning to have your children present, we would like to share some points we consider important. In order to help children, whatever their ages, feel truly comfortable with birth, three ingredients seem essential: good preparation and education geared to the children's levels, sensitivity to and absolute acceptance of the children's wishes and needs, and the presence at the birth of a nurturing caretaker whose *sole* responsibility is the children.

Preparation can take a number of forms: viewing books, slides, movies (some should be in color); role-playing the coming birth with emphasis on the sounds laboring women make (children love doing this!); accompanying Mom to her visits with midwife or doctor; and attending with parents selected parts of childbirth-education classes. Cathy Romeo, a childbirth educator, plans one class of her series just for the children. They view birth slides, ask questions, role-play a bit, draw pictures, share feelings and concerns, and generally feel very important to the family unit. Cathy believes that such preparation is just as vital for siblings not planning to be present at birth; she says that the children will be far more peaceful knowing and understanding what is happening.

Despite parental desires, however, children's wishes need to be sensitively respected. Some children choose *not* to be present. Children should be free to leave the birth room whenever they desire.

Children generally take their cues from trusted adults; if the adults at a birth are calm, undisturbed, and smiling, the child will most likely assume that all is well and feel the same. Thus, the caretaker you choose for your children would best be someone they know and love. However, she (or he) must be someone who can totally and unselfishly focus on the children's needs, even to the point of leaving at the pinnacle moment of birth if the children march out the door! (Would your mother turn her back and follow your children? Your sister? A friend?) Children would also do better with a calm, responsive adult they know only slightly but who shares your philosophy of birth, than they would with a beloved but hand-wringing anxious auntie who doesn't really trust in the normal childbearing process.

Nancy's children were well-prepared and were enthralled by their sister's birth. Elissa's eyes were as wide as saucers, and she held her newborn sister before Andrea was minutes old. Eric thought the baby was neat, although he later told everyone, "The placenta was really gross!" Heather decided at the last minute that she wanted her twin sons (age 6) to be present. They had had no formal preparation. "They loved being there," says Heather. "Nathan said, 'Hey, Mom, that's a great baby you have, but the extension cord sure is weird!'"

Obviously, many factors will contribute to your decision: the ages of your children, the time of day, the length of your labor, for example. What are the needs of the child? What would the effects of his presence be—on himself, as well as on you and your mate? The decision whether or not children should be present at birth is an individual one, based on a variety of personal, practical, and societal factors.

Preparing Children for the Birth of a New Sibling

Children learn about birth through conversation, but also through nonverbal messages and the "vibrations" they receive. Children are continually absorbing incoming signals, decoding them according to their individual process and methods, and adding the resulting messages to information already stored.

We believe that it is of utmost importance when explaining birth to children to come from a point of view that birth is a *healthy, normal, and safe experience*.

We must come from a point of view that women were designed to have babies, that their bodies know how to "get their babies born," and that babies themselves know exactly how to be born naturally. *Without these basic premises, without instilling these views and having them integrated into our children's belief systems, we will continue to produce more and more cesarean parents.*

There are several books available that explain cesareans to children. In our opinion, any book about cesarean deliveries directed to children should make absolutely certain that the child is familiar with birth as a normal experience and has integrated this information before citing exceptions. Any children's book that is discussing birth should also start teaching cesarean prevention. Pictures of women walking during labor, eating and showering, and smiling(!) should be associated with birth. Pictures of husbands and wives holding each other close during contractions, or hugging each other—these are the pictures that will assist children as they integrate the thought that birth is a normal and loving event, not pictures of beds, I.V.s, machines, and hospital jonnies!

Using accurate terminology (for example, "sperm" and "ovum") is important. But using these words without others, such as "love," "caring," and "special," contributes to our society's view of childbirth as a technical phenomenon. In our "sophistication," we often teach children reproduction apart from human feeling. This contributes toward making birth a scientific, medical event.

As a society, we believe that birth is an abnormal event requiring tools, tubes, chemicals, and machines. No wonder so many birthing women become surgical patients. To children, the excitement and drama of the operating room must seem far more intriguing and appealing than a man and woman and perhaps a birth attendant or two.

We believe that children's books about birth can be useful and appropriate. Occasionally, however, they miss the mark. For example, we take issue with one explanation to the child that because babies are often so "big and strong" they sometimes cannot fit through the birth canal. The child who is born by cesarean may then believe that she alone was responsible for her mother's surgery. What we know, of course, is that the inability of a woman to accommodate her baby has less to do with the size of the baby and the size of the pelvis than with the woman's own beliefs about birth, with mismanagement of labor, and with a general lack of support and knowledge in this country about what really helps babies to be born.

The authors of children's books about birth must work through their own feelings about their births, since their unresolved feelings can affect the children for whom they write. A woman's positive internalization of her birth experience (regardless of external events) is important for her children because of their natural intuitive powers. Claudia Panuthos tells us that if a woman feels competent, adequate, and affirmed by the birth experience, these feelings will be reflected in the baby and other family members. If a woman feels inadequate, guilty, or lacking in relationship to childbirth, *these* feelings will be reflected in her offspring. "It is encumbent upon women to create positive birthing within our own hearts because we deserve to feel good about ourselves and about childbirth, and because our children deserve to feel good about their beginnings."

For those of you who are concerned that your child is too young to be present at the birth or would be too much of a distraction, we respect those concerns. We suggest that you talk to others whose children have been present, talk to your child, do some reading, be flexible, and make the decision when you are ready. If you decide not to have your children present, we urge you to have them visit you and the new baby very shortly after the birth and frequently thereafter.

Cathy Romeo shares a belief: "Birth can and should express values in human relationships that are really important to us, so that birth then becomes an affirmation of all that is right and good in human experience." Whether our children are present at birth or not, their integrations of our birth experiences are what really count. If birth is truly a positive event for the parents, that will bring positive feelings about life to our children.

Friend (or Foe?)

Friends can be a wonderful source of love and strength to birthing women. It is interesting that many women who are planning VBACs or purebirths do not find friends and family to be supportive. They don't get the unconditional love from them that they need and deserve. "Oh, you'll never have that baby normally," people say. "Your uterus will rupture!" Everyone seems to be an authority on birth. "My friends seemed to be just waiting for me to have another cesarean so they could wiggle their tongues at me," said one woman sadly. Maybe it's sibling rivalry revived. Perhaps friends are jealous of your confidence, strength, and determination. Perhaps they harbor thoughts that you might have a "better" birth than they did.

It may be that other women have a personal "stake" in our less-than-perfect births. Without even knowing or understanding on a conscious level, they "use" our imperfect experiences to work on healing their own childbirth-related hurts. It may also be that they really care, and, out of ignorance, are frightened.

Most pregnant women in our country have enough of their own self-doubts and fears and don't need anyone else's. We recommend that when you plan your VBAC or purebirth, you tell only the people you know will support you. You don't need to spend three-quarters of your pregnancy educating people about "natural childbirth" or VBAC, or trying to convince them about uterine dependability: it's tiresome and often fruitless. Your purebirth or VBAC itself and your intact incision will do more than hours of discussion to educate people.

"I chose VBAC and lost most of my friends," said Dale. "It was almost as if they were choosing sides! Doctor—10; Dale—2."

We wonder about friends who don't support you—who are judgmental and withdraw their warmth and approval when you've made a decision with which they do not agree. We have heard too often of friends who don't understand. "My friends humor me. They really think that this time I'm going off the deep end." We hope that those close to you will accept you unconditionally, that they can love who you are and continue to support the person you are, even if supporting the decisions you make is difficult.

For those friends or relatives who are genuinely concerned, perhaps you can allay their fears by telling them that your doctor won't let you have the baby until you go into labor! Tell them it's not good for the baby to be born without labor. Remember that by giving a dissertation on the horrors of medical intervention you may be striking sensitive spots in your friends and family. Many of these women have had medicated deliveries; and no woman wants to be told that she didn't do the very best for her baby. You may also be programming yourself counterproductively. "I told so many people I was going to have a VBAC that if I'd had a cesarean I wouldn't have been able to show my face. The pressure during labor (to do it so I could *prove* it could be done) was *awful!*" said Eileen.

Talk to your friends. Tell them you need their support and faith in your ability to choose what is right for you. Seek out other VBAC women. There is support out there, so focus on the positive. There's a wealth of positive support within your own being; let it out. You are the best person to decide what is right for you. We also ask you to remember that there is an unlimited number of positive birth experiences to go around. One woman remarked that eight out of eight women in her class had already had VBACs and it was likely that the "VBAC tickets" were all gone. Listen again: there is no limit to the number of VBACs to be had, and no limit to the number of good births. There is an infinite potential for such births. And it isn't luck that determines the ticket holders but determination, information, confidence, and support. When the golden ring has been grasped by a nimble rider, the other children don't get off the merry-go-round. They keep reaching for the next golden ring, knowing that there is always another. Learn a lesson from the children: GO FOR IT!

Beyond Labor Assistants

We'll say it again: women need love, confidence and trust in themselves and those around them, food, and support, in changing order. Beyond that, each woman must choose what will help. Women have written to us about rebirthing, polarity therapies, flower essences, and many other suggestions that have proved valuable to them prior to and/or during labor. Chiropractic adjustments have benefited many of the women who have written us. Janet Leigh tells us that labor is a symphony that needs to be orchestrated by the woman, not the medical staff.

Many women question us about ways to get through labor. One wanted to use hypnosis. One woman thought masturbating during early labor might help her feel more open. Another heard that learning a particularly difficult verse and repeating it over and over again would take her mind off of the labor and allow her to birth naturally.

We agree with Janet again when she says, "Although every laboring woman knows what is best for her, I generally discourage any method that serves as a distraction." When help is needed, Janet offers herself, not a syringe. Remember that there is no greater contrast than between the moment before birth and the moment after. If a woman uses a "gimmick," she's never certain that she could have done without it. She must find the ways and means to cope that foster her strength rather than distract from it. Past that, what "works," works!

When the contractions get very intense, the woman needs to call on all of her resources. If she's learned to release parts of the body that are tight or tense, this may prove helpful. If she's learned not to complain during her pregnancy, but rather, to find her own solutions to her problems, it will help. If she has learned how to ask for what she needs, that will help as well. If she has "made friends" with her body, it will certainly help. One woman said, "My body aches and feels heavy and I've got all these little discomforts, but I feel blessed and proud walking around in it!"

A woman must be reminded that the pain of labor is normal and healthy. Otherwise, she'll be filled with trepidation and fear. *Spiritual Midwifery*[6] reminds us of a teaching in Buddhism, which says that the antidote for fear is courage. Courage, we are told, comes from a word meaning "heart," and "heart is at least as contagious as fear" (p. 355). If you surround yourself during your labor with people who have "heart," you can borrow or "catch" some of theirs if yours seems temporarily misplaced.

During the time that a woman's body is opening to its full capacity, she may feel unconfident and want to give up. Again, Ina May encourages us: "Assure her that this is temporary and that her brains will return shortly—they are currently in her bottom" (p. 353). At this time she needs confident, uninterrupted touch, and lots of loving, verbal support. She needs to give up struggling and let it happen.

Ina May[6] reminds us, too, that if you can remember your sense of humor, the mother may be able to remember hers. "An amused lady stretches much better than a scared one." Smiles are contagious. They're warming. Bring party hats with you to your birth. They lighten everything up. Ask anyone entering the room to put one on. It's amazing how the atmosphere and energy change when everyone has Big Bird, a Smurf, or Garfield on his head. It helps everyone remember that this *is* a *birthday party*. People smile more, and then you and your body smile more. (Ina May says: "If you can't be a hero, you can at least be funny while being a chicken.") "And always, let the mother's smile be the brightest light in the room."*

If music relaxes the woman, let there be music! (Why not try "Comfort Zone" by Steven Halpern, during labor, or anything else that suits your fancy. Robbie Gass's "Welcome to the World, Dear Child" is the all-time favorite in Nancy's classes for playing at birth.) Singing during labor can be relaxing and fun. If a friend's (or several friends') presence is the key, let that friend be present for the woman. If she needs time alone, or private moments alone with her mate, let it be. Let there be pillows, lots of pillows, so that all her body parts can be supported. Perhaps she needs her mate to hold her, or she needs to put her head in his lap. Sheila Kitzinger tells us that every time a man tells his woman he loves her, and really means it, she'll open another centimeter! She needs calm, gentle, loving voices around her. She must trust her body and accept her labor. She must trust that her body knows exactly how to birth this baby and that her baby also knows how to be born. A woman needs to stop asking why, to stop struggling with it, to let go of her friend's labors, or her mother's labors. She needs to let go of her own fantasy birth and to let this birth *be*. She needs to put as little physical energy into the labor as possible, and to *surrender* to her body's work.

She may need help putting her feelings into words. It's all right to feel lightheaded or confused or frightened. She's normal. These feelings, these pains, *are normal*.

Claudia Panuthos suggests a leg and foot massage for a woman in labor. Tension pulls everything upward. "Massaging the lower extremities in a downward stroke helps ground a woman to the earth. It gives a message to her baby that the earth is a safe and secure place to come to." Dr. Eva Reich, world-renowned natural childbirth educator also believes that massage is important. She sees it as an alternative to drugs, a healing power. She believes that babies should be massaged from birth.

For thirst during labor, we recommend "Labourade," an electrolyte-balanced drink that helps prevent and/or alleviate exhaustion, dehydration, and nausea; it's especially useful during long labors.†

We don't use the word "transition." All pregnancy and birth is transition.

---

*David Gerrold, *Moonstar Odyssey* (New York: Signet Books, New American Library, 1977), p. 13.

†Labourade is basically the natural equivalent to Ringes Solution with dextrose, which is commonly administered intravenously in hospitals. More information can be obtained from ACHI, P.O. Box 1219, Cerritos, Cal. 90701.

One woman who wrote us calls the most active phase of labor the "RR" phase: "Really Rosie." Gina was in "Really Rosie" labor and was handling her contractions beautifully. She overheard the word "transition." "Transition? Am I in transition?" she asked. When she was told that indeed she was, she immediately began huffing and puffing and hooing and blowing. "I freaked right out," she said. Fortunately, she unfreaked when she realized transition wasn't going to bowl her over or knock her down dead.

Norma said, "When labor got really difficult, I thought simultaneously: 'I want general anesthesia right now; I was crazy not to have opted for a repeat cesarean; this is definitely my last kid.' But not too long after that Dana was born, and it was all *most definitely* worth it!"

Women need to be reminded that the contractions at eight–ten centimeters are often no stronger than those at six, seven, and eight; they seem more intense because they last longer and are more frequent. The birthing woman needs to imagine things that open, and to let her body open at the same time. Doors open. Flowers open. Children's eyes open wide when they see Mickey Mouse. A woman opens her mind and body to receive her lover. Open, spread, let go, give in to it, move into it. *Let it happen.*

We believe that, given the right support, and with the right attitude, every woman can accept the energy of birth, feel proud of it, and go with it. The woman can surf on the waves, swim into them rather than override them. She needs praise, encouragement, and a "Yes, you can" attitude surrounding her. She doesn't always have to feel relaxed, but she needs to respond in as relaxed a manner as possible. When the pushing phase begins, she needs to feel free to make noise. ("No one seems to think you are out of order grunting while you attempt to push your car out of a snow bank during a blizzard; it is only natural to make comparable sounds when you work to push your baby into the world.")*

Ed Barna wrote a poem, "Chant for Transition":†

> . . . It hurts because you're doing it
> the more it hurts, the more you're doing it
> of course you can do it, you're doing it
> just do it . . . stay with it
> you can do it! . . . .
> the more it hurts the sooner you're through it . . .
> there's nothing else to do but do it!

Mr. Barna reminds us that we ate for two, we slept for two, now we hurt for two—*but we have the strength for two.* "Just do it."

A woman may need to squat or kneel. If she has a posterior baby, she may need lots of back rubs, compresses, counterpressures as well. She may need to

---

*Marion Myers, "Convention Notes," *Pacesetter Newsletter*, September–October 1982.
†Reprinted from *Mothering* Magazine, with permission of the publishers.

be massaged. She needs to urinate every half hour and have something to drink. She needs to think loose, limp and open. Perhaps she'll need to sit on the toilet for a while, a place that is associated with opening and letting go. She needs candles glowing, or her old quilt wrapped around her, or friends singing to her. She needs whatever she wants, short of drugs or alcohol, to help her. She needs to believe she *deserves* the kind of birth she's dreamed about.

Above all, she needs to maintain a knowledge of her own strength. She needs to be aware that even without all this wonderful, caring support, her body would help her have this baby. Her "locus of control"—her location or focus of responsibility and strength—must rest within herself: she must believe that *she*, not the doctor or the midwife, will have this baby. Fernand Lamaze himself remarked that a woman must be imbued with the thought that she is essentially responsible for the success or failure of her own childbirth. When she "gets" that, she can then remember that she's not alone. She can call upon her baby and her body to work right along with her. What a team!

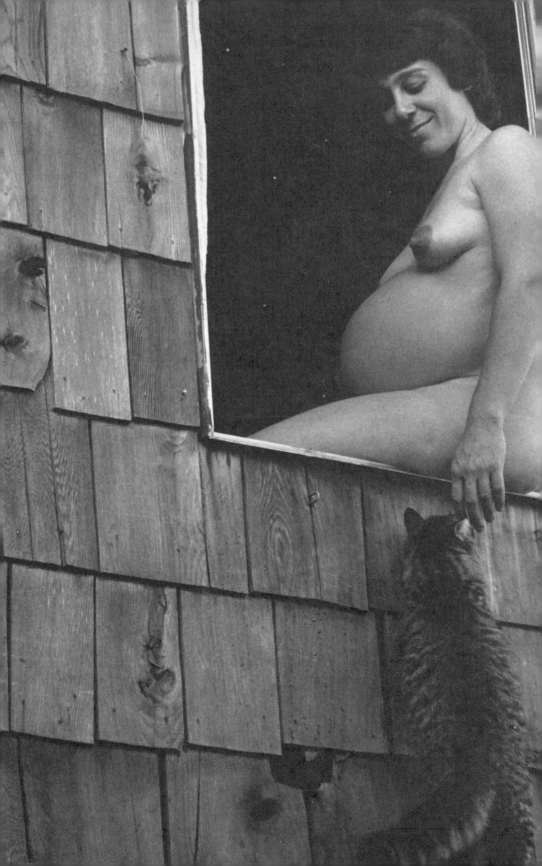

12 ⚬ Mindscapes

It's Friday, thank goodness. You've had a really rough week at work and you can't wait to take a hot shower and curl up in bed with a good novel. (How about *Heartsounds* by Martha Weinman Lear or *Midwife* by Gay Courter?) As a matter of fact, you think, you're probably coming down with a cold. You feel achy and tired, and you're even sniffling. On Monday, your boss wants to speak with you. There's a slowdown at work, and you're certain she's going to give you your walking papers. Just as you step out of the shower, the doorbell rings. It's your neighbor, the one who sometimes drives you a little buggy: she needs your help moving some furniture. You show her that you are already in your robe and have just taken a shower. You tell her that you aren't feeling very well. "Gee, I'd really love to help," you say, "but I'm coming down with a cold." Your eyes begin to tear, and you sneeze. You make yourself a bowl of chicken soup, and crawl into bed to take care of yourself. By the next morning, you've come down with a full-fledged cold.

Let's replay the scene with a few significant changes. You're tired and achy and feeling slightly ill. So you take a shower and prepare to get into bed early. The doorbell rings. Surprise! This time it's an old friend you haven't seen for two years. She's only going to be in the area for the night. She's bouncy and energetic and has the night all mapped out—an enjoyable evening with other good friends you haven't seen in ages. You think, "Hey, this is lucky! I'm already showered and my hair's washed!" You think about the good times you used to have together. What a treat to be with the old gang again! You tell her you won't be a minute. You toss on your clothes. Just as you're leaving, your boss calls. She's decided not to wait until Monday to tell you about your promotion. You leave the house feeling euphoric, and you have a wonderful evening. You haven't laughed so much in weeks. You've completely forgotten that you were tired and planning to stay home, pamper yourself, and come down with a nice cold.

The mind and body work together. All the time. Like Rogers and Hammerstein, the Lone Ranger and Tonto, and Snoopy and Woodstock, your mind and body are constantly interacting, giving each other cues about how to feel, react, behave.

We all know people who work in competitive, stressful office jobs. After a while, some of them begin to lose hair, or their color pales, or the texture or color of their skin changes. Some may lose their appetites; others overeat.

Ellen's mind affected her body. She wrote,

> I had a good cesarean. I felt it was necessary. I was supported by my loving husband and a caring physician. Just short of four days I was home. At the time, I didn't feel I had anything to "work out" from the birth.
>
> Six months later, I started feeling very emotional about having needed the cesarean. The emotions that I was feeling I knew were ones that I suppressed at the time of the birth and postpartum. I rarely get sick but at this time I got a cold. The next three weeks my energies were not up to par and I could feel a major emotional release was in the making. Then one evening I got a terrible stomachache and during the night I got very ill. By the next morning I had the following symptoms: stomachache which caused enough pain to make me have to bend over when I walked, backache, headache, low grade fever, distended abdomen because of gas, swollen and pale face. On top of all this I got my first period since my pregnancy. All these symptoms correlated to ones that I had after the cesarean, with even the period being the lochia. I also craved applesauce, which I ate while in the hospital.
>
> I cried through the night over my disappointment that I didn't deliver my baby vaginally, and continued for most of the next day. I believe I created all these symptoms so that I could relive the birth experience again, this time experiencing the full impact of my emotions. This realization was clarified and supported by a friend and was accompanied by a very cleansing sob.
>
> The next day I woke up with no symptoms whatsoever, but a deepened sense of well-being.

Panuthos believes that there are five mental attitudes which are necessary for positive birthing: self-love; the intention to succeed; an attitude of responsibility (seeing yourself as the source of each of your life's events); open-mindedness (willingness to experience new thoughts and new events); seeing birth as an opportunity for self-discovery and self-expression, and general enlightenment ("You must birth 'in lightened mind' "). When the mind embraces these attitudes, she says, the body is well on its way to normal birthing.

The Body and the Mind

Your body influences your mind. We describe (Chapter 7) how exercise affected our bodies, which in turn affected our thoughts about ourselves. A friend of ours insists she can't think clearly until after she's had her morning run.

We've all heard "You are what you eat." When you've eaten a nutritious breakfast, your body feels good. You can think clearly, and your production level is high. Studies done on children prove that their capacity for retaining what they've learned is greatly increased if they eat a nutritious breakfast before school.

In "Befriending Our Bodies," Peter Michaelson tells us that the body is the basic truth or reality of a person's existence in the world.[31] Our physical self is the sum total of all our thoughts about ourself. In *Positive Birthing*, Panuthos and Silva remind us that what we sow in the mind, we reap in the body.[36] Since "thoughts get results," positive thoughts "can produce a different outcome than negative thoughts." Your mind and your body are *parts* of the *whole* of you; so when you respond to life, all of your parts are continually influencing and affecting one another. Together, your mind and body determine what your response will be.

Why, for example, does one cancer patient get well and another die when the medical prognosis has been identical for both? In the book *Getting Well Again*, Dr. Carl Simonton and his wife Stephanie document their "whole body" approach to fighting cancer.[45] They support traditional medical treatment of the disease, but they combine with it "treatment" for the mind as well: techniques for learning positive attitudes, relaxation, goal-setting, managing pain, exercise, building an emotional support system, and most notably, visualization of body healing. Their remarkable results tell the story: the Simontons' patients have a survival rate twice the national norm. Their records tell of many cases of dramatic remissions or even total cures when medical science alone has offered little hope. All of those fortunate patients learned to heal their bodies with the help of their minds. This is accomplished through visualization and imagery work alone.

Holistic medicine—indeed, holistic *anything*—teaches us that you can't ignore any part of an individual's make-up. You don't just treat symptoms, overlooking causes or contributions from all aspects of the person's life. You don't assume that medicine is the only cure for "what ails ya." Indeed, *within* the individual there are keys to wellness. Physical or mental stresses alone can place a person in a state of disease (*dis-ease*).

The Power of Beliefs

Your beliefs about yourself, your partner, your body, your baby, your life, your power, will influence your birth. If you see your body as a well-functioning, trusted partner in birth, your experience will be different from that of someone who is confused, self-conscious, and insecure about her body. Your mind will influence your body.

H. Deutsch, a psychologist active in the 1940s, knew that at the time of birth it is not just a vagina that is opening: the woman's entire psyche is open and vulnerable. She states that we all come to our birth experience with a set of beliefs from which we govern and guide our lives. These beliefs form from earliest impressions. For example, if we were held lovingly and securely as infants, we would probably begin to develop a belief that the world is a safe and secure place in which to live. If, as infants, we weren't fed when we were hungry and were left to cry or "work it out" ourselves, we might have adopted a belief that there isn't enough food (or love) to go around, and that "when I am in pain there will never be anyone there for me." Our beliefs form our view of the world. They are messages that are integrated into our person and influence how we live our lives. According to Mehl and Peterson, a belief is an assumption made about the world that may or may not be conscious. It has a great deal of emotion associated with it and determines the interpretation of sensory perception.

We applaud the work that Lewis Mehl, Gayle Peterson, Claudia Panuthos, and others like them are doing on the psychophysiological-emotional-spiritual aspects of birth. We regret that their work is almost totally ignored by physicians and childbirth educators. The mind and body cannot be separated. An *entire* woman, and her entire lifetime of thoughts, impressions, and experiences, are present at birth. There is an entire man and *his* thoughts, impressions, experiences, and events, as well. Taken together, these ingredients blend into a labor and birth and season the outcome.

The fact that our beliefs, our thoughts about ourselves, affect our births helps to explain, for example, why many women with an "inadequate" or questionable pelvis give birth to 8, 9, or 10 pound infants, while other women with totally adequate pelves have difficulty or are unable to deliver their 6½ to 7 pound babies. A woman who believes that she is adequately designed to give birth will birth more easily than a woman who doesn't understand how "anything that big can get through something that small." Ina May tells us that "since mind and body are one, sometimes you can fix the mind by working on the body, and you can fix the body by working on the mind." When a VBAC woman gets "stuck" at a particular point in labor, it is often at the same point when a decision was made to do a cesarean with her last birth. By working to free her mind, her body is freed to resume opening.

We collect and integrate beliefs. A belief *system* is a series of messages that combine to form attitudes and influence behaviors. They are, in a sense, a series of "tapes" that we play and replay throughout our lives. Understanding our belief system is important because, as time goes on, the individual supporting beliefs accumulate and the system strengthens. We begin to view the world via our "system." Our belief system becomes a code by which each of us lives, a way in which to bring external events and internal impressions into harmony.

As children, we developed certain beliefs and reinforced them as we grew to adulthood. We continue to keep our lives "in sync" with our beliefs. Our perceptions and our experiences shape our attitudes and beliefs. They are constantly in operation. We use them to make decisions, and they determine our reactions to situations. We continually work to keep our beliefs intact. We see our original beliefs as the ultimate truth, the foundation on which we build all our other "truths." Mehl and Peterson repeatedly remind us that a woman's belief about herself and her labor can determine the course of the labor. ("As a woman lives, so shall she birth.")

Lester Hazell tells us that we must make a distinction between beliefs and truth. She gives examples of beliefs: Birth is hazardous. Labor should be shorter. Fetal monitors are essential to safe birth. She says that birth is a spiritual experience when we are totally present to it, as it is without the imposition of our beliefs upon it. Truth needs the test of time, along with a sense of universality to all mankind. Ms. Hazell gives examples of truths: Each birth is unique. Each and every birth and each and every child creates change in the world. Each labor flows with a pattern that is unique and yet common to all humankind. Each birth involves the mind, the body, and the spirit of everyone present, whether we are aware of it or not. Above all, the process of labor and birth as it exists, unmodified, has evolved to be the best way for human beings to be born: otherwise we would not be here, as we are, and what we are.[22]

Here's an example that will help to illustrate the strength of beliefs and the way in which they operate to create similar, supportive experiences. Pam always wondered why she had a cesarean. "Why me?" she asked over and over. She spent time blaming the doctor, her childbirth educators, the hospital, and herself. She heard about belief systems. She searched to uncover beliefs that would lead her to a cesarean.

Pam realized that one belief she had was that her body was not her friend:

This belief must have started when I was very young, and it was reinforced by several uncomfortable experiences as a child, such as wetting the bed at my grandmother's house and soiling my pants at school in the first grade.

Rather than seeing the early onset of my menstrual cycle as an exciting affirmation of my body's ability to work appropriately and well, I again believed that my body was not my friend. A "friend" wouldn't show up completely by surprise and embarrass me. I never believed my body was a partner. I always considered it an adversary. I dieted during my teenage years but didn't lose much weight. I convinced myself that broken cookies left at the bottom of the box didn't have calories. I now see that if I had stopped eating the cookies and had lost weight easily, then the belief that I had developed earlier—"My body isn't my friend"—would have been inaccurate. I would have had to change a whole set of beliefs that were based on this one. I guess it felt more comfortable to struggle with dieting and affirm my belief than to accept my body as a friend, lose the weight, and have to change the beliefs!

Another belief I had was about hospitals. When I was three, my mother went to the hospital and gave birth to premature twins, who died. She went in to have her babies and came home without them. When I was six, my grandmother went into the hospital, came out with cancer, and died a few months later. Of course she had cancer when she went into the hospital, but, as a young child, I didn't understand that. She looked fine to me before she was admitted but was very sick when she came out. How could that be? I thought hospitals were supposed to make you better! So, at an early age, I set up a belief about hospitals: they didn't get you better.

When I was eleven, my grandfather died—in a hospital. If he had gone to the hospital earlier in his illness, he might have gotten better. I chose to ignore this fact and interpreted his experience as another reinforcement of my negative belief about hospitals. I myself had several personal, unpleasant, experiences related to hospitals, which confirmed my beliefs about my body and hospitals.

I also had a belief that doctors, not women, deliver babies. I had a basic mistrust of gynecologists, since my first vaginal exam was performed minutes after the doctor told me it wouldn't be necessary for him to examine me internally at this visit. I had a belief that my relationship with my mother was better when I was not well— based on times of closeness and understanding that seemed to occur when I was ill. When I went into the hospital to have Jenny, I brought these beliefs with me, as well as "My body isn't my friend" and "Hospitals do not get you well." I was not aware of these beliefs at the time! *I was enthusiastic, if not a little insecure, about the actual birth. I was excited about becoming a mother. Now I see that these beliefs were presences in the room, as real as the nurses and doctors. I now see how difficult it would have been for me to have had a normal birth, given the beliefs that I had adopted.*

In order to have my belief system continue intact, I made each belief come true. Indeed, I went into the hospital feeling fine, and came home, after having had major surgery, weakened and sick. My body certainly hadn't worked for me: it wasn't a friend. The doctor, very pleased with himself for the beautiful incision he had made, had done the delivery. I no longer trusted him, since he'd always told me I had an adequate pelvis. My mother rushed to the hospital to make certain I was alright. All my beliefs stood firm.

I know that my physician's beliefs influenced the birth. I believe his practices were inappropriate, unsafe, and not conducive to normal childbearing. My childbirth educators' beliefs also were an influencing factor; their focus on fancy breathing patterns rather than other, far more important issues detracted from the birth. My husband's beliefs also influenced the birth. But I know now that given my particular beliefs, I could have chosen any physician, any childbirth educator, or any husband, and still I'd have ended up with a cesarean. I now take full responsibility, without guilt, for what happened. I had cast all the players in the play to keep my beliefs intact.

It is our opinion that *most* of us have beliefs about birth that are not conducive to normal childbearing. We live in a culture that views birth as a dangerous, pathological situation. This is evident in many ways.

An afternoon television special for children that is repeated several times a year focuses on birth. Although the actual birth is not shown, there are scenes of a mother on her back, with her feet in stirrups, unable to move, covered from head to toe with green sheets. Everyone is wearing a mask. The popular television show "Eight Is Enough," which is viewed by thousands of impressionable teenagers and children, aired an episode last year during which one of the daughters needed an emergency cesarean. Lo and behold, the baby was saved by the doctor's swift actions and medical technology. Soap operas haven't had a normal birth in twenty years, all for the sake of dramatic appeal. These stories portray birth as a dangerous, abnormal situation. They elevate doctors to positions of power and might, and lower women's bodies to a place of inadequacy or malfunction. They are a reflection of our society's views on birth. They also reinforce these views and perpetuate them.

The impressions that many of us form are that women are totally unable to give birth normally. We believe that birth often results in a serious emergency situation, that it is always a life-or-death situation. We integrate these impressions early on, as children, and continue to believe them as uninformed teenagers. They are reinforced every time we watch a program or hear a story about a problem at a birth.

On one soap, the father of the baby heard that his baby had been born and that the mother (his *former* girlfriend) and his baby were both clinging to life. He rushed to their bedsides and proclaimed everlasting love and devotion. There probably wasn't a dry eye in a home across America that afternoon. The message rang out loud and clear: create a cliff-hanging birth and win back your lover; get yourself into a mess and come out smelling like a rose.

Such television programs perpetuate our society's myths surrounding birth, reinforce them, and contribute to another whole generation of abnormal birthers. We watched many of these programs as young people ourselves. If a girl doesn't believe women's bodies are capable of giving birth, she'll grow into a woman who *isn't* capable. If a boy integrates messages that birth is dangerous and difficult, he'll grow into a man who has difficulty lending total calm and support to his laboring woman. For both men and women, reeducation is essential.

"Little House on the Prairie"—a nice family show, right? After a particular episode aired, we received a letter from Terry:

> *I was so angry! Here is a prime-time family drama supposedly taking place when childbirth was natural and at home, and they manage to work in a cesarean! I can't remember the reason for the c/sec, but it was a new doctor in town, and he was black, and the only way the town finally accepted him was when he pulled off*

this cesarean right in the woman's bedroom. The daughter could have had an easy birth and shown everyone how safe and joyous childbearing can be. Michael Landon, you should have stayed at the Ponderosa!

Even in the rare situations where a television program portrays a natural birth, you hear nurses yelling "PUSH! PUSH! PUSH!" like a cheering squad. You see doctors' faces behind sterile green masks—never mind that birth is not sterile and that masks are useless after five minutes—looking worried and fretful. You see the mother, looking exhausted, bedraggled, puffing up her face, holding her breath, and gasping for air. You see the father, looking at his watch and half-heartedly saying, "You can do it, Marge."

"Is that natural childbirth?" one teenager asked us. "It looks like a football game." So many impressionable young people are being propagandized. But after all, there's more drama to a cesarean than to your normal everyday, run-of-the-mill birth, and after all, drama sells.

Our Beliefs Influence Our Births

Beliefs influence births in many ways. For example, if a woman perceives pregnancy as the only time that she is pampered, she may be reluctant to give it up. She may have a prolonged pregnancy, prolonged labor, no urge to push, or perhaps a retained placenta. Lois felt very special when she was pregnant the first time. She kept a daily journal and cherished every moment. Everyone made a fuss over her, and she felt and looked wonderful in the later stages of her pregnancy. Her labor, when it finally began a week late, was slow and erratic. Her baby never dropped, even though she was almost fully dilated, and she later saw that only a cesarean could end her pregnancy.

If a woman believes herself still a young girl, rather than a woman—if she is not ready to grow herself up—she may fail to dilate. Laboring and delivering a baby is a growing-up process if ever there was one. Women who are not ready to do the birth themselves often manifest "failure to progress" which may be better termed "successful rescue."*

Sandra's belief that life is always a struggle was never more clear to her than at her son's birth, at which time she struggled for hours. "I have to work hard for everything I get," is a common expression in women we see. "Nothing comes easy."

---

*C. Panuthos, *Positive Birthing* (Boston: People Place Press, in press).

One woman wrote to us that she had a VBAC after an especially long and difficult labor. In her birth report she wrote:

In retrospect, this was a good birth, even though I knew it would be impossibly difficult . . . The problem is, my body just didn't want to let go of the baby. For me, there is no way to have a baby easily. My feeling is that I either pay in advance or afterwards. My fear of surgery is greater than my fear of pain, so if we have a third child, I will opt for a vaginal birth, even though it was harder than a cesarean section. I guess I'd have to convince myself that next time it could be easier.

She went on to say that the birth was ideal for her because "it couldn't be improved upon." This woman's belief that nothing will ever come easily to her also affected her labor and birth. Having an easy time would have blown her image of her life: what it was all about, and how it worked.

Another woman who planned a VBAC and had a repeat cesarean used the word "cesarean" in her birth report *every time* she meant VBAC. Her first sentence read, "The birth was not as I expected, as I was expecting a cesarean. I'm sure cesareans are easier—I'm still recovering from the section." It seems clear that she had not firmly integrated beliefs that she would be able to birth normally.

We would like to share a few examples of negative beliefs that women have uncovered and that may have contributed to their cesarean births.

"I'm certain I integrated a belief that childbirth was difficult and left one incapacitated," said Ellie. "My mother had a rough birth with my younger brother, followed by a severe hemorrhage. My own cesarean met my belief that birth was difficult and required a great loss of blood." Friends of hers always spoke about their difficult births. Sarah had a belief that pregnancy was woman's work.

I was told that men just didn't belong at births. Having a cesarean provided a way for me to have a baby without my husband, since our hospital did not permit fathers in for cesareans. If the hospital had permitted fathers in for cesareans, somehow I probably would have required general anesthesia, so that he would not have been able to be there. I love him, but I was told that no man should see his wife in that condition.

Carla, believing "an eye for an eye," uncovered that her cesarean had been her self-imposed punishment for an abortion she had had at eighteen. Carol identified a strong belief that she couldn't hold on to good things. She had had two premie babies born by cesarean, and after identifying some negative beliefs about childbearing, she had a full-term VBAC. Maryellen's observation that she never finished anything important that she started ("college, work assignments, projects, even sweaters I begin knitting!") translated into a belief that she was unable to complete anything satisfactorily; "True to form, I let my doctor finish the birth."

Several women who have contacted us have had difficulties becoming pregnant after traumatic cesareans.* Bernadette wrote, "I'm having trouble conceiving. I do think that the fertility specialist will be helpful, but I realize that I have to be healed of my first birth experience so I can move on to the next one. I'm so afraid of not being able to do it, of my body letting me down again, of being terribly disappointed, that I'm sure this is influencing my fertility."

Denise wrote, "I finally became pregnant—five years after my cesarean. It seams very coincidental to me that I became pregnant just weeks after I faced the last experience and began to deal with it."

Sarah, who had had a particularly difficult cesarean, wrote, "What little conceptus would want to implant in my body knowing what kind of birth awaits it two weeks before it is even ready?"

Several women with histories of infertility had very difficult births that resulted in cesareans, although no apparent structural problems were evident. If a woman is unable to make peace with her body, normal birthing may be affected. Similarly, if she chooses a physician who doesn't believe that women's bodies work, normal birthing will be negatively affected.

One cesarean woman who had an eight-year period of infertility said (after her VBAC), "I did it! I can't believe it!! It worked! I worked!" and began to cry. "For eight years I haven't thought about my body as normal. And it is. It works like everyone else's."

Women whose belief systems include "tapes" (messages that keep replaying in our heads) about the normality of their bodies, the normality of birth, have a much better *opportunity* for birthing normally. We have found that a high number of sectioned women with whom we work do not have beliefs that are conducive to normal childbearing. Most of them did not have trust and confidence either in their bodies or in the childbirth process. Panuthos tells us that a common thought pattern among cesarean mothers is the belief that birth is unsafe. Many women believed that the doctor would get the baby out for them. Many were not ready to give up their pregnancy or to grow themselves up. Many were "needy," and they were able to get what they needed by having a cesarean (more on *that* in a minute!). By the time they had their VBACs, they had identified some of their negative messages and replaced them with positive messages. These messages (for example, "My body is my friend"; "I deserve to have a good birth experience"; "My life 'works'!") were *conducive to normal birthing*.

---

*An excellent organization for information and support for infertility is Resolve, P.O. Box 474, Belmont, Mass. 02178. Resolve has affiliates all over the country.

Identifying Beliefs

> "Your life has been a perfect teacher
> Since you were but a child . . ."
>
> —R. Gass

How can we identify beliefs that may influence our births in a negative way? Sometimes, just talking about birth is enough. We can also be aware of our body language, or misplaced giggles or gasps, while discussing the subject. (In class, we ask individuals to note how they are feeling as they watch particular parts of a movie, or as we discuss various topics.) In an atmosphere of love, trust, and understanding, we can begin to discover and share beliefs about our bodies and about birthing.

Perhaps you and your mate can write down as much as you remember of what your parents taught you about birth. Many of our attitudes and beliefs about birth come from our parents and other close adults. Did Auntie Chloe swallow a watermelon seed, perhaps? You may recall accurate descriptions of conception and birth, or you may have really thought that storks deliver babies. If the subjects were never discussed, that, too, is a message.

You can also ask your mother and father, separately, to tell the story of your birth and the births of your siblings. Be very aware of the ways in which the stories are told. Watch your parents' eyes and hands. Notice the tone of voice, the inflections, the feelings. Don't interrupt, just listen. If you live quite far, ask them to write down their remembrances of your birth or to tape them for you.

A few weeks later, you can ask particular questions of your parents about your birth. "Hey mom, how did you feel when you found out you were pregnant with me? What was the pregnancy like? Tell me what I looked like as a newborn!"

We can learn a great deal about our own beliefs by questioning our parents about our births. Their views and attitudes, which may have changed somewhat with the passing of time, laid some of the groundwork for our own attitudes, feelings, and beliefs. We can learn as much from silence as we can from elaborate description. A parent who finds it very difficult to discuss birth, who cannot or does not use appropriate terms for various parts of the body, who gets embarrassed or defensive, or who thinks this whole thing is silly, is giving information that is as valuable in many ways as another parent who gives a moment-by-moment description of the birth from the first contraction to the last. Our father's attitudes, as well as our mothers', shape our thoughts. A father who takes no interest in birth beyond getting the baby "planted" sends messages to his sons and daughters about fatherhood, sex, sexuality, partnership, and responsibility. Although it wasn't a part of a man's experience to be *present* at birth many years ago, a father's presence at birth was his caring, his love, his support, his understanding. The kind of role he assumed at that time can give us some hints and ideas about how we view birth.

Certain questions may help you identify your beliefs about birth. Once you have identified a belief that may disrupt normal birthing, you can begin to reshape that belief by integrating your *adult* knowledge and awarenesses.

For example: how did you first learn about birth? How old were you? How did you feel about the person who told you? the way in which you were told? How did you feel when you saw pictures of birth for the first time? The spectrum of answers to this last question is astounding: excited, enthralled, ecstatic, breathless, overwhelmed, turned-off, disgusted, nauseated. One of Nancy's strongest recollections about birth involved the movie "Gone With the Wind":

> *In the birth scene, Miss Melanie, frail and shivering, gives birth, while her servant is running around screaming for water and dramatically yelling, "Lordy be! Miss Melanie's going to die, Ah just knows it! Help! Help!" Scarlet comes to Melanie's side and, with her iron will, commands Melanie to deliver or die. Meanwhile, Atlanta is burning. Hardly a joyous depiction of gentle, assured birth. It doesn't matter if my recollection is accurate—what matters is that this scene kept popping up for me whenever I recollected my early exposures to birth. Birth was chaos, and only a strong-willed determined "other" could bring order to the scene; Melanie clearly couldn't have done it alone.*

The fill-in exercise presented on pp. 261–63 was developed by Jay and Marjie Hathaway and appears in their book *Children at Birth.** It provides another opportunity to help you uncover attitudes about birth. Included are some of the responses we hear most often.

There are no right answers and certainly none that is wrong or inappropriate. Your answers are part of who you are. Remember too, that your answers may change during the course of a pregnancy. Accept them and appreciate them, as they provide you with clues to your own beliefs about birth.

Feeling Safe

We've mentioned several times that a woman needs to feel safe when she is giving birth, and that some animals actually stop their labor if they sense danger. It makes sense: if they continued to labor and delivered their babies, both mother and offspring would be easy prey, being in such a vulnerable state. So the animal puts labor "on hold" until the danger has passed. Or she picks herself up and finds a safer place in which to give birth.

---

*Sherman Oaks, Cal.: Academy, 1978.

Fill in your own answer before checking the others.

A woman's pregnant body is _____

Beautiful.   Fat.   Hard to carry.   A miracle.   Wiggly.

The thing that bothers me most about babies is _____

*Nothing.   They spit up.   They can't tell what they need.
The crying.   Changing diapers.   That I'm on call 24 hours.*

Watching movies about birth makes me feel _____

*Entranced.   Enthralled.   Sick   to   my   stomach.   Teary.
Happy.   Very sad.   I've   never   seen   one.   Very   scared.
Hey! I can do that!*

Right now, if I was given a choice as to the sex of my healthy baby, it would
be a _____

When I see my wife in pain I _____

*Want to take the pain away.   Want to leave the room.   It depends
on what the pain is from.   Get scared.   Start getting the same
symptoms.   Would rather have the pain myself.*

What I will enjoy most about the baby is _____

*Nursing it.   The first smile.   Those first weeks when it is so
little and dependent.   The time when it can play on its own for a
little bit.   Holding it.   Cuddling it.   Snuggle time.*

What scares me most about having this baby is _____

*That it won't be healthy.   That my firstborn will clobber it.
Having time for another one.   That it will be cesarean.   Its
complete dependence on me for those first months.*

What I like most about babies is _____

   Their bottoms. Their toes. The top of their heads. Their total openness to life. Their smell. Their innocence. Their dependence.

The sight of blood makes me feel _____

   Squeamish. Terrified. Faint. Blood doesn't bother me. That it can be normal if it's during birth. It depends on whose it is and where it's coming from!—and how fast!

I think labor will be mostly _____

   Fun. Very difficult. A breeze compared to a c/section. Terrifying. A means to an end.

The thought of a normal birth with no interventions makes me feel _____

   Ecstatic! Nervous. Very nervous. Terrific. Apprehensive.

My mother described her births by saying _____

   She never talked about them. They were very painful. It was worth it. She had natural births. Her births were all cesarean. She had seven of us and we just popped right out.

How I think this baby will affect our relationship is _____

   I don't think another will change it very much. A lot. Give us less time for each other. Bring us closer together, especially if the birth is good.

What I want others to do for me during birth is _____

   Leave me alone! Tell me what to do. Keep reassuring me that I'm doing fine. Love me a lot. Tell me my wife is okay and that the baby's fine.

In my childbirth fantasy, our labor takes _____

20 minutes.   Just as long as it takes to get to the hospital. Oh, about three hours.   Eight hours sounds good.

My obstetrician _____

Doesn't exist!   Is terrific.   Isn't supportive of VBAC.   Does lots of natural births.   Won't listen to me.

When I think about pain in labor I _____

Freak out.   Look forward to it because it will mean my baby's coming.

If I was all alone giving birth _____

I'd not know what to do.   I'd let instinct take over.   I'd die; that'd be better than having my old OB!

What I expect to enjoy most about the birth is _____

Being in control.   The pushing.

This is only a sample of questions. Examples of other questions we use are:

When I think about the birth, I usually _____
The biggest change this baby will make in my life is _____
The three best things about having the baby are _____
The best way to show a baby love is _____
The three yukkiest things about having a baby are _____
Pregnancy means _____
What pregnancy does to our sex life is _____

We know this is true for women as well. If a woman doesn't feel safe at a particular point in time, she'll stop her labor, too, to protect herself and her child. This is a protective measure, an instinct that takes precedence over all other human needs and guarantees endurance of our species. "I love you, my infant, so I won't let you into this world unless I am certain that it is safe to do so."

Those of you who were sectioned for failure to dilate, uterine intertia, or lack of progress: how safe *did* you feel during your labors? Was there anyone or anything present that frightened or alarmed you? If you perceived any cause for fear, your deepest, most instinctive response would have been to protect your baby at all costs. Remember, instead of berating yourself for needing a cesarean, honor the decision you made to keep your baby protected!

Perhaps, as some suggest, the *baby* needs to feel safe as well:

I WON'T HATCH!

by Shel Silverstein

Oh I am a chickie who lives in an egg,
But I will not hatch, I will not hatch.
The hens they all cackle, the roosters all beg,
But I will not hatch, I will not hatch.
For I hear all the talk of pollution and war
As the people all shout and the airplanes roar,
So I'm staying in here where it's safe and it's warm,
And I WILL NOT HATCH!

Montagu,[32] Schwartz,[44] and others [1,8,17] urge us to be more conscious of the life of the unborn child, and to recognize that the baby is affected by the emotions and "daily rhythms"[44] (p.15) of its parents.

If the marital relationship is in question, or finances are a serious problem, a mother's instinct to keep her baby inside may conflict with the body's readiness to labor. Half-way up the mountain, the climb seems too high and the fall too steep.

Because we believe so strongly that a woman must feel safe in order to give birth, we can support couples who want to have their VBACs at home as well as women who want to deliver in the hospital. For each individual, her perceived location of greatest safety will be the safest place for her to birth.

Remember: the mind and body always work together. Mickey and Minnie.

Cheech and Chong. Ernie and Bert. When a conflict exists, the mind and the body will both be affected.

Several women who are overweight have discussed with us how their weight problems contributed to their cesareans. They never felt comfortable with their bodies. It is difficult to give birth easily if you are not comfortable with your body or its functions. Many of these women worried about not achieving a respectable waistline soon enough after the pregnancy. They believed that pregnancy helped them look feminine and normal rather than just fat. "It's no wonder that I stopped dilating," said Dorie. "I didn't want to have to start dieting." Her next baby was a VBAC, born after nine hours of labor.

In *Special Delivery*, Rahima Baldwin discusses "psychological dystocia."[1] She tells us that any of the following can slow or stop labor: your own or other's expectations that you "perform"; trying to control your labor; resisting sensation; feeling uncomfortable because of someone in the environment; feeling restrained because of photos; feeling tensions between you and your husband; feeling negated by an insensitive birth attendant; experiencing unresolved fears; inhibition or modesty. We have seen each of these cause problems. When the concern or distraction was removed, labor proceeded with no further problem. Other articles on maternal stress and pregnancy outcome substantiate that psychological state affects physical "performance."

We all have conflicts about pregnancy. Is it the right time? Can we afford it? Will the baby be healthy? Will I have enough time for both of the children? Is our relationship strong enough to include a child? Conflicts are normal, but when they are not addressed, not released, their bound-up energy can unbalance the labor and birth.

Some parents are afraid they won't love their second baby enough. They are also afraid to talk about this fear. One woman said, "This baby was planned— but now that I'm pregnant, it feels like an intruder! I'm going to miss the special time I have with my firstborn." After she had talked about it for a while and learned that her feelings were normal and okay, she said, "Phew! I feel better!"

Remember, it is not necessarily a *solution* to a particular conflict that brings release, just a *recognition* of the conflict. It is unacknowledged and unaddressed stresses or fears that are likely to spin cobwebs in the nooks and crannies of a uterus or cervix. Uncovering the conflict depletes its energy, its power to restrain you. Like bats, conflicts fare better in darkness; so shine some light on them! You needed far more energy to keep the conflict hidden and in check. Just saying, "Yes, I do feel that way . . ." enables you to step away from the conflict ANYWAY, to go beyond it for a time. You can sweep it aside and clear a passageway for normal birth.

In other words, awareness of a problem dissipates the anxious energy that is used to suppress the conflict. Suppression takes energy, energy that might be needed at your birth. And suppression causes tension.

The Pressure to Perform

In the article "Neurophysiology of Letting Go," Rahima Baldwin points out that relaxation is the key to labor. "One must be able to surrender to the force that is driving your body and birthing your baby." It is difficult to relax and surrender to labor if significant conflicts or stresses are present.

One pregnant woman was in conflict because having the baby meant giving up her job. Our information and expereince have shown that career women often have difficult births or cesareans. It's hard to open up and let a baby out when you sense that the baby may interfere with your life. It's so much easier to be pregnant! A news journalist recently had a baby by cesarean. Before she was even a few months pregnant, we prophesied that it would be difficult for her to birth normally. Besides having her blossoming career threatened, we imagined that she felt pressured into being a role model in the hospital. She needed to be the well-informed, self-assured, dignified, sophisticated person everyone expected her to be.

Many artists, writers, and actresses have cesareans. The list is astounding. Can you really believe that all these women are designed incorrectly? Of course not. These women are behind the eight ball to begin with. They have careers. They are public figures and in the limeligtht. They have to "perform" during labor. Their lives are woven with color and drama, and birth presents a creative drama all its own. For many women, it may be easier to expose their bellies than their vaginas. It's not "professional" or "ladylike" to birth normally.

Nurses, woman doctors, male doctors' wives, and other females with connections in the medical establishment also often have difficult births. Their orientation is medical, not normal. There is a belief in technology that supersedes their faith in the birthing process. If these people birth in institutions where they know others on a professional level, they feel as if they have to be good models, good patients. As soon as a woman in labor feels pressured to act a certain way, or to dilate at a certain speed, she's in trouble.

In class, Nancy gets her stopwatch and a knife and says, "Okay, the males in this room have two minutes to get an erection and ejaculate. Those who fail to do so will have the tips of their penises cut off. One, two, three—go! Okay, who's getting an erection? Anyone? Not yet? Hurry, hurry, or you'll be cut!" A little dramatic, you think? As we've already mentioned, thousands of women are threatened with a cesarean if they don't dilate more quickly, even though the baby is fine and the labor has only been twelve or fifteen hours.

Many doctors find it difficult to trade in their stethoscopes and support their wives as loving husbands. Delivering at a hospital where everyone is a colleague is "a bummer," according to one doctor whose wife had a cesarean. Interestingly, many childbirth educators have difficulty birthing. "The pressure!" said one. "I'm going to disappear when I go into labor. I have 125 couples waiting to see how I do." Birth is *not* a performance. *When we can give up, when we can let go of our inhibitions and fears, we can allow our bodies to do what they absolutely, positively know how to do.* One psychologist suggests: Drop your ego and you'll drop your baby!

Birth, Death, and Pain

There is a connection between birth and death. Many women are afraid to "drop" their babies. They connect the pain of labor with death. In Elizabeth Davis's article "Energy Cycles in Pregnancy and Childbirth," she states, "The entire first stage of opening up, or dilating, is a process of ego dissolution, and many women find it akin to what they imagine the experience of dying will be."[8] In order to birth freely, perhaps we must open ourselves to the possibility that birth encompasses many small "deaths." There is the "death" of the pregnancy, for example, and the "death" of the family structure as it was. In each death, however, there is a birth, a *re*birth. A different body. A new family system.

There is pain in childbirth. What we believe or how we are feeling will affect the amount of pain we experience. Richard Stevens, in his article "Psychological Strategies of Pain Management," states that the mental state of the individual significantly alters incoming pain impulses, increasing or lessening them.[46]

Many of us are familiar with Grantly Dick-Read's fear-tension-pain syndrome. Pain is subjective. For example: A child's hand is barely tapped by her mother to stop her from running into the street. The child is disconsolate and bursts into tears. "You hurt me! My hand hurts soooo bad. It's all red and it hurts!" That same child, in a more defiant mood, might never even flinch when the mother firmly spanks her behind the second time she ventures into the street. She even smiles smugly and says, "I will *too* go in the street. I'm big enough and you can't stop me."

Barb recalls cutting her finger. She was on her way to get a bandaid when she stubbed her toe. She forgot all about her finger. Pain is subjective, and discriminating, as well!

As you know, we are in total disagreement with childbirth education that teaches women to distract themselves and disassociate from the pain. This is nothing more than running away from childbirth. Davis[8] reminds us that our bodies know what to do. They know how to breathe if we don't interfere by using arbitrary, preconceived patterns.

We need to let the pain flow. We need to adopt a concept of childbirth pain as *healthy, normal* pain. Childbirth pain *is* healthy, normal pain. The duration and intensity of pain for each of you will be different. If you integrate that belief, you will be free to let the pain work for you. The pain of labor is the body's healthy work to deliver the baby.

It may be that we have some recollection (albeit subconscious) of our own birth experience.* If, indeed, there is some memory of that time activated as we give birth, the perceptions that are present may influence how we give birth. If we know or judge our own birth as being extremely painful, we may judge our own birth as being extremely painful, we may "hold back" (out of fear, or to protect our own child from experiencing what we believe to be a hurtful experience). Lewis Mehl, M.D., reminds us that "a healthy fantasy in advance can compete with contrary experience."

We recommend that women begin to get a sense for their strength during pregnancy. Find your own way to deal with normal aches and pains, rather than looking for sympathy and attention. If you see yourself as a problem solver, you'll be able to see yourself in this role during labor. If you *believe* that the pain is benign, you'll accept it more readily, and experience your might.

"During my birth *I* was the source of power and strength! Everyone else helped, but I was the source!" said one woman. Remember that, in a sense, fear is a decision, based on information and feelings. You can *decide* not to fear labor and birth.

Stress, fear, and anxiety are known to counteract the work of natural hormones that help labor progress. Newton states that premature labors are more likely to result from stressful pregnancies.[33,34] Crandon concluded that high anxiety levels during pregnancy increase a woman's potential for encountering obstetrical difficulties.[7] Other studies substantiate that maternal anxiety negatively affects progress in labor, or the baby's well-being. Uddenberg et al. believe that repressed conflicts may inhibit the psychological process of birth.[47] We know this to be true. We have seen women who have expressed interest in VBAC for no other reason than fear of cesareans. We also know women who have had cesareans because of their mate's fear. There are also many women who are sectioned because of a doctor's fear. It is important for you to work to decrease fear and stress through education, self-confidence, and loving support.

Birth as a Sexual Experience

Birth is a sexual experience. The parts of our bodies involved in lovemaking are also those that create life. The parts of a woman's body involved in sexual

---

*For those of you interested in the subject of pre- and neo-birth memories, or in releasing birth-related trauma, we recommend *The World of the Unborn*, by Leni Schwartz (New York: Richard Mareck Pubs., 1980); "The Perinatal Continuum," in *Brain/Mind Bulletin*, Feb 16, 1976 (Box 42211, Los Angeles, Cal. 90042); *Rebirthing in the New Age*, by Leonard Orr and Sondra Ray (Millbrae, Cal.: Celestial Arts, 1977); and *Transformation Through Birth: A Woman's Guide*, by Claudia Panuthos (Bergin & Garvey, 1984).

intercourse are also part of the birth experience. The beliefs that a woman has about her body as a sexual being—about sex, lovemaking, her breasts, nudity, and sexuality—will influence her birthing. Often the noises a woman makes during birth—assuming she is allowed free expression—are strikingly similar to those made during lovemaking. In "Childbirth: Alternatives to Medical Control," Shelly Romalis tells us, "If we choose to be mothers, our pregnancy becomes, perhaps more than any other time in our lives, [a] period of fully confronting the meaning of femaleness."

Sexuality has to do with the joy and pride a woman feels about being a woman. It encompasses her confidence, acceptance, and appreciation of her physical and emotional self. It has to do with the joy and pride a man feels about being a man. It has little to do with macho or sexist feelings or a battle between the sexes; only that it feels good and right to be *this* person in *this* body.

Are you glad you were born female? Was it fun growing up in a girl's body? Did it feel rewarding, or did being a boy seem more appealing? Did boys succeed more often or get special privileges? What do words like "feminine" or "womanly" mean to you now? How you feel about your own sexuality is partly related to how your parents felt about theirs. You can go back in time and picture yourself as a child. You can remember what messages you perceived about women's bodies, menstruation, blood, childbirth. As children growing up, we were like sponges that soaked up what was around us. We were constantly identifying, assimilating, and modeling. Remembering the kinds of attitudes your parents had may give you some clues about what you have integrated. A woman who feels comfortable with her body and comfortable about the things it does can call upon these positive feelings at the time of birth.

How did you feel when you first menstruated? Embarrassed, horrified, surprised, relieved, delighted, excited . . . all of the above? Was the information about this normal function (assuming you were given information) provided with love and care, support and pride, or with indifference, fear, tolerance, or disgust? One woman remembered her mother yelling, "Don't go getting yourself pregnant now, or I'll kill you." Another remembered her mother presenting her with a hug and a beautiful hand-embroidered handkerchief that had belonged to her grandmother.

Women (and men) can learn by remembering what information and thoughts they may have integrated and now carry about their bodies. It may be helpful to consider the influence of each of your parents concerning sexuality, sexual performance, nudity. For example, how was nudity treated in your home? Was the atmosphere relaxed? Too relaxed? Stringent? Stifling? Birth involves at least one totally naked body—your baby's—and the partially or completely nude body of the birthing woman. (Many young children who are present at birth seem quite surprised that their little brother was born "bare naked, Mommy!")

Our parents' relationship, or lack of one, will influence our thoughts about sexuality and sex. We recall one class discussion during which two women

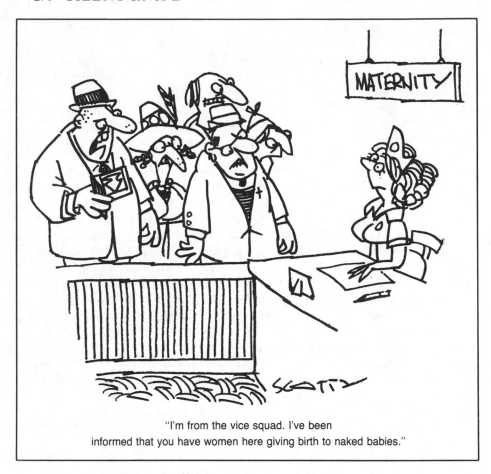

"I'm from the vice squad. I've been
informed that you have women here giving birth to naked babies."

revealed that their fathers often "grabbed" their mothers. For one, these "grabs" were viewed as hostile assaults resented by her mother. For the other, the "grabs" were delightful and playful. "She even grabbed back when she thought I wasn't looking!" These two environments produced very different beliefs and attitudes about touching and about the boundaries or "space" we set for ourselves. In one class a man stated, "My father never, I mean *never*, touched my mother in a loving way." Another man told us that the love, warmth, respect ("and occasional lust!") his father and mother had for each other was a legacy left to all the children in the family.

How did you learn about "sex"? From books? From friends? From a loving mother who answered all your questions? From both parents, or just one? From parents who were ill at ease about the subject? In the streets? From your first boyfriend or girlfriend? The attitudes that were present as you grew and were exposed to the "facts of life" may have influenced decisions you made at your births! Were you taught that your body was clean and wonderful and normal and well functioning? Were you given messages not to ask question and not to talk about "those kinds of things"?

How was affection expressed? Did people touch each other easily? What verbal expressions of love were present? Helen Wessel, author of *Under the Apple Tree*, says, "Anything that embarrasses or inhibits the mother's free expression of her sexuality adversely affects the progress of her labor, for childbirth is a sexual experience."[48]

Unfortunately, most women in our culture don't feel very "sexy" when they are giving birth. Yet, think about the parallels: sexual intercourse is an intimate expression of oneself, and it results in another intimate sexual act: birthing a baby. We believe childbirth can be and should be sexually satisfying; women can feel great pride in their own sexuality. For a couple, it is a time when mutual respect and pride for each other's sexuality can be paramount.

How a woman births her baby is a statement of her feelings about herself as a woman, wife, lover, and mother—an expression of her sexual self. (How those attending the birth view women and sexuality will also contribute to the energy at the birth.) Normal birthing can heighten a woman's appreciation for her body and reaffirm positive sexuality. Ina May[17] suggests that women remember to notice the sensations of muscle release following orgasm, as this will be the ideal condition of the same muscles during the second stage of childbirth. She believes that relaxation of the muscles of the pelvic floor has more to do with a sexual acceptance of the energy a woman is feeling than with a need to expel a large object.

We are sexual beings. We need to remember how our sexual inadequacies, inhibitions, concerns, and insecurities affect birthing; conversely, we need to remember how our feelings of sexual acceptance, confidence, and pride can enhance our giving birth.

"Lucky you," people say to cesarean women. "You didn't have to go through labor. You took the easy way out. Don't you just love how cesarean babies' heads are so nice and round? No labor pain, no pushing your guts out, and your medical insurance covered every cent! What a way to go!"

Is it really? For those who choose to be mothers, pregnancy, labor, giving birth, and lactation are each a part of that choice. A woman who accepts her total sexual functioning welcomes each of them. Like menstruation and menopause they are part of the harmonious flow and rhythm of her female life. Each provides her an opportunity to experience her sexuality.

We learn that everything coming out of our bodies is dirty. Urine, feces, mucus, wax. No wonder so many women hold back their babies or see birth as an "aggressive expulsion"[16] of something huge. No wonder some women have difficulty producing enough milk. It's the psychological, not the physiological, that interferes with normal functioning.

Accepting the responsibility of labor and birth, taking the pain and the pleasure, and learning to work with one's body, can be a profound learning and growing experience for us. One woman likened labor to an amusement park she had often visited as a child. "The rides were too fast, the fun house was scary, and I usually threw up. Nevertheless, I yearned for that fair!" Another woman said, "I felt so completely awed by my body's strength and power." These positive statements and other similar expressions are commonly offered by women who birth consciously and purely.

Compare these to many of the letters from cesarean women, which call up feelings of self-doubt and discomfort. Our beliefs about sex and sexuality are present at all times and are powerfully effective—and affective—at our births.

We have reason to believe that sexual readjustment after a cesarean is more difficult than after a vaginal birth. Hundreds of women have described to us feelings of inadequacy about their bodies that boil over into their bedrooms: "I didn't feel feminine." "I just didn't feel like a woman." "I was afraid to make love." "I might get pregnant, and I couldn't bear going through another cesarean." "Looks like a Mack truck ran me down." One doctor, newly out of medical school, had visions of his wife's belly ripping open if he made love to her. A limited number of women have commented positively about their sexual readjustment after a cesarean. For example, one woman said, "Sexually, things are all right. After all, I didn't have an episiotomy."

For some women, appropriate expressions of sexuality are always demure, quiet, and controlled. Many childbirth classes perpetuate the myth that femininity and silence are equal: we should not be loud and powerful, only "controlled." Control is equated with dignity. Nonsense! Control is *not* essential, it is counterproductive: it *produces* body tension. A quiet, subdued woman can be *less in control* than another who is excited, noisy, or crying. Lynn Richards writes:

> Acceptance of our inability to control birth is so important! The force that pushes our baby has nothing to do with control. I felt the strength of that power when I was pushing out Zac, because I wasn't doing it. Something so much stronger than I could ever be grabbed hold of my body. There was certainly no thinking, no doing, no conscious act or thought. Just that incredible force that has given me faith I never thought I could have. We must let "control" out the window, just let it go.

The Force will be with you, too!

Territorial Primacy

In some species of the animal world, male and female pair up for life. If an intruder ventures anywhere near the female, war is declared. No matter that the object of these affections has hair on her nose and serves him raw lizard for dinner. Territorial primacy—"owning" your mate—is instinctual.

We believe that something similar to territorial primacy goes on subconsciously with men at births. Doctors know they are in someone else's "territory" and mask their intrusion by covering their own bodies and women's as well. Husbands intellectualize by saying, "After all, he's a doctor," but we believe that the woman's mate still harbors an intrinsically deep discomfort when another male is involved in "that area" of *his* female's body. We can't imagine that any man can stand by dispassionately while another man pokes or explores the most intimate parts of his mate's body.

Sally shares the following story:

> *The intertwining of territory, sex, and birth became more clear to me when Fred was operated on in 1979. Knowing what I do about anesthesia, I would have been frightened no matter what part of him was being operated on. But the fact that Fred was in for a hernia repair made it worse. I kept thinking, "What if the knife slips? What if the surgeon didn't have a good breakfast? What if the doctor is in a bad mood because he just found out his wife is running around with the anesthesiologist? I mean, that's a very special part of Fred he's going to be working on, and it's mine! It's a part of him that no one else shares! I don't want anyone fiddling with that part of his body except me."*

Sally concludes, "For me, it would have been worse if the surgeon had been a female. Another woman just didn't belong in that area of his body, doctor or not. Call it irrational. Call it proprietary. Call it whatever you like. But I'd have called her off."

When we discuss territorial primacy with the couples in class, some men do not agree. "Now you're going too far!" George told us. "He's just a *doctor*." Others do agree. Norman said, "Every time he did a vaginal exam my wife screamed. I didn't like him doing all those exams, and he certainly didn't have to be so rough." Another man said, "He kept joking about sex. After he stitched Elaine, he put his arm around me and told me not to worry: now she could have multiple orgasms again." Another husband commented that the physician did not make eye contact with him at all during the entire labor.

Some women "love" their doctors. Years ago, when C/SEC was working to get fathers into the operating rooms for cesarean deliveries, we asked women to use only doctors who supported father-supported cesareans. Many women looked at us aghast. "Change doctors? But I *love* my doctor!" Some stayed with physicians even though these doctors refused to permit fathers to attend the births. Perhaps the choice is a deliberate attempt to keep a man away from his child's birth, since there are many competent surgeons who encourage a father's attendance at a cesarean section.

Maybe we have to "love" our male doctors in order to make what they do to us acceptable. They squeeze our breasts and scrutinize our vaginas. If we have a "love" relationship with them, it may ease any anxious thoughts: it's all right to be this intimate with someone you *love*. Sandra said, "I acted like a little girl with my OB. I saw him as a father. After all, my 'dad' would never do anything to hurt me." Pat said, "My relationship with my OB was strictly business. 'Good morning, Mrs. G.' 'Good morning, Doctor.' Then he'd slip his hands up my vagina." For those of us who were given messages such as "Your slip is showing, pull it up," and "Keep your legs crossed on the bus," it is not always easy to walk into a strange man's office and spread our legs. So we may act in ways that decrease embarrassment. We may support a thought that because we are in a "love" relationship, what we are doing is all right.

Marilyn Moran, author of *Birth and the Dialogue of Love*,* tells us that when there is a period of physical change and development, social interaction can be affected with lasting consequences. She discusses imprinting behavior and remarks, "Human beings are subject to the same laws of nature as are lesser creatures. The moment of birth is the magic moment for the woman to fixate on a preferential someone." Moran asks the question: at this critical period in her life, what visual stimulus is the woman offered as she gives birth in the hospital among strangers? Whose smell, whose touch, whose voice? "The answer is obvious. The Doctor's!"

From Daughters to Mothers

Deutsch[9] believed that at the time of birth, repressed, suppressed, or avoided conflicts regarding our own need-to-be-nurtured can resurface. We believe that the way women birth is in many ways connected to their thoughts about their own mothers. Perhaps we need to reconnect with our mothers in order to connect with our children. Perhaps we need to make peace with our mothers or separate from them in a healthy way.

Some of us have a need to be loyal to our mothers. If your mother told you that birth is difficult, and you feel best when you are being loyal, you may have supported *her* thoughts about birth when you labored. Many cesarean women were born by cesarean. We believe the reason for this is psychological, not anatomical. Women who have a strong need to bond with their mothers may create situations that will put them on common ground with their mothers, to help them relate, rebond, reconnect. These women need to know that they don't have to please their mother or do the birth *her* way in order to show their love for her.

One exercise we find helpful for everyone goes like this:

---

*Leawood, Kan.: New Nativity Press, 1981.

Close your eyes. Release . . . release . . . Let a recent image of your mother come to you. . . . Allow this image of her to become younger and younger . . . until she's at the age when she was pregnant with you. . . . Imagine her feeling you kick for the very first time. . . . Imagine her anticipating labor and delivery, just as you did with your child. . . . Imagine her birthing you. . . . Remember that every decision a woman makes during labor is an act of love. . . . Your mother birthed you the very best way she knew how. . . . Take a minute to appreciate her and thank her for your birth . . . Imagine that you are being placed in her arms. . .

To you, dear woman of the Earth,
Whose act of love gave blessing to my birth:
You gave your blood and breath that I might come to be
Then from your womb you worked to push me free.
To my mother who taught me what it means to give:
You gave yourself that I might live.
I honor you, the being that you are . . . in the
    temple of my heart.*

Those of you who are angry with your mothers might try some forgiving. "I forgive you. I forgive you. I *do* forgive you," just as we hope our children will forgive us for whatever mistakes they judge we have made along the way. It feels wonderful to have forgiven, and to have freed up some of that tension you walk around with. Forgiveness is a path to harmony, inner peace, and more positive birthing.

Here's another thought: There's quite a bit of evidence that, given an appropriate opportunity, we can remember our own births, that somewhere deep inside of us there is a memory of our own birth experience. In his book *Birth and Before: What People Say about It in Hypnosis,*† David Chamberlain claims that many of his clients have remembered their births and then complained bitterly about being separated from their mothers and handled roughly. Several recent articles have described two- to five-year-olds recalling vivid and accurate memories of their births.

Deutsch[9] believes that during childbirth, a kind of altered state of consciousness occurs, which makes unconscious material more accessible. This is due to the tremendous energy involved in birth. If your own birth was difficult or traumatic, that memory may be activated as you are birthing your own child. If you experienced birth as difficult, you wanted to save your child from that experience. A cesarean seemed the best alternative. Once again, remember that out of love, you protected your child from being subjected to an experience you perceived as dangerous.

---

*From "I Honor You," by Robbie Gass. From the album *Trust in Love,* available at Spring Hill, Ashby, Mass.
†San Diego, 1981.

Opening the Heart

Many cesarean women say that they have difficulty feeling close to their babies. Studies have shown that attachment is more difficult in abnormal births. A woman from Pennsylvania writes:

> I would like to tell you the most precious thing that has happened to me. It has to do with my son, Joshua. He was a scheduled cesarean delivery. All I kept telling everyone was how wonderful it would be to pick my baby's birthday and for my husband to conveniently know what days to take off from work. If I felt so wonderful, why did the pictures of me in the hospital look as if I had been diagnosed with some incurable disease? I looked like an expressionless blob. Once home with my new baby, to whom, by the way, I didn't really coo or talk like my first, I kept thinking that the baby didn't really like me. I would say things to my husband like, "Joshua doesn't like me to hold him close," or "If Joshua is crying and I pick him up to talk to him, he just cries harder," or "Why is Josh so content when you hold him?" I just never bonded to him. The awareness I now have finally helps me to understand what was happening. I was very angry that I had allowed my baby to be brought into the world in such a cold manner. I can't help feeling what it would be like to be yanked out of my nice, cozy, warm, safe environment into a cold sterile room with no warnings at all (I guess I feel that labor is nature's way of telling a baby that change is coming). Joshua was not rejecting me, I was rejecting him because I didn't want to face the thought of him having such a traumatic birth experience. I have worked hard to resolve these feelings, and I finally feel good about myself and my relationship with my son. I am finally celebrating his birth. I can't tell you how long I held him and cried. It felt so good. It was all those tears of joy that came with the experience of childbirth. He is my baby, and I do love him very much, and he loves me. Words cannot express how much this experience has changed our lives.

We know that this mother's ability to open her heart and love *this* child will free her to love her *next* baby more easily as well. Love multiplies. Love will also help her baby feel ready to be born. The baby senses that all those good hugs are on the outside waiting, and yells, "Wait for me! I want some of those!" (A wonderful book for the whole family is *Baby*, by Fran Manushkin. It's an enchantingly illustrated story about an overdue baby. Only the daddy can figure out how to entice the baby to be born!)

Love: Birth's Most Precious Assistant

Loving yourself enough to believe you deserve a good birth experience is important. However, in this section we'd like to talk about couple-love.

We have worked with several single mothers who have had VBACs. Being in a relationship with a man is certainly not a prerequisite for a good birth. However, drawing on the strength of a relationship, *any* meaningful relationship, is a boon for pregnancy and birth. Since most of the women who have contacted us are committed maritally or otherwise, we will share our experiences of ways to use that relationship to increase your chances of birthing joyously. Dr. George Wootan remarks, "Our children won't be as healthy if our marriages aren't good."

We know that birth has the potential to bring people very close together. In *Spiritual Midwifery*[17] Karen says, "We got to places we had forgotten we could get to . . . going through the birthing I felt his love very strong. It was like getting married all over again." Michele, a VBAC mother, said, "Peter hadn't really been there for me with our first birth. But he was there, every cell of him was there this time, for me, for us, for our baby." Peter said, "I loved her more at that moment than ever before. She was so strong, determined—and so beautiful! That image will be with me forever."

We also know that birth has the potential to separate couples, to create a chasm that takes a great deal of patience, time, and energy to cross. Many couples express frustration, disappointment, and bitterness that seemed to begin right at the time of the birth. We are concerned that our culture ignores the man's and woman's relationship and how it affects childbirth. On the surface, men are included, in childbirth by being encouraged to attend classes, to learn how to be "coach," but the important issues involved are either skimmed over or completely neglected.

Each pregnancy encompasses a myriad of feelings: fear, joy, excitement, exhaustion, loneliness, strength, dependence, irritation, eagerness, peace. Often, for varied reasons, couples do not share many of their feelings. Even good communication patterns occasionally slip away from us. Maybe she wants to tell him she's afraid of labor, or of dying, but she's worried that he'll think she's silly. Maybe he doesn't want to tell her that there's a part of him that isn't getting enough holding; after all, she's been so tired. It would be selfish to complain. Maybe she wants to describe to him exactly what it feels like to be pregnant, but she is afraid he won't understand. Maybe he wants to tell her how insecure he feels; financially things aren't as good as he would like, and he works so hard and wonders how ends will meet. But if he tells her that, she'll be upset; and she's pregnant, after all, so why burden her? Maybe she feels undesirable, and he's so preoccupied! Maybe he's afraid to touch her—after all, there's a baby inside!

So perhaps she goes out and buys some maternity clothes, hoping that maybe he'll find her more desirable if she has some pretty new things. When she brings them home, he tries to be enthusiastic, but he feels concerned and anxious. "How am I going to pay for this?" he wonders. She senses "disapproval," and it confirms her suspicion that he doesn't like the way she looks anymore. In defense, she puts a wall up around herself and seems distant. In turn, he thinks, "She's wrapped up in this baby and pregnancy," and, to cushion himself, he gets busy in a project or hobby. "He's having a great time," she thinks. "He'd rather be out in the garage working than here with me." Out of loneliness, she begins yet another sweater for the new baby.

Pregnancy is a catalyst, not just for issues about babies, but for issues about love, caring, affection, finance, security, sexuality, and a multitude of other topics. We find that all too often couples do not communicate their innermost feelings, for fear of not being understood or for fear of being hurt. Pregnancy is a time of great strength and also of great vulnerability. There are many couples who become close during this time, but our experience suggests that pregnancy is also a time when old patterns of stress response are activated.

Couples who have had a cesarean are often very anxious during a subsequent pregnancy, not knowing if they'll find support for a VBAC and worrying that they'll have another upsetting birth. Ina May[17] tells us that sometimes a couple isn't very together when their first baby is born because they weren't prepared to be as open and compassionate as they needed to be at birthing. Couples that learn from experience, she says, are a good team for their next birth.

"Through the woman's capacity to intimately know the baby—whose life she totally supports—a man comes to know his child." Men form the relationship with their unborn children, using their woman as a channel of information and love. The more a woman communicates to her man her experiences of their new life, the more the man comes to know his child. The more receptive the man is to listening to his partner about that new life, the more he is able to feel participation and emotional connection. "This communication exchange forms the psychological and spiritual cradle of love that infants seek to be born into."*

There are many ways couples can feel close and continue to communicate openly during pregnancy. This is one of several exercises we ask couples to do in class:

> *Face each other . . . Women, please remain completely silent . . . Men, take your wife's hands . . . Look directly into each other's eyes. . . Men, think for a moment, and then share with your mate the qualities about her that first attracted you to her. . . Now, share the one quality that is most endearing about her at this particular moment. . . Wives, just say, "thank you," nothing more. . . Okay, let's switch. Women, take your mate's hands. . . Look at him right into his eyes. . . Tell him the qualities about him that are most special to you . . . and now, the one quality that is most endearing to you at this moment in time . . . Men, simply say, "Thank you," nothing more . . .*

The exercise is done between each couple privately. No one is required to do it. It is presented gently, and couples may decline. Some individuals are

---

*From *Ended Beginnings*, published by Bergin & Garvey, 1984.

eager to take part—it has been such a long time since they have heard how precious or special they are to their mates. It is interesting to note how many people have difficulty making direct eye contact.

We ask each couple to reminisce (privately again) about the first moment they knew they wanted to spend their lives together. We then ask them to recall specific occasions when they felt especially close to each other and to discuss these times in detail with each other.

In the discussion that follows, we talk about the exercises. How difficult or easy were they to do? How do you feel when you look directly into each other's eyes (the pathway to the soul!)? How do you express love and affection now, and are these expressions different from those of years past? How do you feel about being able to reach out and touch your mate lovingly in a room full of people?

One man said he didn't do the exercise because, "She knows I love her. I don't have to tell her," whereupon his mate responded, "Yes, you do! I never hear it anymore!" There are often tears in an exercise like this: it's wonderful and cleansing and healing to be able to let them out. There is also laughter and sharing.

These exercises and others like them are helpful for both the man and woman. Love really does help a baby be born. As a conscious act of love, a woman opens her body to receive her mate. So, too, decisions to love and displays of affection will help her to open to let her baby be born. Spiritual leader Hazrat Inayat Khan once said, "With love, even the rocks will open."

Couples have said that after these exercises they feel "bouncier" inside than they have for a while. One woman told us that she and her husband made love that evening for the first time in many weeks, and her nausea permanently subsided that night. We see many couples holding hands or sitting closer after the exercises.

We also see couples who are silent, or distant. Perhaps for some, these exercises open a can of worms. We only know that love does help a baby get born (have we said it enough?!) and that childbirth classes are a place where love needs to be discussed and affection encouraged.

We ask that each morning the couple share with each other the quality about their spouse that was most endearing to them the previous day. One woman said this helped her day start with a smile. One man told us that he didn't like being told when to express affection to his wife. "I don't like being told what to do," he said. "I didn't like being told what to do for my last birth," his wife blurted out. "I was told when I had to have an enema, when I could roll over. It was awful." This common feeling—of not liking to be told what to do—provided a new understanding on the husband's part about the frustration and hostility the wife felt about her cesarean.

We ask that couples use a list of questions (see Appendix C) designed to explore areas that may influence the birth experience. This list may also help to insure that important areas of discussion are not neglected or treated nonchalantly. For those of you who decide to use the list, we ask that only one question be discussed per evening. Be sure to focus on your feelings. A feeling is a state of mind, body, or heart. It follows the words, "I feel _____." (If you say "I feel *that* _____, you are expressing an opinion or judgment, not a feeling.) Feelings are neither right nor wrong, they simply exist.

Remember that any honest sharing lovingly expressed from one person to another, whether you agree with it or find it difficult to hear, is a gift. During the sharing, remember the qualities that you love and respect about each other. Try to bring back the feelings of closeness and warmth and love that you felt so strongly during your courtship.

Another exercise we suggest in class is as follows: We ask each couple to write a love letter to their mate, and to exchange them at a point during labor when they'll be most appreciated. Each person then writes a love letter to her unborn baby, and one to herself—also to be read during labor. "Reading my own words—those written at a much calmer time—was very powerful," said Kay. "It helped me relocate my perspective, and remember why I was doing this [laboring and having a baby]. It helped me continue, far more peacefully, with my labor."

We also recommend touching exercises and massage to strengthen coupleness. Set aside time, a private time, with no interruptions. (One woman met her husband for lunch, brought a blanket to his office, locked the door, and put out a sign that said, "Important meeting in session. Do not disturb!") These exercises are designed to create a comfort with touching and an appreciation of your bodies. Ina May tells us that touch is the first language we speak. Babies learn about the universe through touch. She mentions that she has cured babies of colic by helping the mother to hold her baby more lovingly. Once the baby knows his mother is really *there* for him, she says, "the baby gets over his bellyache."[17]

For both men and women, touch exercises can soothe weary bones and quiet aches, too. They can give both of you a chance to become more at ease with your pregnant body, and they can be an opportunity to communicate with the baby as well. Mothers often communicate love to their babies just by a touch or a pat on their belly. These exercises will encourage fathers to do so as well. They can also help to ease discomfort with nudity that can negatively influence birth.

In the privacy of your home, set aside time to be nude with your mate. One at a time, touch or cuddle the other, but refrain from intercourse or genital contact. Some couples have little difficulty with this. It's a wonderfully soothing and sensual experience; a time for appreciating pleasure that comes from both giving and taking. Other couples find it impossible to refrain from intercourse.

Our society is certainly "open" about physical intimacy and sexuality, but only on the *surface*. Talk shows discuss all the hottest sexual subjects. Although these discussions leave little to our collective imagination, intimacy in the flesh is a whole different concept. Many couples consider themselves totally open and free with each other, very comfortable with each other's bodies, *but* their intimacy is always bounded by lovemaking. In other words, they can be intimate as long as they're sexually involved. Apart from the sexual act itself, many couples feel embarrassed, restrained, and inhibited with each other. Out of bed and in the light of day, they may rarely touch. All this is *fine* if it feels right and comfortable. Yet, examining sexual attitudes and all they encompass can help smooth a couple's way for giving birth. We ask only that each couple be very aware of how they feel about their bodies, how they touch and do not touch, how they feel about being touched, and what they have learned from doing or not doing the exercises. In *Spiritual Midwifery*,[17] Cara reminds us that one of the best ways to get a baby out "is by cuddling and smooching with your husband. That loving, sexy vibes is what puts the baby in there, and it's what gets it out, too."

When was the last time you took a walk together? Packed a picnic lunch? Ran through the leaves? Had a candlelight dinner at home? Played in the snow? Keeping romance alive and well is wonderful! *And it can influence your birth.* Of course, many women with no mate or no romance in their lives birth joyfully and normally. Some women birth better without a man present. The thoughts presented here are for those of you in relationships who want them to be more meaningful.

We enthusiastically recommend a Marriage Encounter weekend. When people first hear about this, they get visions of a weekend orgy, or they think we are recommending marriage counseling or group therapy. "We already have a good marriage," some people say, or "We're not into *that* kind of thing." Marriage Encounter is not an orgy, nor a religious experience, nor a marriage counseling session. It is a weekend designed to give you time for each other, to put you in touch with feelings you had when you first discovered that you loved each other and wanted to spend the rest of your lives together. It's for couples who have good marriages and want to make them better, or for relationships that are struggling but committed. It is a completely private, non-threatening weekend. Although there are many other couples on the weekend, you only have time to meet them at mealtimes. The rest of the weekend, is spent listening to presentations about different aspects of married life and communicating with your own spouse.

Going away to a hotel for a weekend is always nice, but three days after you return, it hardly seems as if you have gone. You slip right back into daily pressures and routines. But weeks after your Marriage Encounger weekend, the weekend will still be alive for you.

Marriage Encounter weekends are sponsored by many church organizations. The fee is minimal, and no one is ever turned away for lack of funds. It's an opportunity for rediscovering and enhancing your love for each other. Both the Cohens and the Estners know that the new communication techniques we learned and the feelings of love and warmth we experienced profoundly influenced us as we birthed our VBAC babies.

One other suggestion we give to the couples in class: Make one list of five things you can do to make your mate "Number One" this week, and another list of five ways he/she could make you feel as if you were also a "top priority." Share your lists and use them. Not only is this exercise fun, it's good to feel special and to help someone you love feel special, too.

Creating a Cesarean

Robert Frost tells us, "Our very life depends on everything recurring until we answer from within. The thousandth time may prove the charm." Every experience in life has a lesson to teach us. If we learn from the particular experience, we won't have to repeat the experience to learn it. In this context, repeat cesareans are another opportunity to learn something that you need to know in this life. We ask that you make a list of ten positive things you gained (or will gain) from having a cesarean—besides the baby. "Are you nuts?" some of you are asking. "I got nothing that was positive from that horror show besides the baby." The sooner you can begin making a list, the sooner you will begin your path to VBAC rather than repeat cesarean section. We suggest that you make your list before reading on, even if it takes a few days. We *know* the exercise will be of value to you. What did you get from your cesarean that was positive besides the baby? What did you learn about yourself that you didn't already know? How did you grow from the experience?

Nora said:

> When I was first asked to make this list, I was furious. "You think having a section was a picnic?" I said. "You try having major surgery." I scribbled and doodled for a whole week. "I got **nothing** from the cesarean except the baby," I thought. "And besides, it was enough that I got him." But a list formed, and it grew. "Well, I did get some attention from my mother, I mean a different kind of attention than I would have gotten if I had had a regular delivery. And come to think of it, Joe stayed out of work an extra few days. That was nice; I really loved it when he was home. He was so good with the baby and so calming. I learned how determined I could be: I actually demanded my baby!" I continued, slowly and reluctantly, to see that there **were** positive factors that had come from David's birth. In addition, I had reinforced many strong beliefs about my life that I had set up. The list kept growing!

Couples in the classes bring in and share their lists. They share what beliefs influenced their births, what was positive about the cesarean, or what they have learned: "We hadn't felt very close to each other before the delivery. The cesarean was a real emergency, and it made us realize how precious we were to each other." "I gave up a baby for adoption at seventeen. I wasn't going to let another baby out only to be taken away again. I know now I hold back even my love, thinking it'll be whisked away and not returned." "I think I am a better nurse for having been through this. I'm certainly a better childbirth educator." "Now I *know* what it is like to have major surgery, to be a patient, and this knowledge benefits me in my work. Also, when I tell a woman I understand, she can believe me." "I got to hold the baby first, even before my wife did. I'd always been worried that the baby wouldn't love me as well." "I learned what a high pain tolerance I have." "I had had two abortions. I didn't feel I deserved a good birth experience." "I realize now I'd become quite independent from John. Having a cesarean meant that I truly needed to lean on him again." "I wanted my husband to be close to our baby, since my father never was close to me. When I had the cesarean, he had to take full responsibility for Andrew's care and I know that helped them bond." "I wanted a girl so badly. The amniocentesis said I was having a boy. I labored twenty-six hours and had a section. I guess I didn't want to open for another boy. My little boy was a 7 pound pound baby girl." (This woman subsequently had a homebirth VBAC after two cesareans.) "I had had two miscarriages and I resisted labor, thinking I'd lose this baby too."

What did (do) *you* need to learn that a cesarean birth could provide? What would you get from a cesarean that you need in your life at this time?

Pampering? A closer relationship with your mother? Sympathy and attention from your husband? A change from housework? An opportunity to see how strong you were or how much pain you could withstand? Did you have a cesarean to punish yourself? To reinforce old beliefs?

Ask yourself the following question: Do I need these things still?

If you do, you might create another cesarean in order to get them. We suggest that you find a way to get what you need without having another section (or a cesarean in the first place). One woman said, "I knew I needed my mother to help out. I told her I needed her and that I wanted her to take off from work for a few days to give me a hand. I told her I didn't want to have major surgery in order for her to feel that it was acceptable to take time off."

If anyone had told us years ago that in a sense we *create* our cesarean births, we would have punched him/her in the jaw. What a ridiculous, uncaring, insensitive thought! But we know know that our beliefs influence every one of our life experiences. (One psychologist has suggested that as a culture, if we integrated a new belief that women over 40 do not necessarily produce genetically defective babies, we might in fact, note a decrease in abnormalities in this age group.)

Birth is one of the most profound teaching experiences life offers. It touches us in the depths of our souls, the most private recesses of who we are. It requires that we respond with more creative energy, more conviction, more trust, than almost anything else we do. Birth requires an intensity that is rarely demanded by other experiences. And through it, we can learn more about ourselves, our strengths, our weaknesses, our relationship patterns, and our needs than through almost any other experience we will face in our life.

"Why Me?"

Some women do everything "right." They eat well, exercise, refuse interventions that can lead to a cesarean, clear our negative beliefs, work to get their locus of control centered within themselves, find an excellent support system—and still somehow find themselves the (reluctant) recipients of a cesarean. Why?

We don't know for sure. We do believe that approximately 3 percent of the time, nature needs a little assist. For example, women with maternal conditions that years ago would have made it practically impossible to carry a pregnancy to viability are now often able to carry longer and can resort to cesarean section to help assure a live and healthy infant. With the help of fertility specialists, women give birth who years ago might not have been able to.

Sometimes there is no earthly explanation. Linda said, "I did everything right, uncovered all of my garbage. I guess I'll have to keep sorting through it." Perhaps this will help, perhaps not. Occasionally, the answers aren't ours to discover.

One philosophy is that the baby herself may have needed to be born by cesarean to work out her own "karma." "Karma" is a Sanskrit word meaning "acts" or "deeds"; for our purposes, "karma" refers to the sum total of an individual's conscious and unconscious acts and deeds. It also refers to that individual's paths in life, both worldly and spiritual. Perhaps you were the person that could provide the kind of birth your baby needed to begin learning what *she's* supposed to learn in this lifetime. Perhaps your baby chose you because you were the very best person to work through her own life and discover her own paths. She looked at all the available homes, saw yours, and said, *"That's where I want to be!"* (Adopted babies find a way to get where they want to be, too!)

Karma is a part of Eastern philosophy. Western holistic thought has some related concepts (mind, body, and soul or spirit). Perhaps these approaches can offer you some new ideas, and your own path to peace concerning the birth. You can search as long as you like to discover why the birth you dreamed about was not yours to own at that point in time. At some point, when you are ready, you'll discover why, or you'll let go of the search.

"But I'm Due on Tuesday!"

We want you to know that if you came to us late in your pregnancy, you would not get a ten-day course on belief systems, sexuality, or marital counseling. Women have been birthing their babies for hundreds of years without detailed psychological presentations. We would help by asking that you eat very well, take some walks, and make certain that you have a good support system (changing doctors or hospitals if necessary).

We would also recommend that you begin to say some affirmations. Affirmations are present-tense, positive statements about ourselves that may not feel true at first, but which become integrated into our thoughts and begin to come true: I am a strong and capable woman. My body is working for me. I am designed to give birth. I am giving birth normally. I am invincible. I am woman! (For more affirmations, see Appendix E.)

We'd ask you to remind yourself over and over again that your body was designed to have babies. We'd give you our "If you were in the backwoods of New Hampshire and you were in labor and your car wouldn't start, you'd have your baby and be fine" routine. And we would give you lots of support and plenty of hugs. *Family Health Magazine* tells us that four hugs a day are necessary for survival, eight for maintenance, and twelve for growth!

However, we hope that you do have some time before your birth. We ask you, then, to take a look, however brief, at your beliefs. Your beliefs about yourself and your life *will* affect your labor.

You can learn about yourself through suggestions presented here, therapy, reading, or visualization. In addition, Mehl and Peterson have designed a risk screening evaluation procedure (to assist instinct and judgment) to predict a woman's potential for normal birthing. The procedure is 98 percent accurate and 85 percent correct in predicting complications (and often *specific* complications!).

Some women are turned off or frightened by the psychological approach. One woman said, "I wonder if putting so much emphasis on the psychological might actually create obstacles for some people." A childbirth educator said, "I'd never discuss *this* stuff in class. We're not supposed to be psychotherapists, and I'm not opening cans of worms!" Edith was confused: "First you say birth is a completely natural event, then you say we can make it go wrong if our head isn't on straight."

However, most couples and educators alike are excited and fascinated with the discussion of psychological aspects of birth. They can see how feelings influence outcome. "If, indeed, I did make my cesarean happen, then I can make one *not* happen!" said Alice. Sharon wrote:

> The emphasis on the internal—on the sacredness, complexity, and connection be-
> tween my head and my body—I am most grateful for, for it has profoundly affected

me. I was given license and finally exhorted to look inside myself—and there I found not only some answers, but also some very lovely places that I've been able to spend time in. There was a kind of peace available in there that seems to emanate out from some eternal woman place—a wonderful place!

So, if you like, you can begin to look inside yourself, find all the good things, and change any negative beliefs. You can begin to trust your body to bring this baby into the world safely, in your own unique way. We have noticed that as a woman takes responsibility for her birth experience, so is she able to take responsibility for other areas in her life. She is able to change the way she views herself and to make active decisions about how she will live. She is no longer a passive victim of life's twists and turns, but an active road-mapper. Jane said, "After I birthed my daughter, I knew there wasn't anything in this world I couldn't do."

13 ❧ Planning Your Birth

"Only in America does a woman have to plan her birth!" —First-time mother, who would have preferred to sun herself during her pregnancy, but who was later very glad she had taken time instead to plan her birth wisely

The time you spend preparing for your baby's birth can be a time of peace and purpose, or it can be a time of frustration and tension. There are many decisions to be made. You will need to think about what kind of childbirth education will be best for you, where you will feel safest giving birth, and whom you will want to have attend your birth.

No doubt you will encounter some people who do not understand the heavy investment you are making in your birth plans. "Just find a doctor you trust," they will say, "and leave everything up to him."

"Just take a Lamaze course at the hospital. You'll learn everything you need to know."

"What do you mean, 'No anesthesia?' Everyone is having epidurals now. Don't be such a martyr!"

"Don't ask so many questions. Why do you need to know so much?"

"You won't need to bring your own labor support person to that hospital. The nurses are *wonderful*."

"HOME BIRTH?! Are you crazy?!"

In all such comments, the underlying messages are the same: Don't challenge the authority of the medical establishment. Don't make waves. Don't upset the status quo.

If it is a VBAC that you are planning, you might be made to feel downright irresponsible. Some people will act as though you are endangering your baby's life for your own selfish fulfillment. They need for you to validate their choices by doing things their way. "What's good enough for me is good enough for you," they will say, in so many words.

You need to do things in a way that is right for *you*. Your baby's birth will profoundly influence the rest of your life and all of his. It is crucial that you make choices that are right for both of you.

If you are a person who is used to taking responsibility for your actions and making your own decisions, then you will do so now. If you are not, we suggest that this is a good time to start. Childbirth is an intensely personal experience. The decisions and choices you make in preparation for it should be equally personal.

The first thing you will need to decide is what kind of childbirth education will be right for this pregnancy. If this is not your first child, chances are that you have already graduated from one of the traditional childbirth-education courses offered in your area. Chances are, too, that you found what you learned to be less than adequate. This will be especially true if your last birth was a cesarean or a less-than-satisfactory vaginal birth. You will need to do some rethinking before you begin to make choices for this birth.

Childbirth Preparation

Can you imagine women in African villages leaving their laundry to soak in the river while they take a childbirth-preparation class? Can you envision the men coming home early from hunting to practice timing contractions? Can you visualize the Pilgrims cutting short their harvesting on Tuesday to attend an evening of films on birth? Maybe the Indians caught buffalo mainly to serve at break-time at their classes on Wednesday night?

Women have been birthing babies without formal classes since the beginning of our species. Every one of you knew exactly what you needed to know to birth a baby before you even opened the cover of this book. Women don't need classes to give birth. Nor do they need hospitals, instruments, tools, drugs, chemicals, or doctors. None of these is a prerequisite for bearing children.

In Jarara, South Africa, women birth in a shelter in full view of everyone. There is no concern over this matter. Childbirth is considered a normal phenomenon, a fact of life. "Classes" for those lucky women were held throughout their early lives, as they grew up among women who birthed close by, and as they learned from them. Present-day childbirth preparation provides information that used to be integrated over a long period of time within the context of family living. It seeks to familiarize women with pregnancy and birth, since we now live in nuclear families and are not exposed to these processes frequently enough to give us confidence and reassurance. It makes sense to us that childbirth education begin before pregnancy, and we are concerned about formal classes that do not permit participation until the sixth, seventh, or even eighth month. Those last months of pregnancy should be filled with confidence and peace and free time; instead, women in our culture are rushing to get through with dinner and out the door to classes.

Gordon and Gordon[16] tell us that disturbances in childbearing are more likely to occur in women who have recently moved away from relatives and friends. In our transient society, it is common for women to be removed from relatives and friends; during birth *most* women are "recently removed" from loved ones. In *Lying In: A History of Chidbirth in America*, Dorothy Wertz tells us that birth in our country is not only a time of alienation from family and friends, but "from the community and even from life itself."[45] Thus, childbirth classes must fill additional needs no longer filled by the family and community. In addition to information, they must provide the love, care, friendship, and strength that women need at their births. Too many classes focus on the information over and above the other, more vital, "lessons" to be shared.

A survey done in one county in New York found that the hospital with the highest number of prepared couples also had the highest section rate.* In *Mal(e) Practice*, Robert Mendelsohn tells us that prepared couples are a delight for doctors.[32] Prepared women, he says, are prepared to listen to the doctor, prepared not to question, and prepared to trust him completely. They are sent to prenatal classes "presumably to be informed and reassured, but actually to be softened up for all the needless interventions that their obstetricians have in store for them." Another "how to" lesson: how to be compliant, good little girls. Marieskind adds that, interestingly, most classes are markedly uncritical of the rising cesarean rate.

In an article entitled "Natural Childbirth—A Review and Analysis," Beck remarks that despite numerous claims about the efficacy of the psychoprophylaxis method, "even a cursory examination of the literature" reveals errors in methodology. "Many of the studies did not even meet the most fundamental and basic requirement of the scientific method—the utilization of appropriate control groups."[5]

We believe that unless childbirth preparation makes some drastic changes, the rate of unnecessary interventions and cesareans among "trained" couples will climb. That the rate of intervention is already so high is attributable to many factors. For example, Madeleine Shearer, editor of *Birth*, points out that most couples who pay for childbirth education are generally "more affluent,

---

*1979 *Survey of Suffolk County Hospitals*, by the Mothers' Center of Suffolk [New York], Inc.

better insured—and therefore 'sitting ducks' for all the interferences that lead to surgery." We hope the factors will continue to be identified and resolved.

We believe that childbirth preparation can be useful. We also believe it can be counterproductive. Unfortunately, many of the classes taught in our culture are more misleading than useful. Fortunately, that is changing; unfortunately, it is not changing fast enough. Childbirth education has such *potential!*—and much of it has not yet begun to be tapped.

Traditional Course Content

Many years ago, in a lecture on childbirth preparation, Sheila Kitzinger stated that childbirth education must go beyond uterine activity and what can be done to tolerate it. "Instead," she said, "*relationships* and *feelings* must be paramount." We agree. From strong and loving relationships grow the feelings of strength and love for our babies and our bodies that contribute to normal birthing. From communicative interactions with physicians and staffs, more positive birthing can result. By exposing, sharing, and releasing feelings, we clear ourselves for joyful experiences with birth. A spring cleaning, if you will. Childbirth classes must help by providing the equipment to begin the cleaning. Until childbirth education speaks to the *psychological* we will produce less-than-satisfactory results.

"Puff, Puff, Pant . . . Help!"   Far too many instructors spend a lot of time on breathing and biology.

Teaching breathing is a waste of time. It aims to distract the woman rather than help her focus *in* on her labor. It is physically exhausting and mentally fatiguing, as well. Mehl and Peterson tell us that dissociation of mind and body is *not* helpful. Dozens of couples have shared that they *argued* about doing their breathing exercises! Couples often feel tense because *he* didn't want to do the breathing, or he kept pushing her to do it better; or *she* felt discouraged because she didn't feel competent at it, or she refused to do it altogether. Are not those precious few minutes each day best spent talking to each other, holding each other, and sharing the day's events instead of practicing how to breathe?

Many classes teach that proper breathing will negate pain and allow the woman to stay in control. If the breathing does not meet these expectations, it is likely that the woman will become very discouraged. We've been breathing our whole lives: must we be *taught* to breathe for labor? We have not taught breathing to any one of the couples who have come to us for childbirth preparation. Not once did anyone not breathe during labor or stop breathing while giving birth!

Breathing exercises do not have to take up more than a moment of class time.

The following are examples of the only breathing instructions we have found necessary: "Take a breath. Let the oxygen flow through your body right down to your cervix. Let the breath help to open your cervix as it passes through and opens your lungs"; "Breathe. Let the oxygen go where it will to release any part of your body that needs releasing"; "Enjoy the inhale! Expand your ability to take in a good breath! With it, take in anything and everything you need (love, comfort, peace). Then let gravity take the exhale, and with it, let out anything you don't need (tension, tightness, anger)." Breathing should be a way of achieving relaxation and peace; instead, it often produces exhaustion and tension during difficult phases of labor.

Pain: A Four-Letter Word   In many childbirth classes, words such as "discomfort" and "pressure" are used in place of "pain." "Pain" is considered a four-letter word. It is believed that this reconditioning is appropriate and helpful. We disagree. The couples we teach are graduates of these classes. They feel cheated when they get into active labor and feel *pain*, not just discomfort or pressure. They begin to think that something is wrong. They become tense. Tension inhibits the body's normal, natural work of labor. The more pain they feel, the more frightened they become.

As the pain increases, the special breathing patterns often don't work. Sometimes they make things worse. "I got up to level four and had no place else to go, but it wasn't helping. I panicked," said one woman.

"I was so tired from all that hoo-ing and ha-ing that I had no energy to push," said another.

"All that counting and breathing did nothing but make me tired and thirsty, but no one would give me anything except some ice chips," said a third.

"I must have been doing it wrong," said another. (*"There is no such thing as doing it wrong,"* we told her, *"if you do it your way."*)

Melzack et al. found that 81 percent of the prepared mothers in his study asked for epidurals. The authors conclude that prepared childbirth was insufficient to reduce pain enough to decrease the patients' needs for anesthesia.[29] Childbirth educator Penny Simkin comments that epidurals must have been "terribly available!" She remarks, "It may be time to study the effectiveness of different curricula, attitudes, and methods taught in childbirth classes, and their relationship to the goals of both educators and parents."

The infamous "focal point" is another suggestion given in many classes to reduce pain. "I found no distraction, no matter how hard I concentrated," said one woman. One father shared, "I was talking in her ear. 'Don't think about the pain! Think about the beach. No? How about our dog?' " When nothing worked, he threw up his hands in desperation and yelled "Sex?" One woman distracted herself so completely that she completely missed the birth. "I had no sense of having participated at all. I was separate from the whole labor."

We suggest that if a focal point is to be used, it should be for support, not distraction. It should be someone else's eyes, or one's own body, or the contraction itself, or an image of the baby. Pain is a healthy part of birth. To accept it, to welcome it as the energy that will allow your baby to be born, requires an attitude of faith, trust, and confidence. Janet Leigh reminds us continually to say "Yes." Say yes to your strength, yes to your contractions, yes to your pain, yes to your baby.

Biology 101 In many childbirth classes a great deal of time is spent describing "the architecture"! All the bones and muscles of our anatomy are described in great detail, as are conception, implantation, and fetal growth. It is our opinion that this is basically a waste of your time and your money. There are countless books describing your anatomy and the processes of conception, implantation, and fetal development written at varying reading levels. Anyone who is interested can find materials that describe in full detail the scientific aspects of fertilization and pregnancy. Precious time should not be wasted on information that can easily be obtained by couples who are so motivated. We have come to believe that detailed, scientific instruction about the processes of conception, implantation, and fetal development is *not* the responsibility of the childbirth educator.

We believe that childbirth classes should take childbirth *away* from the medical and the scientific. Although specific information about how the birth process "works" can be useful, couples should not have to hear all the scientific terms, the exact times at which particular organs develop, or every detail of conception, implantation, and development. If they want this information, then the childbirth instructor can be an excellent resource and direct them to the information. But many couples have shared that they find their childbirth education to be little more than a series of biology lessons and they often feel incompetent, overwhelmed, or bored, and continue to lack confidence about the upcoming birth.

In our classes, we show just enough charts during the "biology" discussion (which lasts only ten or fifteen minutes) to explain basic terms. There are fundamental beliefs underlying every statement that the whole process is wonderful; that it is very special (but also unique for each person); and that it *works!* There's an overriding theme throughout the discussion, indeed, throughout all the classes, that *bodies are incredibly wise.* They know how to produce the sperm and the egg and get them to meet and make love all over again to form the baby; each uterus knows how to grow and protect the baby and not let the baby out until the time is right; each placenta implants nice and high. That's just what placentas do! The amniotic sac fills with clear sterile fluid that surrounds and protects the baby. The baby's head is heavy so that it just sinks down into the uterus. The cervix effaces and dilates. The pelvis opens. The perineum stretches. The umbilical cord is just the right length. The placenta separates from the uterine wall after the baby is born. The breasts produce colostrum and milk. Everything knows what it's supposed to do and does it. The perineum doesn't produce milk, nor does the placenta efface. These unique and special parts of our bodies do just what they have been doing ever since they were created to do them.

Men are able to see what they've got. Women aren't. Part of our childbearing anatomy is inaccessible to us. We don't know exactly what we have inside or if our equipment is "top quality." For example, at your very first vaginal exam, how many of you had a doctor who said, in a nonsexual way of course, "Hey! Wow! This is a WONDERFUL PELVIS! I mean, it's really dynamite!" No one? You mean, not one of us was told we had a magnificent pelvis? What, then, *were* you told?

- "That it seemed adequate."

- "That it was a little narrow, but not to worry."

- "That my muscles were tight, I should relax."

- "That I shouldn't have a problem."

- "That I could probably accommodate a 'normal'-sized
baby without too much difficulty."

God in Heaven! How many of us want to be told that our body SEEMS adequate? How many men want to be told that their penis SEEMS adequate? Your muscles are *supposed* to be firm! And how in the world are you supposed to RELAX when someone has his fingers in your vagina? We want to suggest to all of you that the seeds of doubt about your bodies, which in some way may have led you to a cesarean, were planted a long time ago—and that one of the seeds that took root probably did so at the time of your first vaginal exam, when no one told you what a *marvelous, perfect-for-you,* childbearing pelvis you had.

Your pelvis will open as you give birth. In labor (labor activated by your body, not by the doctor or some chemical), your hormones change, and this relaxes the ligaments that support the pelvis. In turn, the pelvis, which is flexible and "gives," releases. From the comments made to us by physicians, we'd never know how wonderful nature is and how *infrequently* a pelvis is inadequate to its job.

You never questioned that your vagina would open to accommodate your mate's penis. Why question whether your pelvis will open for your baby? Everything knows the plan and follows it. Your hormones change. Your baby's head molds. Your placenta stays exactly where it's supposed to until just after the baby is born. Your uterus directs your baby out of your body. This has been happening successfully from the beginning of humanity. Sometimes your body is given confusing messages about what it's supposed to do, and we'll learn about those. We'll learn how to help your body if it's in need of a little assistance at any point. But first must come the belief that the process is wonderful and that it works. The process of giving birth must be appreciated, exalted, *honored.*

We believe that women were designed to have babies. We believe that babies were designed to experience labor. We believe that just as your body opened to receive your mate and conceive this child, your body is equally able to open and release your infant—given the right set of circumstances. The atmosphere for lovemaking had to be right. Your mate wouldn't have been able to get an erection if people had been sticking I.V.s into his arm, telling him he wasn't doing it well enough or fast enough. . .and women can't help their babies get out, either, with tubes in their arms, or under pressure to do it faster. But more on that later.

For now, *appreciate your body.* It is healthy and wise. Take good care of it. Respect it. Trust it. Respect the beauty, intricacy, and intimacy of the act that places your baby inside. Marvel at the process that has gotten babies safely *outside* their mother's bodies for generations. Believe in it. And believe, with us, that your body is perfectly capable of birthing your baby. That is the very best preparation you can have for your baby's birth.

Is There Such a Thing as "Failure"? There is no right way to have a baby, we are told. We are cautioned not to project our own values on to someone else's birth experience. However, we consider it a primary responsibility of all childbirth educators to help all women share strong values about the importance of pure birthing.

For a long time, childbirth educators were afraid to talk about pain; now, childbirth educators are afraid to talk about "failure." Is it a "failure" to take medication? Is it a "failure" to have a forceps birth? Is it a "failure" to have an unnecessary cesarean? We think not, for childbearing must be free from suffering and guilt, but it *is* a sadness. We have a whole country of weeping mothers and infants to prove how sad it really is. Panuthos and Silva, in *Positive Birthing,** tell us that childbirth classes must teach couples to ground their hopes in realistic expectations of positive outcomes without the burden of ideal birth scenes that even the most well-adjusted couple would have difficulty achieving. We'd take an inch and ask that you aim for the stars. You may not reach them; but, oh, what an experience on the way up!

Cesarean Classes Classes for "cesarean birth" have become fashionable. For the few women who require a cesarean, there should be information and

---

*Arlington, Mass.: People Place Press, 1982.

support; but for the countless thousands who could and should deliver vaginally, cesarean classes are a great disservice to women. Cesarean-birth classes keep many childbirth educators, anesthesiologists, hospital staffs, and obstetricians well fed and happily employed. Most women attending these classes could have their babies vaginally with no problem whatsoever. We were once proponents of cesarean-birth classes. However, we now believe that they are an insult to us all. Only in America would a group of women be instructed in "How to be cut open unnecessarily and keep smiling through it all."

Some instructors have commented that since no one in the area will allow a VBAC, they are providing a service by making cesareans a better experience. Others say, "I discussed VBAC, but no one wants one." It's no wonder no one wanted one. With words like "rupture" and "anesthesiologist present every minute," Mother Earth herself would run for cover. Because a cesarean can be a good experience is no reason to put a women and baby on an operating table without first making the safer alternative more appealing.

We do believe that the issue of cesarean section needs to be addressed. We hope it is done in a way that gives couples the incentive to avoid the operation, if possible, and the strength to avoid interventions that will increase their chances for the surgery. We believe that after accepting the popular premises of cesarean-birth classes, one-quarter of the students in such classes will have c/sections. One childbirth educator in Boston had a 25 percent cesarean rate for five years. "Then I started teaching cesarean prevention. Now the rate is five percent or less."

Hospital VBAC Classes   One hospital in the Boston area is teaching "VBAC" classes. The instructor, a nurse, has never had a VBAC. She teaches more about "Getting ready for a cesarean, just in case," than she does about cesarean prevention. L.A.s are not permitted in that hospital, so the concept of a labor assistant is not even mentioned. Food during labor is not permitted, so the virtues of I.V.s are extolled. The worst insult is that couples taking the class must have written permission slips from their doctors. Unbelievable!

Finding the Right Instructor

David Stewart of NAPSAC tells us that parents have the right to choose, what may seem to a professional, a wrong choice. Since we aren't even going to learn what all of our choices are from the medical professionals, we are going to have to take responsibility for learning them ourselves. We hope that childbirth educators will see it as their responsibility to teach these choices to us as well.

Drug companies don't need our business. Amnio hooks, surgical knives, and catheters are selling fine. The fetal monitoring business is not only thriving but supporting thousands. Childbirth educators do not have to lend support to these companies or sanction the use of their mostly unnecessary pieces of equipment. Nor do childbirth educators bear any allegiance to physicians. Obstetrics is one of the largest and most lucrative specialties in United States medicine (although doctors who oppose midwifery do not often speak of one reason that may be on their minds: money).

What childbirth educators must do, first and foremost, is to be an *advocate for our unborn babies*. They need to provide an atmosphere where enthusiasm and joy are abundant and where accurate, consumer-oriented information is presented. They need to teach couples to protect themselves against unnecessary interventions, impatience, overestimation of technology, and human meddlesomeness. In the words of an educator from the Midwest, they need to "inspire self-confidence and stimulate the woman in such a way that she considers the reproductive task not a burden but a creative deed." They need to help women find fulfillment and satisfaction through a conscious commitment to pure, normal birthing.

Childbirth educator Liz Belden Handler remarks that the role that is perhaps *most* important for each childbirth educator "is that of a *birth activist*."* And Marilyn Moran tells us, "The revolution has begun!"

Childbirth educator Debra Evans writes:

> I am sorry for the women who create a great distance between their bodies and their thoughts, their children and themselves. As a childbirth educator, I work to bridge the gaps; I strive to eliminate facades; and I seek to nurture the innate strength and courage that each woman often buries under layers of cultural pretense. Preparing women to give birth requires nothing less than the most transparent kind of sharing, so that pregnant women can be convinced how important 'opening up' can be.

Lynn Richards, a midwife who shares her views on conscious childbirth, tells us that childbirth classes must support "exercises for the body, information for the mind, release for the heart, and mediation for the soul." In *Childbirth Educator*, Sherry Lynn Mims Jimenez writes, "I used to be a Lamaze instructor. Like an army drill sergeant, I gave orders and watched over my class as they practiced. Now I am a childbirth educator. Instead of giving my knowledge to my clients, I help them find it themselves."† We hope you'll find a childbirth educator whose philosophies match Debra's, Lynn's, and Sherry's. We rather doubt you'll find them within a hospital, but if you do, you've found a rose among dandelions. Consumer-oriented classes are rarely found where fetal monitors are as abundant as wildflowers.

---

*From the *Clarion*, the CPM (Cesarean Prevention Movement) Newsletter, (Summer 1982), no. 1, p. 5.

†"My Way: The New Lamaze," *Childbirth Educator*, 1 (Winter 1981–82), no. 2.

You can contact local NAPSAC groups for names of instructors. You can contact the American Academy of Husband-Coached Childbirth for instructors who teach "Bradley." You can contact the Association for Childbirth at Home, or HOME (Home Oriented Maternity Experience) or Informed Homebirth and take a homebirth course, even if you plan to birth in the hospital. You can also contact ICEA or ASPO. Be very selective about the classes you choose, and screen your instructor carefully.

Educators Who Don't   We'd like a penny for every childbirth educator who has told us she either wouldn't or couldn't recommend the many good consumer books and publications available. Either they aren't on her "Approved Reading List" or she is worried that she'll be fired if she talks about certain issues (the dangers of fetal monitoring, for example, or the value of eating during labor). So they protect the doctors, the hospitals, and their pocketbooks, and once again a potential advocate for safe, normal birthing—*and for the baby*—has defected.

Sometimes an instructor tells us, "These women are not ready to hear that stuff." We think it's her job to get them ready. Must women have cesarean sections before they are radicalized enough to hear consumer information?

There are several approaches that childbirth educators can take, but far too many simply help women adjust to their community's obstetrical policies. These educators are advocates for the doctors and hospitals, not for the parents. Some childbirth educators believe that as they become respected and liked by the professionals, change will occur; but, while they are taking time to woo the medical community, women are being dragged in, drugged up, and put under. It is our belief that childbirth educators have a responsibility to get consumer information to pregnant women and couples as quickly as possible and let them, as consumers, use it to influence the medical community.

Hospital Classes?   We rarely recommend classes that are taught within a hospital. The very location of the classes draws healthy couples to an institution devoted to illness. Robert Mendelsohn[32] tells us that a group of ten thousand nurses was questioned about hospital preferences. One-third of them said they would not choose to be patients in the hospitals where they worked. Most would not want to birth in them, either. Often course material and content must be sanctioned by the obstetrical staff, and the instructors are usually medically trained. Teaching hospital policy is not childbirth education! *Any instructor teaching what pregnant couples should know would be barred from teaching in most hospitals in this country!*

Many hospital classes distribute materials put out by formula and drug companies, as well as their own propaganda. New parents are impressed by the wealth of printed matter they get for their money, but we find that most of the material brainwashes these individuals by providing only one point of view, the hospital's. Consumer-developed materials are sorely missing from the mounds of literature extolling the virtues of fetal monitors, supplements to breast milk, and all the latest technological devices. Coffee and pastry—no suitable snack for anyone, let alone pregnant couples and developing babies—are often served. In this social atmosphere, the hospital becomes a friend. But "friends" don't withhold information that is essential for your baby's well-being.

Consumer Classes The childbirth experience must be an opportunity for women to believe in themselves and their bodies above and beyond technology and apart from doctors. Classes should provide the spark that ignites positive energies so they will spread, and be a place where love and support are in abundance. Peterson[36] remarks that classes must foster acceptance of the unknown: "To forget about plans and expectations and to trust to the unknown is the source of yielding, an attitude of primary importance prior to birth." Additionally, it is the responsibility of every childbirth-educator to stop the rising rate of unnecessary cesareans and to challenge outmoded and outrageous obstetrical practices.

Jay and Marjie Hathaway, directors of the American Academy of Husband-Coached Childbirth, present a list of questions to determine if the classes you are considering give a consumer point of view. Included in their list are such questions as: Is class size limited? Do parents receive reprints of articles? Do classes prepare couples for unmedicated, natural birth? Are couples taught to "tune in" to their own bodies? Is avoidance of drugs during pregnancy and birth (unless absolutely necessary) taught? Is breastfeeding not only encouraged, but fully supported? Is continuous contact between parents and baby advocated? Are consumerism and positive communication taught? *Is the instructor independent of outside pressures that could compromise your birth experience?* Is she supportive of alternative birth centers and homebirth? Is she respectful of the couple's right to choose their place of birth and is she supportive of that decision (even if she doesn't necessarily agree with it)?

To Marjie and Jay's questions we would add: Are there at least 25 hours of class time? Is the atmosphere one of caring and support? Can any thought or concern be expressed without censorship? Is nutrition stressed? Is the concept of psychophysiology ("mind and body as one") introduced? Are the rights and responsibilities of birthing couples taught? Are supportive doctors and hospitals listed? Are couples encouraged to come before pregnancy, or very early on? Are the classes interesting, stimulating, wonderful, and fun? Are birth visualizations and relaxation exercises used instead of traditional "labor rehearsals"? Are the subjects of medical interventions and their consequences thoroughly investigated? Do you learn how to create a positive environment (within as well as without) for birthing? Is *pain* discussed? WHAT IS THE RATE OF PURE BIRTHS PER GROUP?

Last but not by any means least, prepared-childbirth classes need to prepare couples to birth their babies. Is there a discussion on "What to do if the baby comes before anyone else does"? This is essential so that women come to understand that they need not depend on others (doctors) to birth their babies for them.

Choosing Your Birthplace

Some women find it difficult to feel relaxed in a hospital setting, even when they are just going to visit a friend. Other women feel safest in hospitals, where they are surrounded by predictable routines and efficient-looking caretakers. If you are one of the latter, and a hospital birth is right for you, then you need to take a good, careful look at the options available in your area, to determine which facility you will patronize.

For Those Who Choose a Hospital Birth

One hospital in our area has attractive, softly flowered wallpaper and matching drapes. It boasts the newest in "borning beds," a bed that does virtually everything but roll over and play dead. There are several prints on the wall, including an "oil" of a basket of fruit. The fruit is a tease, because this hospital does not permit a woman to eat while in labor. Nor are friends permitted, nor siblings. This is their birthing room. Another boasts "excellent lighting": their entire labor unit is underground and there are no windows. As Julie Butler, editor of the *Partial Post* remarks, "A potted plant doth not a birthing room make."

Another hospital has small, Kermit-green rooms. There is a token picture on the wall, an inexpensive farm scene. There is no borning bed. The curtains are wispy and, true, the view from the window is no prize. But there's plenty of love and nourishment and support. Friends and siblings are welcome.

Women are lining up for birthing rooms. "But of course we were in the birthing room," they say; "where else?" Some birthing rooms cleverly disguise an atmosphere not at all conducive to purebirth. You can just about see the fetal monitors peeking out from behind the fancy drapes.

Whatever room you happen to be in when you birth your baby is your birthing room. The color of the walls or the style of the wall hangings is insignificant. The energy, love, and support are what make the difference.

However we feel about birthing rooms, we do not believe a woman should be denied them because she's had a previous cesarean. Many women who have had VBACs have birthed in birthing rooms. Remember that emergencies for VBACs are rarely, if ever, more urgent than any other obstetrical complication—and if you have refused unnecessary interventions, you are even less likely to encounter any problems. It is common for articles about VBAC to insist that VBAC women give birth in fully equipped hospitals complete with full staff, blood bank, lab facilities, anesthesia services, and a ready operating room. We agree that these facilities "represent essential services for proper management of many emergency obstetrical situations such as cord prolapse, placenta previa, and abruptio placenta."* Anyone who has that philosophy toward VBAC probably believes that all birthing women must be in fully equipped hospitals. We do not. (And of course we ask again: What kind of hospital is *not* equipped?)

We hear from women every day who have had disappointing and upsetting hospital birth experiences. One woman called from California this week and said, "All of us are having 'cruddy' births. What can we do?"

Another woman called today. She felt sore from pushing and wanted to know if we had a sitz bath for rent. "They only have one sitz bath for this whole place. It's being used. Central Supply can't locate any either. This is a maternity hospital. Where are the sitz baths?!"

Check out the hospitals in your area. For each, what is the rate of *normal* births? How many monitors do they own? Do they have showers? As many showers as monitors? Is 100 percent rooming-in encouraged? What is the cesarean rate? One woman was delighted by her hospital. She wrote to them and they printed her letter in a publication advertising their facility: "I was in the maternity ward where I found the patient services excellent—even better than I expected. While I was there the whole maternity ward was full, with almost half being cesarean births, which take twice as much care. Even with the overload of work, everything still ran perfectly. I couldn't have been more pleased with my entire stay." If we were that hospital administrator, we wouldn't have been so proud of announcing a 50 percent section rate on *any* given day. If the hospital you have selected has a high cesarean rate, watch out.

We have been informed about several hospitals that require that a potential VBAC sign a special form, releasing the hospital from any responsibility. A community health plan in New England has a similar form that mentions death no less than twice. On the next page is a reproduction of an actual consent form from an East Coast hospital. You can see why many women don't even consider VBAC an option when they are presented with this form or something like it. We would like to know why similar forms aren't presented for cesarean section.

---

*M. P. Donnelly and K. T. Franzoni, "Vaginal Delivery Following Cesarean Section," *Obstetrics and Gynaecology*, 29 (June 1967), no. 6, p. 871.

If women had to read all the possible consequences of *that* choice, they would surely do their best to deliver their infants normally. (We also wonder why consent forms are not presented for each and every one of the interventions, with all of the potential consequences of each clearly spelled out.)

MEDICAL CENTER

INFORMED CONSENT

FOR VAGINAL DELIVERY AFTER PREVIOUS CESAREAN SECTION

I, _____ consent to vaginal delivery after having the risks involved explained to me by Doctor _____. I understand that the risks involve both my baby and myself should any serious situation arise such as rupture of the uterus. I have been informed that the infant may experience severe distress or even may not survive. I have also been informed that in such an emergency, I may require blood transfusion, possible hysterectomy, and may subsequently be infertile. I am also aware that I may require Cesarean Section because of fetal distress, failure to progress in labor, abnormal presentation or other severe complications of labor.

SIGNED: _____

WITNESS: _____

A top priority of every hospital should be to make their birthing units as homelike as possible. A couple's decision to labor and birth away from the hospital should come from a genuine belief that the alternative location fosters the best (safest) environment for them—not because they are frightened or concerned that the hospital will sabotage their plans. Making the hospital like home includes welcoming friends and/or siblings at birth.

This consent form provided by Jane Szczepaniak, Linthicum, Maryland.

Ask about giving birth in the labor room. For VBAC labors, indeed for any labor, it is unneccessary and disruptive to have to be thrown on a bed and rushed to the delivery room as your baby's head is crowning. If your scar were going to give way, it would most likely have done so long before you began pushing your baby into this world. Do not agree to comply with any requirements that discriminate against you because of your scar. As we've mentioned, McGarry* says that a VBAC labor should be managed "as if the scar didn't exist."

In fact, VBAC labors do not need to be managed; nor does any other normal labor. Every spontaneous VBAC is one more victory, first for our babies and then for ourselves. Gretchen writes, "Finally we were told we could use the birthing room. It was a first for our doctor and that hospital."

Marylou said, "After sitting with ten previous cesarean mothers through their labors, our doctor said he wasn't going to treat us any differently than anyone else! He said he'd check in every now and then and keep track."

A woman from Massachusetts said, "I finally screamed, 'Get that #!?#!& anesthesiologist away from the door. I'm having this baby and it's not going to be a section and I won't have any anesthesia!' " Everyone thought it was funny, but he doesn't hang out with VBACs anymore."

Having a baby is not "risky," although it is viewed as such by most medical personnel. We are reminded of David Corbin's tongue-in-cheek article, "High Risk Sex":

> The American Medical Organization contended that sex in the home should only be performed on specially designed tables provided in hospitals. These tables have been shown to reduce the incidence of overstraining . . . patients should never have sex unless they are monitored to determine whether the sex is becoming too strenuous . . . Susan and John Eros (speaking against the AMO) note an example of drugged hospital sex: anesthetic ointment placed on the genitals—against the patients' wishes . . . "to slow things down." "Furthermore," stated the Eroses, "the hospital practice of separating partners immediately after sex is contrary to what researchers suggest is desirable". . . [7]

Make certain the hospital you choose welcomes L.A.s. One husband was told there wasn't enough room in the labor room for an L.A. He noted that two residents were cordially invited (by the physician) to attend the labor. Make sure that your mate can be with you if a c/section becomes necessary during a VBAC labor. In some hospitals, fathers cannot be present for the cesarean if it is a "failed trial of labor for VBAC."

Birthing chairs are becoming very fashionable these days. They are expensive (we consumers will, of course, absorb the cost), and they are designed, once again, *with the convenience of the physician in mind*. One model has already been recalled because electric shocks were caused when amniotic fluid leaked

---

*J. A. McGarry, "The Management of Patients Previously Delivered by Cesarean Section," *Journal of Obstetrics and Gynaecology of the British Commonwealth*, 76 (February 1969), 137.

onto the wires and controls. Although a few women have found the chairs comfortable, we urge you to remember that they are not necessary for birthing. They restrict changes in position, especially when they have been elevated three feet off the ground. In many positions, the woman is tilted no better than if she were on her back, and an episiotomy (or undeserved tear) is inevitable.

Making a Hospital Request List   We recommend that you design a request list either for your own use or for that of your doctor and hospital. Some physicians and nursing staffs find this very helpful. After attending birth after birth they find it useful to be able to make a quick check of the couple's wishes. Others feel extremely threatened by the request list. Some women paste copies on the labor room door and on the bottom of the bed, to remind their physicians what they have agreed upon. It would be nice if the requests were general hospital policy in most hospitals; unfortunately, they aren't.

The hospital should be agreeable to your requests and should do all that it can to satisfy them. All of the requests are reasonable for healthy, normal birth, which of course includes VBACs. Request lists should be designed according to your particular needs. It is important for everyone to realize that this is a request list, not a list of demands, and that it is intended to assist your physician by clarifying policies and procedures ahead of time.

In *Labor and Delivery: An Observer's Diary,* Constance Bean remarks that emotions of laboring couples tend to be more open during birth than other times. "Yet, women and men restrain their feelings of fear, joy, desolation, doubt, depression, and excitement in order to conform to what they feel is expected of them in the hospital." Bean also remarks that couples "are often short-changed in the hospital in terms of both emotional and physical care."[3] We believe that creating a request list—whether or not you actually use it—will help uncover many feelings and serve as a catalyst for discussion. In doing so, it may help to keep *everyone* more open, aware, and alert to the emotions and needs of couples at birth. *

REQUEST FOR OUR CHILD'S BIRTH

TO:

PARENTS:

APPROXIMATE DELIVERY DATE:

OBSTETRICIAN:

PEDIATRICIAN:

MIDWIFE OR L.A.:

---

*Our list has been adapted from "The Optimum Birth Letter," by Kathleen Matthews (Putney, Vt.: Homecomer) and "Birth Plan" by Norma Shulman, *C/SEC Newsletter,* 5 (Winter 1979).

Because it is difficult to hold discussions and make decisions during the involvement of labor and delivery, we have carefully discussed our concerns and expectations in advance, and would like your staff to be aware of our requests. We expect to rely on the normal physiological processes of labor and delivery to the maximum extent possible. By withholding routine interventions and respecting our hope for a natural family-centered birth, the medical professionals involved can enable us to achieve our optimal experience. The health and well-being of our baby is of utmost importance, which is one of the reasons that we have taken the time to explore the safest options. The following listings are important to us, and we rely on the sensitivity of the hospital staff, as a joyous and personal birth experience is something we long for, and hope to achieve with this delivery.

OR

We are deeply commited to a philosophy of birth that wholly relies on the normal and natural physiological processes of labor and delivery, and helps insure the safest beginning for our child. Thus, we fully expect our child's birth to be normal and free of medical intervention; in the unlikely event that complications occur, we shall confer with our obstetrician, whose medical judgment we respect and trust. Therefore, we ask that routine interventions ABSOLUTELY be withheld for our child's birth. Of great importance to us is that we maintain an aura of personal intimacy throughout labor and delivery, so we ask that interruptions to our privacy be restricted to an absolute minimum. The health and well-being of our baby is of utmost importance, which is one of the reasons that we have taken the time to explore the safest options. We will depend on the sensitivity and cooperation of all involved as we anticipate joyfully welcoming our baby.

Labor:

Use of birthing room requested
Husband and nurse remain with mother
No routine prep, enema, fetal monitor, I.V., or artificial rupture of membranes
No labor stimulants
No medication
Minimum of internal exams
Mobility unrestricted
Use of bathroom
Camera/tape recorder permitted
I.V. placed high, mobile stand, by doctor or his specific orders
Water (or my own honey, tea) as needed during labor
No visitors unapproved by mother
Deliver in own clothes or nightgown
No routine confinement to bed or labor room (or hospital!)

Delivery:

Husband and L.A. present
Flexibility in table/bed set-up and delivery position
No routine episiotomy
Dimmed lights
Camera/tape recorder allowed
Immediate and sustained contact between baby and parents (breastfeeding)
Cord allowed to finish pulsing
Placenta to deliver spontaneously (no Pitocin)
Allow vernix to remain (no bathing)
Suctioning only as needed
No silver nitrate (waiver enclosed)
No anesthesia to examine uterine scar
I.V. removed as soon as possible
Anything unexpected: full information
Any medication or anesthesia: administered only with our complete knowledge and consent
Deliver in labor room (if not in birthing room)
Siblings included as soon as possible
Husband and L.A. present if anesthesia administered
Vitamin E oil and hot compresses for perineum
Father help deliver or "catch" baby, or mother gently lift baby from body
Father cut umbilical cord
Mirror for mother (during pushing)
Baby placed on mother's abdomen immediately
Choice of delivery positions (including squatting)
Baby warmed by mother's body heat
Baby to hear *our* voices first (we wish to be the first to speak to our baby)
Early discharge (approximately 4 hours after birth); if not, 24-hour rooming-in
Children present at birth
No residents or interns

Recovery:

No recovery room unless necessary
If so, husband and baby go as a family
Vitamin K decision will be made at this time
Breastfeeding as baby desires

Postpartum:

No bottles
No routine separation of mother and baby if maternal fever or neonatal jaundice

Private room with bath requested
Sibling visits with baby

SCN:

Parents' visits unrestricted
Contact with baby
All procedures, medications discussed with parents
Totally breastfed or mother's milk (will pump)

If Cesarean is necessary

No demerol or other medication
Choice of anesthesiologist
Spinal anesthesia—husband present
Husband present if general anesthesia is necessary
Shaving only as necessary
Husband and L.A. present
Camera and tape recorder allowed
Mirror available (if not, permission to bring our own)
No curtain to obstruct mother's view (if necessary, we will wear masks)
Mother's hands free
Contact with father and mother as soon as possible
Breastfeeding as soon as possible
I.V., catheter removed as soon as possible
Fluids and food (yogurt, honey, etc.) as soon as possible
Use of same incision, if possible
Special-care nursery only if absolutely necessary (and if so, contact with parents before)
Helper to stay with mother 24 hrs. (Husband or relative)

If baby requires ICU:
Birth attendant or husband to go along
Baby to receive only my pumped breast milk and to begin nursing as soon as possible
If baby is transferred to another hospital, family to go as a *unit*

If complications arise at birth:
Father not asked to leave at any time
L.A., midwife, or attendant present at all times
All previous requests to be honored to the extent possible

cc:Doctor
    Covering Doctor
    Coach, L.A., or Midwife
    Pediatrician
    Chief of Staff
    Chief of Anesthesiology
    Director of Nursing
    Director of Administration

What about Homebirth?

We've mentioned several times that a woman must feel safe in order to give birth. Midwife Carol Leonard tells us that when the woman isn't feeling relaxed in her surroundings, she may not have F TP ("failure to progress"), but the baby may have WCO—"won't come out!"

Cynthia planned a homebirth. After a very long and difficult labor, with little progress, she finally agreed to go to the hospital, presumably for a cesarean. Cynthia wrote, "Upon arriving at the hospital, much to everyone's surprise, the baby was at the vaginal opening, through the cervix, and ready to be born!"

Pamela said, "I'd get to the hospital and my labor would slow down. I'd go home and it would pick up fast and furiously. I went back to the hospital, and the contractions petered out agian. This happened three times!" It seems Pam and her baby were checking out the hospital to see if they felt safe enough to birth there before they committed themselves.

Anne wanted a homebirth but was afraid to stay at home. In her eighth month of pregnancy, she decided to birth in the hospital. Her 45-minute labor produced a beautiful 7 pound daughter in her living room before she had time to close up her bags and be on her way.

As you know, we have worked with many women who have planned homebirth VBACs. Most have had their babies at home. Several VBAC homebirths were after more than one cesarean. There were three hospital transfers: two women birthed vaginally at the hospital and one had a repeat cesarean. One woman decided to birth in the hospital because she was several weeks overdue. As we have already stated, *there have been no complications whatsoever in any case.*

Most doctors are opposed to homebirth to begin with. Most are opposed to VBACs. Imagine their hysteria at the very thought of a homebirth VBAC. However, it isn't their decision. Not one of the couples we have worked with has made any decision without considering their baby first; they are all responsible human beings who have educated themselves, assessed risks, and chosen the place of birth accordingly. Professor Kloosterman, whose authority we have already cited in this book, remarks, "Before beginning of labor, it can be ascertained with high degree of accuracy, if the labor will conclude without any outside interference and also if the condition of the baby will need hospitalization." He also goes on to say that in rare cases where difficulties arise during labor, mother and baby can still be transported to the hospital.*

We will not spend time extolling the virtues of homebirth. We know, however, that some VBAC women who go into their hospitals are considered so high-risk, and are treated with such caution and fear, that they *become* high-risk. For these women, homebirth can be a safe alternative. When someone asks what we think, home or hospital, we answer by asking, "What do *you* think? Where will *you* feel safest and get the best care? What is best for your baby?" We ask mothers who are in conflict to find a quiet time to reflect upon these questions.

Although they are few and far between at this time, there *are* doctors who support homebirth VBAC, or who are willing to provide medical back-up in the hospital if necessary. One doctor told a VBAC hopeful, "The staff is still scared of VBAC. They either hover around like buzzards, or treat you as if you had leprosy. If I were you, I'd probably stay home." There are many doctors who encourage VBAC women to stay home until labor is well established. Many midwives also encourage VBACs to stay out of the hospital as long as possible or to birth at home.

Muriel, a midwife from Minnesota, speaks for several midwives who have contacted us:

> Women who had had previous cesareans for nonrepeating reasons place themselves at high risk for another section by going to the hospital. From that standpoint, I feel home is a safe place for them to give birth. Midwives are making a "mistake" by refusing homebirth to previous cesarean moms. They are virtually asking them to place themselves at very high risk by forcing them to return to the hospital for birth.

Chris, a midwife from Toronto, writes:

> As a birth attendant, I feel comfortable attending VBAC women wherever they wish to birth, be it home or hospital. I have a supportive doctor to work with at home-births. Most of his colleagues would call him crazy, but I'm confident things are changing. The other day an OB who accepts referrals from me for hospital VBACs suggested to one of my clients that she might want to birth at home! I was privileged to attend two VBAC births last week—one, on Christmas Day, was the first VBAC at home in Toronto, I believe. There was no worry about THE SCAR . . . from all appearances it was your usual homebirth—with the father and a friend helping and big sister climbing into bed with her mother and the new baby moments after the birth—but Hilda's smiles as she gave birth were for more than just herself. She was thinking also of other women with a previous cesarean who might now begin to see homebirth as an option for themselves. Mainly, I attend VBACs because I'm so impressed by the women and men I work with. It's very exciting to see these people achieve something they've worked so hard for and to be part of it. There is

---

*NAPSAC News, 4 (Summer 1979), p. 3.

*a support network growing, and doctors are learning from these women. I'm glad
to be able to give support when it's needed.*

In *Mal(e) Practice*, Robert Mendelsohn suggests to those of you who choose
to birth at home: "If an irate doctor asks, 'Do you want your baby to die?' you
can reply, 'No, that's why I want to have it at home.' "[32]

A growing number of VBAC couples has chosen to be at home to deliver
their babies privately, without assistance. This requires love, trust, confidence,
some practical information about birthing, and someone knowledgeable who
can be contacted if necessary. If cab drivers "deliver" babies, certainly the mother
and father of the child are more than capable. It isn't for everyone, but for some
couples it is the most fulfilling way to bring their child into the world. A book
called *Birth and the Dialogue of Love*,[33] as well as the *New Nativity Newsletter*,[34]
can assist those of you who choose to birth privately.

Julie Butler writes that "homebirth is real 'whole wheat' birth."* Ruth, a
VBAC homebirth mother, agrees, although her analogy differs slightly: "Our
healthy *baby* was the 'ice cream'. Having a VBAC was the hot fudge. Having
him *at home* was the whipped cream and cherry plopped right onto the top!"

There are no guarantees. Life is a risk. Living is a risk. Just breathing is risky,
when you consider what's out there to breathe. Even the best of plans can fall
through. In one situation, a couple planning a hospital birth went into labor
when their doctor, their doctor's back-up, and both their midwives were all
either out of town or at another birth. In another case, an ambulance that was
"standing by" for a VBAC homebirth wouldn't start. A back-up ambulance was
called and got stuck in the snow. (Neither was needed, but in this case, their
old trusty, forgotten car would have served them just fine.) Cover as many bases
as you need, but remember: the best-laid plans occasionally get stuck in the
snow. Many couples who have planned VBACs have concluded that birth itself
was far easier than all the preparation.

Roadblocked?

Occasionally when a woman is planning her birth, she finds herself worrying
about possible complications. This is not a book about complications; however,
because so many women ask about breech and herpes, we are including some
information about these situations.

Breech Presentation

Many of the women who contact us were sectioned because their babies were
breech. Most of these women were informed during their pregnancies that the

---

*Circle News, 1 (March 1982), no. 3, p.3.

baby was "bottom-down," but very few were told that there are exercises that can be done to encourage a breech baby to turn. (Lois had never heard of the exercises when she had her cesarean.) In the situations when the women themselves asked their obstetricians about the exercises, the responses were often similar: "Oh, yes, *those* exercises. They don't work. Don't waste your time."

We know twelve women who would disagree! Of the fifteen women with breech babies with whom we worked this year, twelve had their babies turn between the 35th and 40th weeks of pregnancy as a result of the exercises. Some babies turned within hours after the exercise program had begun. Most others turned within a week. One woman's baby turned two days before birth.

At the 1977 World Congress of Gynecology and Obstetrics, Dr. DeSa Souza reported that 88.7 percent of a series of 744 breech babies were successfully converted with the use of postural exercise.[57]

One exercise is called the breech tilt: Lie down on a hard surface with your pelvis raised on pillows nine to twelve inches higher than your head for ten minutes, twice a day. Wear loose clothing. A heavy meal prior to assuming this position is not recommended, but we suggest a short walk outside or a few breaths of fresh air before you lie down. For maximum effectiveness, the exercise should be started between 30 and 36 weeks, and practiced a few times daily for four to six weeks—or until the baby turns. Three-quarters of the babies turn within two to three weeks. Even if they fail to turn, they are often dislodged for easier external version. Getting on your hands and knees for a few minutes several times a day can also help turn a breech baby (or rotate a posterior baby).

Another exercise: Rest an ironing board at about a 45-degree angle on your couch. Put chairs on either side for balance. Lie on the ironing board, legs elevated, your head down and supported by a pillow. Bend your knees and bring them slowly up toward your shoulders (as if you were bicycle-riding). Try to press your upper thighs firmly *but gently* in toward your abdomen. One woman did her ironing-board exercise faithfully, even when company was present. Her baby turned, and two weeks later she had a VBAC (classical incision and all, we might add). In "Unnecessary Cesareans: Ways To Avoid Them," Diony Young and Charles Mahan add the following:

> Practice . . . with an empty stomach (before lunch and dinner). If the baby does turn, stop doing the exercise or the baby may turn back to breech again. Once the baby has turned, do lots of walking to help the baby settle further down in the pelvis.[47]

Given that these exercises are often successful, we are appalled that so few physicians are aware of or give credence to them. Most of the women we counsel who had their cesareans because of breech presentation were never informed of the options of the tilt position exercise, nor of external cephalic version.

External version is another technique for turning breech babies. It involves gently manipulating the fetus and turning it to a vertex presentation. It is done preferably between 30 and 36 weeks, or at the beginning of labor if the membranes are intact. Anesthesia is not required, not only because of its effects on the fetus, but also because the manipulative force used on an unconscious mother may be more than what is acceptable for the baby. In one study, of version on 860 fetuses, from 1949 to 1970, initial attempts succeeded in 781, subsequent attempts were successful in 25, with a final rate of breech presentation at delivery of only 1.10 percent as compared with the usual 3–4 percent. Like breech delivery, external cephalic version is an art that is rarely taught in American medical schools and is therefore seldom an available option to the pregnant woman carrying a breech.

The physical and mental relaxation of the mother is important during external version. According to *Myles' Textbook for Midwives*, "warm hands and smooth gentle manipulation are essential"(p. 557) Ina May Gaskin[50] tells us that it is not so much the size of the baby as the relaxation of the mother that makes version possible. In *Williams Obstetrics*, it is said that if the procedure is properly and gently performed, it carries little danger. Ranney[55] believes that successful version may reduce the likelihood of prematurity, which is more common in breech presentations. It also reduces the likelihood of a cesarean. Ylikorkals and Hartikainen-Sorri[58] also concluded that breech presentation warrants attempts at external version.

Some doctors don't know how to do versions. Some do it and use analgesic drugs for relaxation. Some first use ultrasound to confirm the presentation of the fetus and locate the placenta. Some doctors are concerned that version presents serious risks, including antepartum hemorrhage and premature labor. Many have never learned how to do a version. Some consider the exercises and/ or version interferences in themselves—if the baby is breech they believe the baby was meant to be that way. If more physicians were comfortable with breech deliveries, perhaps women wouldn't bother trying to turn their breech babies— but most know that if they don't do something, they face a cesarean section, and are therefore most anxious to have their babies turn.

Even when the exercises and version have been tried and have failed, vaginal delivery need not be ruled out. The NIH report* recommends that "vaginal delivery of the term breech should remain an acceptable obstetrical choice for delivery with an anticipated fetal wight of less than eight pounds, with normal maternal pelvic dimensions, with a frank breech without a hyperextended head, and with a physician experienced in vaginal breech delivery" (p. 14). Even when the first three conditions have been met, most breech babies are born by section. It is time for us as consumers to demand that medical schools once again teach the skills of external cephalic version and breech delivery.

---

*The final report of National Institutes of Health Task Force on Cesarean Childbirth is available from the Office of Research Reporting, Bldg. 31, Rm. 2A32, NICHD, 9000 Rockville Pike, Bethesda, Md. 20205.

Many women whose babies persist in a breech presentation are sectioned without benefit of labor; they are told that it would be too dangerous for them to go into labor. No one tells them that oftentimes breech babies turn during labor, that labor is *good* for babies, and that breech births are not nearly so risky as we've been told, when attended by someone who is competent and experienced.

There are several reasons that women are told they must have their breech babies by cesarean. They are told that the baby's buttocks will come through a mother's pelvis, but that the aftercoming head, being larger, may not fit. They are told that a breech baby may take its first breath while still in utero, aspirate fluid, and asphyxiate. Prolapse of the cord is more common in breech presentations; many physicians routinely resort to a cesarean for this reason as well. Many woman are told that if they allow their baby to birth breech there is a good chance that it will be brain-damaged. One doctor said, "I'll guarantee you a healthy baby if you agree to a cesarean, but not with a vaginal delivery." A cesarean by no means guarantees a healthy anything (unless you consider the hospital's bank account): the physician's own inadequacies, lack of experience, and insecurities about breech delivery can cause him to intimidate his clients.

What mother, given only the risks of breech delivery, will choose to birth naturally? How could anyone ever forgive herself if she "selfishly" allowed herself to go into labor and delivered an asphyxiated baby? Thus threatened, women make the decision to be sectioned *without enough information to make an informed choice.*

A woman with whom we spoke years ago told us that when she was a Peace Corps volunteer in Africa, she attended several births. A breech baby was considered *lucky!* "It had something to do with the baby being born with its feet firmly planted on the ground."

As you may recall, we quoted Marieskind earlier (p. 22) to the effect that most doctors do not know how to assist at breech births. This is well documented. Marieskind suggests that the risks of breech birth may be far less than those suggested: doctors are afraid to do breech deliveries, so they exaggerate the risks. Many women then "choose" to be sectioned, which contributes further to the physician's inexperience in vaginal breech deliveries. The few breeches that are delivered vaginally are then often attended by nervous, inexperienced hands.

Certified Nurse Midwife (CNM) Phyllis Long[52] tells us that breech births can go very well.

> It is even more important in the breech birth to avoid intervention . . . It is essential to avoid pushing until the cervix is fully dilated and retracted. To decrease the urge to push, help the mother assume a knee chest position or in some way elevate the hips in a semi prone or side lying position. The guiding principal in breech as well as in cephalic births is to recognize normal progress. As long as descent of the baby is continuous, there is no need for intervention—just guidance,

encouragement, and patience . . . If progress stops, active assistance is indicated . . . it is believed the baby can tolerate up to ten minutes of this type of cord compression; however, aiming for less than that time without traumatic hurrying is sensible . . . So I don't propose a rule of no intervention—but holding off until there seems to be a lack of progress. Gentle assistance at that time should prevent hypoxia.

One physician in the Boston area is fast becoming an expert on breech births. The women he attends are always in an upright position, either standing, squatting, kneeling, or on all fours. They are given an abundance of support, both physical and emotional. He says that he has not had a single problem with a breech birth in the twelve that he has attended this year.

Some doctors tell us that breech labors "don't work as well" as vertex labors. Having spoken with many mothers of breech infants, we believe that *psychological* factors play the most important role in influencing progress patterns. No woman who thinks she may damage her baby by allowing it to come through her body is going to let her labor continue. She'll just close up shop. Time and time again, *fear* has been shown to slow labor. The fear of breech delivery is so great in our culture that it should be no surprise that so many breech labors appear abnormal. One woman who contacted us was examined when she got to the hospital. She was then nine centimeters dilated. "My doctor screamed at me, 'Oh my God, it's breech!' His voice was octaves above normal." Five minutes later she was seven centimeters dilated. Another woman came in to the hospital ten centimeters dilated and pushing. Before she had time to blink she was sectioned, general anesthesia and all. "I just know I could have had that baby."

In an article by Ettner,[49] we are told that in an attempt to be properly selective in the management of breech presentation—neither to perform cesarean section indiscriminately, nor to attempt a vaginal delivery when this route would be dangerous for the baby—Zatuchni and Andros described a method of studying women prior to labor. An evaluation of certain factors in a patient's history and physical examination enabled them to predict with a high degree of accuracy the outcome of breech delivery. An independent study by Bird and McElin[48] concludes, "We believe it imperative to reject the concept that breech presentation is a *mandatory condition for abdominal delivery*." A study at the Mayo Clinic concluded that cesarean section was justifiable approximately 12–15 percent of the time in breech presentations, not 100 percent.

When a woman calls us and tells us that her baby is breech, we give her several suggestions. First, we check with her about her diet. Her body has the best possible opportunity to open and stretch if she is in excellent health. Second, we suggest the postural exercises and Kegels and/or external version. Third, we discuss whether the physician she's using knows how to assist breech deliveries.

We then ask her to consider whether there have been (or are) any significant conflicts about or during this pregnancy, or if she has any particular fears about having this child. Most women experience some conflict during pregnancy. It has been our experience, however, that women with breech babies (and also women with placenta previa) are often struggling with an important or difficult issue in their lives. For example, nine out of eleven women who called with breech babies during the last six months acknowledged that the baby was not planned, or that there was a significant problem (marital, financial, or emotional). Our thought, which has been substantiated by Mehl, Peterson and others, is that the mother will do what she can to keep the baby inside—keep it protected—if she isn't ready to have this baby, or if she doesn't perceive the world to be safe. Since we know that the mind and body influence each other, we know that the baby's—or the placenta's—position can be affected in some way by the conflict. Perhaps the *baby* decides to set a spell longer. He sits cross-legged, folds his arms, and sings, "I'm a-waitin' for better times!" Perhaps the placenta dramatically flings itself across the cervix and yells, "No one is going to get his clammy paws on this precious little being until *I'm* sure everything's okay!"

We also suggest visualization. We ask the women to find a place where she can stretch out and relax and spend time on conscious relaxation. We then ask her to begin to visualize anything that gently falls (snow) or droops (willow trees or branches of a tree when the fruit is heavy).

Later in the exercise, the woman can begin to envision the baby in her uterus. (If she likes, she can *become* that baby for a while.) She can imagine that . . .

> The head is getting heavy—oh, so heavy—and that it would feel so . . . much . . . better . . . if she could just let it gently droop . . . and droop . . . and droop . . . . At the same time, she can envision the uterus, shaped like an upside-down pear. The bottom is nice and round, just perfect for the baby's head . . . The head continues to droop . . . first onto its chest . . . Then it tucks itself under a little more . . . a little more . . . and then the whole body gently floats over . . . The baby then just sinks down . . . down . . . into the larger part of the cradle where everything fits more comfortably . . . And the baby feels wonderful because she can rest her heavy . . . droopy . . . little . . . head in the cradle of the pelvis . . .

In a letter in the *American Journal of Ob/Gyn News* (March 1, 1981), S. Semchyshyn, M.D., remarked, "I would like to think that a well-trained, not necessarily 'supertrained' fellow in maternal-fetal medicine should be able to manage breech presentation appropriately, including the performance of external cephalic version. After all, there is more to the practice of obstetrics than spontaneous vaginal delivery and cesarean section."

Herpes

Six women planning VBACs who contacted us were told by their physicians that they would not be able to deliver vaginally because they had herpes during the course of the pregnancy. All six had healthy babies—vaginally. One had a lesion at the time of the birth, located on the labium. In the other situations, the virus was inactive. One woman was not certain whether she wanted to go through with a vaginal birth or schedule a cesarean to be "safe." Eleven days before her due date, while she was still deciding, she went into labor and delivered her baby vaginally moments after she got to the hospital. Her labor was just over an hour in length. Another woman had a 45-minute homebirth.

According to Kellerhouse and Esparza, the most prevalent way herpes is transferred to the infant is in the birth canal.[63] If a sore is present during birth and the baby comes in contact with it (directly or through the fluid after the membranes are ruptured), herpes may be contracted. Usually, an active sore has to be present. Herpes can cause brain damage, neurological damage, and blindness to the baby. It can also cause respiratory damage, malformation, and even death.

Kellerhouse and Esparza suggest several methods of warding off herpes or "nipping it in the bud." These include certain foods, amino acids, vitamins, and herbs.

Kellerhouse and Esparza also state that open-minded doctors or midwives who have had experience with herpes in pregnant women do not instantly recommend a c/section unless the sore is in the birth canal. Although cesareans are often performed, the surgery is no guarantee that the baby will not come in contact with the infection; it is possible for the baby to become infected even when a cesarean has been performed on a woman with intact membranes. In rare cases, cultures from the amniotic fluid reveal the presence of the herpes virus, which is believed to travel through the mother's bloodstream and possibly infect the baby in utero. In a situation such as this, a cesarean isn't necessary and won't help.

Sidney Kilbrick, M.D., reports[64] that if the herpes is inactive at term, no special precautions are necessary. The length of time considered necessary between the absence of an active lesion and the onset of labor varies. Some doctors believe that as soon as the lesions are healed a vaginal birth is safe. Others insist on a minimum of one clear (their term is "clean") month before allowing a vaginal delivery. Some midwives swab the lesions with various agents and then cover them to prevent contact during the birth. We have been told that one or two doctors have cauterized the lesions before birth.

We recommend the Council for Cesarean Awareness *Newsletter on Herpes** and *Mothering magazine* for Winter 1981.[3] Both provide information on the subject, as well as bibliographies. The American Social Health Association in Palo Alto, California, distributes a newsletter, "The Helper," for information on herpes. Other sources are listed in the bibliography.

One midwife in our area believes the virus is transmitted transplacentally. She

---

*Council for Cesarean Awareness, 5520 SW 92d Ave., Miami, Fla. 33165.

also questions routine Pap smears. The current protocol, she says, is smear at 32 weeks, 36 weeks, and weekly thereafter. Her question: do Pap smears detect— or *do they cause*—active cervial herpes in women with a history of past active herpes infections? She believes that the more Pap smears are done, the greater the chances of having an active infection. Others disagree.

"Herpes and Cesarean Delivery," an article by Lynn Richards, reports on observations of two infants with neonatal herpes.[67] Neither of the mothers had active herpes at the time of delivery. Both had intrapartum internal monitoring: both babies contacted the herpes virus at the electrode site. Clearly, though not maternally active, or detected by culture, the virus was present and was activated by trauma to a sensitive area, the fetal scalp, at a time of stress. The article reports on a Dr. Debauchea in France, who cited the case of a mother who had an "unexplained fever," which went away and did not return. Four days later her son was born vaginally. The infant was covered with fluid-filled blisters that were already broken and scarring over. The infection had obviously been contracted in utero, and tests showed unmistakable evidence of herpes. Richards writes, "If, in fact, babies are contacting Herpes within the uterus, then perhaps the mode of delivery has much less to do with neonatal Herpes than has been believed. Once again, perhaps cesarean delivery has become the escape hatch for dealing with a complex set of questionable circumstances. The decision of how to handle your own 'Herpes childbirth' can only be yours.

We suggest you read as much as you can about herpes. Talk to women who have had herpes and find out what decisions they made. Talk to midwives. Do some relaxation and visualization work. Get some support. The decision about how to handle your birth *is* yours.

When Purebirth "Fails"

Some instructors are concerned about our approach. "You get people all excited about birthing. What happens when they can't do it? You raise their expectations. What happens when they fall flat on their faces?"

First of all, we don't get people excited about birthing—women are excited on their own. To paraphrase Mead and Newton, birthing, like coitus and lactation, had to be physically desirable for the race to continue. We don't raise women's expectations, per se. We share our knowledge and our joy and enthusiasm, and they are "catchy"! A *woman must raise her own expectations and be enthusiastic and excited; otherwise she will probably* **be delivered** *rather than birth her child.*

There are a few women who have gone through the classes, psyched themselves up, and had cesareans, Yes, they are disappointed. Yes, they would have liked to birth naturally. But they gave it their all. They didn't sabotage themselves by refusing to get psyched up. They did what they could.

These women see themselves with pride. Gayle Peterson tells us in *Birthing Normally*, "Courage to look inside at the unknown country that stretches beyond ourselves is necessary for birthing *ourselves* as well as our babies.[36] Roberta told us, "If I'd gone in and allowed them to section me, I'd always have thought of myself as a coward. I'm no coward, not this time!"

Another woman said:

> This was not the birth we wanted. I eventually reached my limit of pain and endurance and discouragement. However, I feel I did my very best, so there are no regrets on that score, no thoughts of, "If only I had held on a little longer!" I am grateful for all the good parts, for Jon's love and support, and for the fact that the labor was mine. And, of course, the most healing and blessed thing of all is the perfect and beautiful baby who lives with us now.

Another wrote, "I totally accept my experience of this birth. I have nothing 'heavy' to work out this time. The absence of fear on my part minimized the pain, both physical and psychic." Joelle wrote, "I would have liked to deliver vaginally, but I didn't and I gave it my all. I think I'll have a good cry down the road, but *this* time, I think *one* good cry will do it!" Cathey wrote, "Next time, I'm staying home!"

Each planned VBAC, whether completely realized or not, is a success. It insures that the baby will be born according to his chosen birthdate, gets him ready for this world, and gives the mother an opportunity to make decisions about her birth and her body that are denied in cesarean section and shows physicians how unfounded and ridiculous their fear of uterine "rupture" really is. Each and every one of the women who has had a repeat cesarean has stated that she will not be sectioned in the future unless it becomes absolutely necessary. Each one will plan another VBAC and is glad she didn't just get up on the table, lie down, and get sectioned, without first giving it her all.

Choosing a Physician

"Many women find themselves at war and birth at the same time."

—C. Panuthos

Dr. Andrew Fleck's study* of the widely diverse section rates around New

---

*From Gena Corea, "The Cesarean Epidemic," *Mother Jones* (July 1980).

York State led him to conclude, "If you go to a doctor who likes to do cesarean sections, you're going to get sectioned."

The problem is that given the more predictable expenditure of time, the greater glory, prestige, and fee, the supposed defense against malpractice suits, and the climate of approval that accompany cesarean delivery these days, the anti-cesarean physician is scarce indeed. Add to those incentives the fact that many male surgeons have a sexist attitude toward cutting women—"No ovary is good enough to leave in, and no testicle is bad enough to take out"[2]—and we find ourselves on very shaky ground in our search for a physician.

In her quest for a doctor who supports purebirth and VBAC, Charlene from Alabama writes, "It's slim pickin's down here!" Her situation is pretty much universal. The letters we receive from all over the country show that trying to work within the existing system can be extremely frustrating. Women are forced to confront the underlying, all-pervasive, frightening fact that health care in America today is the property of male professionals, that in almost every child-birth scenario in our country, the final decisions rest on someone who never did and never will give birth.

We find it incredible that in an age when women are demanding rights and earning recognition in almost every sphere of their lives, the delivery room remains the domain of the male physician. It sometimes seems that there is an inverse relationship between the strides we have made in every other realm of our struggle and those we have made in the arena of childbirth; that the more control we gain of our day-to-day lives, the more we relinquish on the days we give birth.

"No!" you want to shout. "You've forgotten all the battles we have won: the right to be conscious when our babies are born, the right to have our husbands with us, the right to keep our babies with us, the right to have our older children visit, the right to leave the hospital as soon as we wish." We do remember all those victories, but we agree with Gena Corea when she says, "These changes center childbirth on the woman; cesareans put it back in the hands of the doctors." And as long as we allow the cesarean delivery rate to climb unimpeded, all our victories are hollow ones, and our "power" is a sham.

In "Witches, Midwives, and Nurses: A History of Women Healers," Barbara Ehrenreich and Deidre English stop us dead in our liberated tracks with the information that 93 percent of the doctors in the United States are men, as are almost all the top directors and administrators of health institutions.

> Women are still in the overall majority—70 percent of health workers are women—but we have been incorporated as *workers* into an industry where the bosses are men. . .
>
> When we are allowed to participate in the healing process, we can do so only as nurses. . . [who are] taught not to question, not to challenge. "The doctor knows best." He is the shaman, in touch with the forbidden, mystically complex

world of science which we have been taught is beyond our grasp [emphasis in original].[11]

As conditioned as we are to depending on men for our health care, the stresses of labor make us even more vulnerable to their influence. All a doctor has to tell us is that a cesarean will be better for our babies, and we unquestioningly trust him to cut us open. Dr. Hugh Drummond[10] states that the persona of the physician is the essence of patriarchy. "Whom else would you trust to stick a knife into your body?" he asks. No matter that there are no studies whatever that support the idea of better babies through cesareans. No matter that there is no evidence whatever that the liberal use of cesarean delivery has done anything to raise the mental performance of children. No matter that cesarean babies are more likely to need stimulation to begin breathing, more likely to be premature, and more likely to have fluid in their lungs, low Apgar scores, respiratory distress syndrome or hyaline membrane disease, and depression resulting from anesthesia. None of this matters when your physician decides that a cesarean is best for your baby.

What does matter is that your doctor is not likely to be well prepared for any normal delays in your labor, although he is probably quite skilled in obstetrical technology. It matters that he believes that a cesarean will protect him from a malpractice suit if your baby isn't perfect. The economics and the convenience of a cesarean matter. It matters that your doctor is likely to have little real understanding of the emotional implications of giving birth. Claudia Panuthos tells us that the motivations of most people, including male obstetricians, are not malice, evil, or revenge; and that they are victims of their own inadequacy feelings and technological teachings.

Dr. Robert Mendelsohn[31] believes that only one out of fifty medical students will escape dehumanization in medical school. Dr. Lendon Smith* tells us that over 50 percent of the material learned in medical school is inaccurate: "The problem is, we don't know which 50 percent." Sheila Kitzinger† tells us that the majority of doctors, when queried, describe a good patient as one who "does everything I ask her to do." In "What Medical Students Learn about Women," Kay Weiss writes that all the leading textbooks in obstetrics and gynecology have themes about women: most of the themes are degrading, chauvinistic, and inaccurate.[44] And we all know why residents become animated when complications arise—it's their only way to learn how to treat them.

In *Gentle Vengeance: An Account of the First Year at Harvard Medical School*, Charles LaBaron remarks that eight or ten years after entering medical school, students emerge, realizing that they never had a youth. "What is the hamburger machine that chops up nice kids and turns them into the doctors I know?" he

---

*From an interview in New York in 1978.
†From a lecture given in Boston in November 1981.

asks. He speaks of twelve white coats (belonging to the teachers and to the students) sweeping into rooms, grabbing for the charts, and discoursing loudly over the patients' beds "in technical jargon as if they were dealing with a hunk of beef." LaBaron ponders over how physicians start reacting to the *cause* of their lost sleep and the irretrievable loss of youth—the patient. You treat him angrily, bitterly, resentfully, he says.[24] We believe that medical schools have a long way to go to produce doctors who are not angry, bitter, or resentful.

In "Natural Childbirth and the Reluctant Physician," anthropologist Shelly Romalis says, "Unless labor is short, the woman is well motivated, has a physician who is a real natural childbirth advocate, and is supported by an energetic partner, her chances of 'Making it' are slim." She remarks that it is well documented that when physician support is evident, pain is decreased, and the chances for a positive outcome are greatly increased.[40] Yet many physicians are patronizing, condescending, and even deviant (in their attempt to lure the woman as a patient).

Romalis remarks that many physicians use techniques to gain the woman's confidence, "but at the same time, establish dominance." She uses the following examples:

> *Of course, if you think you can have a natural birth, I'll go along with it. Remember, though, that the most important thing is the baby and not your own wishes or comfort. If complications arise, I'll have to step in.*

> *I have no objections to your taking classes. But they tend to make you feel guilty or like a failure if you don't make it.*

> *I'm in favor of birth without drugs, but women who have set ideas about not having medication usually scream for it when the going gets rough. Do you think you can do it?*

> *The only kind of birth which is not natural is a cesarean, and even those are so simple and safe today they are as good as natural.*

Romalis tells us that the voice of professional authority is hard to counter. The messages the woman receives are that she has limited decision-making power, that childbirth is painful, and that things go wrong quite often. The woman learns that "it is unusual to have a nonmedicated birth, that she might be putting her baby at risk to achieve her goal, that guilt results from trying and failing, that there is nothing unnatural about medication or even a cesarean." Romalis warns that the woman is clearly being primed for "acceptance of a medical definition of birthing" (p. 70).

Childbirth is not a medical complication. It is a healthy, normal function of our healthy, normal bodies. Doctors who like to keep busy doing things should be assigned to emergency rooms, not to maternity floors. In *Immaculate Deception*, Rich Quint, M.D. says, "Most obstetricians will admit it is a bore to deliver at normal births."[1] Robert Bradley, author of *Husband-Coached Child-*

birth, says, "A good obstetrician has been defined as one equipped with a broad rear end and the good sense to sit calmly on it and let nature take its course." Unfortunately, however, men have always sought to control what they don't understand.

Women are beginning to take more responsibility for their care during pregnancy. Many test their own urine and have friends take their blood pressure. We are competent, intelligent beings, capable of taking part in our own health assessment. However, it may unbalance a doctor if he hasn't much "busy work" to do at your appointments or at the birth. One woman said:

> During one of my nine-month checkups, my doctor walked in. He asked for my urine so he could test it. I told him I already had and gave him the results. He went for the Doptone and when I said, "No thanks," he said, "Oops, I forgot." He couldn't find his fetascope, but I told him not to bother, the baby was moving just fine. He began to put on a glove. Once again, I said, "No, thanks." He went to prick my finger, and I told him I'd had an iron count at a local lab, and I was fine. He sat down, sighed, and said, "So, what's new with you?"

And that's what obstetrics should be about! Relationships! Dialogues between human beings! Birth is about relationships! A good obstetrician must enjoy sitting back. He must be patient and gentle, and above all, he must be willing to listen and respect your decision. He must believe that each woman is really the best judge—or at least an excellent source for finding out—about what's going on with her body.

Susan wrote:

> It was time for my husband to change into the required garments, so he quickly left. No sooner had he closed the door when the doctor, trying to hurry the process, reached both his hands inside of me and proceeded to stretch the birth canal. A muffled scream escaped my lips . . . He explained, "It will make the delivery easier for you." Did he really think I was that naive? . . . I looked around for my husband who was just arriving through the swinging doors. He had no idea what the doctor had done to me."

Compare the remarks of the previous women with the following letter from a woman in Missouri:

> On December 2, I gave birth, vaginally, to a beautiful baby boy, almost 20 months to the day after a cesarean. The doctor just stood by giving advice and encouragement and mostly keeping busy with our Polaroid. He helped ease the baby out slowly to avoid tears and immediately placed the baby against my chest. He showed my husband where, and after the cord stopped pulsing, my husband cut the cord. Of course, all this time the doctor is taking more pictures! They left us alone, so we could be together as a family. I am happy for myself and my baby. It was so beautiful and rewarding. I am also happy that I was able to increase the confidence of my doctor in this philosophy.

Another woman wrote:

My doctor ordered an I.V. I told him that I didn't want one. He was very nice as we discussed the situation back and forth. He finally said, "I'd really like you to do this, if for nothing else, then for me. It would make me feel better." I almost agreed at this point, but just as I was about to give my consent, I thought, "Wait a minute! I'm the one in labor. Why do I have to make him feel better?!" I refused, and fortunately, he handled the refusal without getting all bent out of shape.

One couple from Connecticut found a "supportive" physician. All during the pregnancy he seemed "relaxed about all our requests." However, when Candy went into labor:

I was monitored both internally and externally, plus I had an I.V. Just as our son's head was visible, I was moved to the delivery room and put flat on my back with my legs in stirrups. Also, the doctor was so anxious to get the baby out that he took one swipe with the scissors and really sliced me. He told me later he felt terribly stressed during the pushing, poor thing.

Barbara wrote:

We are very angry at the doctor because of the way he reacted when we came in fully dilated. He took my husband out into the hall and blasted the hell out of him for not bringing me in sooner. He said if I hadn't delivered when I did he was going to give me ten more minutes and then do a cesarean. We hope other women will find the determination and courage to say "No" to a medical establishment that demands repeat cesarean.

Susan from New Jersey wrote:

One doctor I called said yes. I was very encouraged by our conversation, so I made an appointment. Fred and I drove an hour to see him. Once we were there he said no. He said there was a 15 percent risk and he didn't want to have to tell my husband that I died giving birth. He charged $30, thank you, and said goodbye. Another doctor told us over the phone that he was comfortable with VBAC. Nature takes care of itself, and I'm tired of the fear of malpractice, he said. We went to see him. He wanted me prepped for a cesarean with an internal monitor, I.V., external monitor, and a spinal at nine centimeters. If I was at all overdue—bang— a cesarean. When we began to question him, he told us to trust him and not concern ourselves with such things. He said we knew too much and we would be better off with less knowledge.

Another VBAC woman wrote:

I had to take the best of the lot. No prize pig, believe me. As he was going to do an episiotomy our midwife said, "She doesn't need it!" He yelled, "I'm in charge here!" Well, I got cut, believe you me. Dr. H. then pulled the placenta out and sarcastically asked our midwife if she wanted to sew me up. He turned to me with the placenta and said, "What do you want to do, fry it?" At my six-week checkup, he admitted he would rather just be a gynecologist.

Many women report that their doctors are rude. A woman in California wrote, "Everything was going fine until I put on six pounds in one month. Then he told me if I didn't keep it down to three pounds per month, I'd never have a VBAC. He said the extra weight would be too much for the scar. I knew it was time to switch."

Julie said, "One doctor I interviewed said, 'Aha! Here's the high-risk woman.' (I can't wait to get my hands on you!) His eyes lit up as if he had finally found his prey."

Letters from women whose doctors are respectful of them and of the birth process are few and far between. As Gena Corea says, it is more common for the demands of birth technology and the medical technocracy to take precedence over the best interests of mother and infant. The rising cesarean rate provides clear evidence of that. In a cesarean delivery, the woman is 100 percent out of control of the birthing, and the physician is 100 percent in control. As Hugh Drummond remarks, the cesarean is the obstetrician's last opportunity to play God.[10]

Some physicians are beginning to descend from Olympus and offer support of purebirth. Some are even working up enthusiasm for VBAC. Most, however, remain staunch interventionists, terrified by the possibility of rupture, and unwilling to witness or permit the slow progress of a long VBAC labor. It has often been said that obstetricians think and act as if pregnancy and labor constitute pathological rather than normal processes. According to Dr. Atlee, their entire medical education is so obsessed with pathology that it is practically impossible for them to think of any woman who comes to them as other than sick.

For that reason, many of the physicians who ostensibly support VBAC are merely paying lip service to it. They stand by, knife in hand. "Doctors have their own myths about how painful labor is, and they see it as an ordeal from which they can rescue us."[35] A woman is monitored, starved, and I.V.ed, right down the line. At the first "sign" of anything going awry, she finds herself being sectioned. The doctor says, "Well, we tried. It just didn't work." He's home in bed long before she is even out of the recovery room.

Dr. Gerald S. Stober, a physician from Queens, N.Y., describes a common occurrence. A woman says, "I want a vaginal delivery," and the obstetrician gets the message that unless he agrees, she is going to go elsewhere. So he says, "Yes, I can do it," and she is deluded into thinking she's found what she wants. The doctor will let her labor a little and then say, "Well, we have to do a cesarean after all, too bad." Stober admits that despite all the rhetoric about VBAC, very few are actually taking place. "The best way to reduce the number of cesareans," he says, "is to be sure the first one is necessary."*

---

*Joan Rattner Heilman, "Breaking the Cesarean Cycle," *New York Times Magazine*, 7 Sept. 1980, p. 92.

In *Our Bodies, Ourselves,*[35] it is stated:

> The fact that the specialized field of obstetrics-gynecology is now claiming that it wishes to be identified as *the* resource for all of the health needs of women needs to be looked at closely. It implies that women can expect to have all of their needs for psychological as well as physical care met by the obstetrician-gynecologist. Yet there are no standing requirements . . . for an ob/gyn to demonstrate any competence in any aspect of behavioral science, human development, psychology of women, or even psychology in general. Every woman should understand that what this means is that just because a doctor is a certified ob-gyn doesn't mean that he is qualified or trained or prepared in any way to give advice or counsel or any other sort of help in any human-relations area of a woman's life [p. 352].

Diana Scully, author of *Men Who Control Women's Health: The Miseducation of Obstetrician-Gynecologists*, reports that "baby catcher" is medical slang for obstetrician, "reflecting the belief that this field is boring and routine."[42] Much of the operative interference into birth is simply a tactic used to convince women that obstetrics are necessary.

Interviewing an Obstetrician

We would like to help you select and interview your physician. Good money and lots of it is being spent, whether you are paying directly or not. You should expect time, honesty, and support for this fee, as well as competent medical care in the event of an emergency. You needn't love your doctor, nor trust him implicitly. (When a woman says, "I trust my doctor completely," we add 10 points to her statistical chances for having a cesarean.) Young and Mahan say that when your relationship with your physician is based on "mutual honesty, trust, and shared decision-making" (p. 1), you have the essential elements for a rewarding experience.

We suggest that when you schedule your appointment, you ask for a time slot when the doctor is less likely to be behind schedule. You can schedule early in the morning or right after lunch. If, in spite of careful scheduling, he is rushed, tell him you'd rather reschedule than feel deprived of the time you need.

Use the time you are kept waiting in his office to see what books he has around. If there's one you are happy to see, chat with him about it when he comes in. You can learn a lot from seeing what he reads or what he wants you to think he reads. Look for Dr. Marieskind's report on cesarean section and the National Institute of Health Task Force Report on cesarean birth, Arms's *Immaculate Deception*, Gaskin's *Spiritual Midwifery*, Baldwin's *Special Delivery*, Mendelsohn's books, and the NAPSAC publications. If you don't see them, ask him if he has read them. If he hasn't, ask him if he will.

Face to Face. . .   If you do not understand an answer, say so. Keep at it until you do. When a statement is made, ask if it is an opinion or fact. If it is a fact, you have every right to ask for references! You can say, "I didn't know that. I'd like to know more. I'd be interested to read about it and would appreciate your references." It's better to find out in an office rather than in a labor room or operating room that the doctor you have chosen becomes easily unglued or defensive.

If the doctor indicates that he does VBACs and is comfortable with them, ask him for a few names of VBAC women he has attended. If he can't think of any, ask his nurse or receptionist. If she can't think of any, you can assume he doesn't attend VBACs very often. (Perhaps he is worried about patient confidentiality. Suggest that he contact the VBAC mothers and ask them to contact you. We haven't met a VBAC woman yet who is unwilling to talk!)

We suggest you talk to the doctor when you are fully clothed, before any physical examination. If you have an internal exam, get dressed before you continue the interview. We recommend that you sit across from the physician, at the same level, and position your chair so that there is no desk between you. Tricky, but possible. One woman picked up her chair and plopped it down in a better position. "I'm hard of hearing," she said. A desk puts miles between you and keeps capital letters on "The Doctor."

Many of you already know that doctors are *different* when fathers are present for prenatal office appointments. Without a doubt, most physicians alter their manners appreciably when the man is present. They seem less harried; they are more conversational and "charming" and less paternalistic. Many physicians put their hand out to the father and introduce themselves by first name. (Rarely does a physician extend his hand to a woman and say, "Glad to meet you. Bob Jones." It's usually *Dr.* Jones.) Invariably, questions are answered more completely. Men: when your woman tells you something about the obstetrician, believe her! He's different, and his attitude and answers are different, when you are there.

If the doctor calls you by your first name, call him by his. If he calls you by your last name, you can still ask to call him by his first name. You probably call your mailman, milkman, plumber, and carpenter by first names—why not your physician? First names change the entire character of the communication. A first name may help to humanize the doctor in your eyes: he may leave the sphere of "authority" or even "impersonal provider" and become a cohort in the achievement of your goals. How much easier and more effective to communicate with an equal than to diffidently approach a "pedestal"!

Ask a personal question or two. You needn't demand disclosure of his bank account or personal affairs, but you can certainly expect to learn whether he smokes or exercises. You can ask what kind of childbirth experiences his wife had or if she breastfed. You can ask him how he feels about birth. You can watch his body language. You can search for a strong enough "human being" to counteract or balance The Doctor.

When asking a technical question, you may want to rephrase it and ask it again. Watch for discrepancies. "I don't like to rupture membranes," followed by, "I think an internal monitor can be helpful in many cases," would make us suspicious.

Your baby's birth is not a time for war or even a quick skirmish. Careful screening ahead of time can keep your birthday party peaceful and happy. Sometimes the interview can take place over the phone. Instead of asking, "Can I have a VBAC?" you can state: "I've had a cesarean. I have a lower segment incision and I am planning a VBAC. I'd like to know if you are willing to support a completely natural birth." Clear, precise, and no one's time is wasted.

If the doctor tells you he is going to stay with you the entire labor, this is a clear indication that he considers you high risk, since we assume he does not stay with all of his clients throughout their entire labors. Chances are his presence at your entire labor will not calm you. Eventually, it will wear you down and cause you to feel as if you aren't dilating fast enough. Most doctors find it impossible to sit without *doing* something (i.e., rupturing the membranes). The women we have worked with, even those with long labors, found it much easier to labor apart from the doctor's clinical gaze. Their L.A.s provided whatever expertise was needed.

One woman who thought her doctor's constant presence would be a *necessity* for her emotional well-being found it instead a distraction. She finally asked him to leave and felt far more relaxed. The physicians we recommend keep in close contact, drop by every now and then, give a word of encouragement, and leave.

Some doctors charge more for VBACs. "I need it to pay for the Grecian Formula to cover the grey hairs I'm going to get while you labor," one said. This practice is discriminatory. Some doctors charge extra because they are planning to stay with you throughout your entire labor. Some hospitals charge extra, as well; they insist that an anesthesiologist be present throughout your labor. We find this completely unnecessary unless you choose to incur this expense for your own peace of mind. The problem is, if an anesthesiologist is there, he may be too difficult to resist.

Partners . . . But Not with You An OB's life isn't always easy. Many are run ragged, and so take on an associate. A doctor who works with a partner can be at the hospital while the clients are having appointments back at the office. This arrangement may work for *them*, but it rarely works out as well for the women. First, although the doctors assure women that they practice obstetrics in very much the same manner, this is rarely the case. Too many women have said, "I was assured that either doctor would respect our wishes. But when I was in labor with the partner, I was told, 'This is how *I* practice obstetrics.' " Second, since there is only a 50 percent chance of being with a woman in labor, a physician's commitment to a particular client is greatly reduced. Third, if you alternate visits with the two, you won't get to know either very well.

The quality of care and caring in a shared practice is rarely as good. This is evident in a local health plan where there is a one in five chance of being with any particular physician. It's like playing Russian roulette. In another health plan, six doctors have six different opinions. Two doctors favor VBAC—one enthusiastically, the other less so. Two others are openly hostile (at least they're *open* about it!). Another gives lip service to it—it is clear that he would much prefer to do cesareans and not be involved in "whims" about natural birth. The sixth is "neutral"—we'll wait and see. Not very good odds. The level of commitment diminishes dramatically with every name added to the door.

We are losing the one-to-one caring that came with a local doctor who knew us well, and really cared about us and our family. In *Immaculate Deception*, psychiatrist Alfred French explains that doctors spend their whole lives trying to do two things at once: to get the intimacy they've got to have and at the same time protect themselves from it. We received a warming letter that renewed some faith from a woman who had a cesarean in New York and couldn't find a doctor who would agree to a vaginal birth. She wrote her old family physician in her home state. He responded, "I delivered you. And your brother and sister (as a matter of fact, a good portion of this community). I saw you grow. I know you can have your baby naturally." She delivered an 8 pound VBAC at home with this physician in attendance.

VBAC women have all the same concerns that any woman has during pregnancy. Will my baby be normal? Will my first born freak out with a new baby in the house? However, many VBAC women have the additional thought (every time there is a normal twitch or twinge) that the uterus will rupture. (One VBAC woman woke up in the middle of the night to a loud "pop" followed by a feeling of wetness. She shook her husband. "Wake up! Either my water just broke or my uterus just ruptured!" He jumped up. "Which is it?" She sat for a moment and said, "Well, I feel terrific, so it must have been the water!") Many also have concern that their doctor will not come through for them. We repeat, the time to find out if the doctor is going to support you is long before your contractions have begun.

The following is a list of questions that can be used when you interview a physician. We do not recommend that you "fire them away" all at once. First choose the ones that are most important *to you*. Make sure that you find out if this doctor has a case of the "in-cases": "I'll just hook up an I.V. *in case* you aren't large enough." Ask what his section rate is. (One nurse wrote, "I work with a very fine group of obstetricians. Though our cesarean rate is 15 percent, I see these physicians weighing many factors before jumping in and resorting to cesareans." Fifteen percent! What "factors"? What time dinner is served? If their rate is 15 percent, you can bet they are jumping in, clothes and all.) Get a sense for who this person is, what his attitudes are about birth, and how you will feel with him or her at your child's birthday party. Find out *ahead of time* what his philosophies and practices are—this is one birthday party that you don't want to be full of surprises!

Questions To Ask Physician Candidates

- Are you accepting more clients at this time?

- With what hospital(s) are you affiliated?

- Are you willing to work with me toward a natural birth? VBAC? Will you treat me as if my uterine scar doesn't exist, or will it be an issue for you?

- Do you believe that women were designed to have babies?

- Have you read the reports by Dr. Marieskind and the NIH Task Force?

- How many VBACs have you attended? Do you suggest VBAC to women or must they inquire first?

- What is your cesarean rate?

- Will you welcome my labor assistant into my birthing room? Friends?

- Is it hard for you to do nothing at a birth?

- Do you insist upon any "prep"? (Shaving? Enema?)

- Do you encourage women to eat, drink, and walk during labor?

- Do you prefer to use a Doptone or a fetascope to check the baby's heartbeat?

- Are you aware of any problems associated with ultrasound?

- Do you require an I.V.? Does the hospital?

- Do you require a fetal monitor? Does the hospital? Are you aware of their restrictions and consequences?

- What alternatives do you suggest for a "slow" labor? (Walking? Changing position? Urinating often?)

- How would you define a "slow" labor? Do you set a time limit for any part of labor?

- Do you rupture membranes routinely? At all? When? Why?

- If the membranes rupture spontaneously, do you set a time limit before insisting upon a section? Do you do any testing to determine if an infection is indeed present?

- What is your policy if there is meconium in the fluid?

- Do you agree with the American Academy of Pediatrics that "No drug is proven safe during the maternal course"?

- What percentage of your patients receives Pitocin?

- Do you know how to attend a breech birth? What percentage of your breech births are cesareans?

- What percentage of your patients deliver in stirrups?

- What percentage of your patients deliver with forceps?

- What is your episiotomy rate?

- How do you help women to birth without episiotomies? (Hot compresses? Vitamin E oil?)

- Do you wait for the natural delivery of the placenta?

- Do you encourage parent/infant bonding?

- What is your policy concerning siblings at birth?

- Does the hospital with which you affiliate encourage the father to stay for all procedures?

- Do you insist upon silver nitrate and vitamin K, or will you agree to waive them?

- When you do a cesarean, do you do so with future VBAC for the woman in mind? What incision do you use? How do you feel about manual exploration of the incision after a VBAC?

- Will you fully explain any procedures I don't understand?

- How long do you "permit" a woman to be overdue?

- Under what circumstances would you recommend x-rays? Amniocentesis? Ultrasound?

- Will you honor a hospital request list?

- Who covers for you? Does that person share your views?

- Where did you go to medical school? Where were you in your class?

- Why did you go into obstetrics?

- Are you familiar with NAPSAC, SPUN, ICEA, La Leche League?

- Do you have any children? What were their births like?

- Will you respect a second opinion?

- Are you able to appreciate the uniqueness and specialness, the wonder and the newness, of each individual birth?

- Whom do you see in ultimate "power": the administration, obstetrician, nurses, anesthesiologist?

- Do you support homebirth? Do you provide back-up? Do you provide back-up for VBAC homebirth?

- Do you mind answering so many questions?

In addition, we would like to share with you a list of questions that Esther Rome, a woman from Massachusetts, submitted to her group of doctors.

- How long have you had a policy of requiring consent forms for fetal monitor (unspecified type) and I.V. in advance of labor and delivery for women wanting a vaginal labor after a previous cesarean delivery?

- Why is consent in advance requested for these procedures and not others which may be routinely done, e.g., amniotomy or episiotomy?

- What precipitated the change in your policy?

- How many women gave birth vaginally after sections without I.V.s and fetal monitors before this policy went into effect?

- How many had complications and of what type?

- How many of these complications could reasonably have been avoided if the I.V.s and fetal monitors had been used? Please explain.

- What is the percentage of uterine rupture in women without previous sections?

- What is the percentage of uterine rupture in women with low transverse sections?

- Is this figure for complete rupture or does it also include anything that could be considered benign rupture?

- In women with low transverse sections who do have rupture, is the rupture always at the site of the previous scar?

- What are the predisposing factors for uterine rupture; e.g., are the following risk factors: low iron count, poor diet, multiple pregnancies, spacing between pregnancies?

- Have you ever had a situation during birth in which you couldn't find a vein to put in an I.V.?

- What are the circumstances under which an I.V. is needed?

- What are the predisposing factors for needing an I.V.?

- In what percentage of cases do these circumstances occur in the general U.S. population? In the hospital population? Particularly, in your population?

- In each type of case in which an I.V. is needed, how much time is there in which to put in the I.V.?

- What is the average length of time it takes to get an I.V. at your hospital?

- What are the risks of using an I.V.? Do they include restricted mobility or bladder distention?

- Would you use a heparin lock instead of an I.V.? Why or why not?

- How is it determined whether an internal or an external monitor is used?

- What are the risks of ultrasound connected with the use of external monitors?

- What are the risks of infection connected with the use of the internal monitor?

- How much is the laboring woman allowed to move around when attached to each kind of monitor?

- Can either type of monitor be used intermittently?

- Are certain laboring positions favored when the fetal monitor is used? If so, what are they and what risks and benefits are associated with these positions?

- With internal monitors, at what stage are the waters broken? What kind of fetal electrode is used? What is the infant scalp infection rate at your hospital? What is the infection rate for the mother compared to other women who have their waters broken but have no fetal monitor, and compared to women who don't have amniotomy?

- Who reads the fetal monitor results? Is there a special monitor team? What are the training and experience requirements for the person reading the monitor?

- How often is the monitor checked? Theoretically and actually?

- If no monitor is used, how often are fetal vital signs checked? Theoretically and actually? By whom?

- What is the section rate on women who have monitors (each type) and those who do not?

- Would you indicate if your answer is based on your own clinical experience, the clinical experience of other M.D.s in your practice or on well-controlled studies? If the information is based on studies, please include references.

Esther writes, "The physicians in the plan I used were very happy to answer my questions, but the bottom line was that if I didn't abide by their decisions on how labor should be managed, then they wouldn't accept responsibility for me as a patient." Her 7 pound, 3 ounce VBAC son was born at home.

"It's a Long, Long Way to . . ." Another concern for VBAC women is that they may have to travel to get the kind of support they want. How far is too far to travel? Some women think twenty minutes is tops, others drive three hours or more. Nan wrote, "My pregnancy is progressing just fine. I wish I could say the same for my doctor. He told me I should be 'grateful' he was willing to allow us to try a VBAC. I let him know in no uncertain terms that a VBAC was our decision. We have decided not to go back to him. We're using a doctor two hours away. Initially, that time sounded too far. Now, for peace of mind, two hours seems quite acceptable."

If at all possible, we recommend staying close to home. Being surrounded by familiar people and places can help relax you. Being in your own home during early labor—being free to open the refrigerator, make noises, take a walk, drip fluid on the rug—helps labor to be much more relaxed than being in a car, in a room at a motel, or laboring at someone else's home.

Changing Physicians

One suggestion for dealing with an unusually chauvinistic or difficult doctor, or one who routinely relies on interventions, is to change. If you don't like the apples at the supermarket, you don't buy them. You either do without apples or you go elsewhere. If there is only one physician in your area and you are unwilling to travel, keep to the forefront thoughts about your own strength and capability. You needn't be intimidated or abused. Bea wrote, "Frankly, the man scared me to death. But I was determined to be able to talk to him intelligently and without hysteria. I kept picturing him as a little boy. Dirty knees, short pants, a cowlick. I pictured him playing with his building blocks and trucks. It helped to humanize him and remind me that there must be a person under that facade."

How late can you change physicians? Right up until your baby is born. One woman switched three days after her due date, and one changed in labor. Ideally, you will have interviewed doctors before your pregnancy, or early on, so you can relax and enjoy the rest of the pregnancy. Unfortunately, some doctors are wolves in sheep's clothing, and you don't notice until you have gone into the woods many times.

One woman wrote, "My doctor was charming—until I started asking questions. He tried to remain charming, but became increasingly upset. My questions were legitimate! After only three questions, he actually began *shaking!* He tried to remain controlled but *yelled* that if I wanted to practice medicine my way, I ought to go out and get myself a license."

Doctors Who Care

To all the doctors who really do care, who respect women and the process of birth, who are in obstetrics because every new life is a constant wonder and amazement to them: You are difficult to find; please tell us where you are and how to reach you. And please don't let the others wear you down.

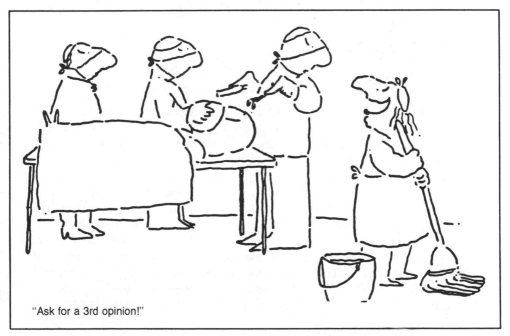

"Ask for a 3rd opinion!"

Some good doctors do exist. They keep a low profile. They often refuse interviews or television invitations. Some of them are scared—not of malpractice, but of their peers. They survived obstetrical training as intact humans, and their humanity is ridiculed, even branded irresponsible by their colleagues.

A word about women obstetricians. Sadly, they are not necessarily "good guys": too many of them eventually adopt and integrate the "male view" about women and birth; they are such a small minority that it is enormously difficult for them to take a stand on personal conviction. In order to receive respect from the rest of the (male) staff, they prove themselves by being "one of the guys." One female obstetrician said, "If you make any unpopular decision, the disapproval is outstanding. The tension can eat you alive." Some female physicians continue to act like interns or residents for years after they have hung out their shingles.

Recently, a couple traveled to another state to screen an obstetrician. They called and said, "We knew we had found the right doctor for our VBAC when we told him that all the doctors in our area insisted upon an I.V., a monitor, and a definite time limit in labor, and he responded with, 'You're kidding!' "

One doctor told us, "At first, the very thought of VBAC was enough to frighten me. But as each VBAC took place, I became more and more comfortable with it. I now tell a woman with a previous cesarean that if she decides to use me as her obstetrician, she will have to understand that I will not do an automatic repeat cesarean, and that I will help her as best I can to have the baby vaginally."

Good doctors like this do exist, although you may have to look long and seriously for them.

Medical Records

Medical records are a one-way street that only doctors are allowed to travel. We are required to pave the way for physicians by making our records available, whereas professional secrecy shrouds the performance records of those who purport to be competent to help us.

In the early part of this century a physician by the name of Codman preached "the revolutionary doctrine that institutions were responsible for the work of their staffs." He called on hospitals to study the work of each physician, analyze his results, compare them with those of others, and actually enable the public to choose the doctors they wanted based on this information.* Too bad Dr. Codman's views didn't sit well with the profession! We'd venture a guess that finding out how many episiotomies, for example, each doctor has done would be extremely difficult. Can you imagine laws that would make each doctor's statistics public knowledge? Yet doesn't it seem we have a right to know?

---

*New England J. Med., 224 (13 Feb. 1941): 297.

Several midwives in the Boston area keep detailed records of their attendance at births. They list the total births, the number of interventions (very few if any), the number of complications (ditto), the number of twins, premature babies, breech births, etc. They record how complications were managed. They record the number of episiotomies (generally none) or lacerations that require suturing (generally none). They record the length of labor, birthweight, number of mothers requiring cesareans (generally 2–5 percent). Why don't more midwives—and doctors—make information of this kind public?

Most physicians insist upon reviewing your previous medical records. Information gained may discourage them from taking you on, or it may help convince them that a VBAC is a likely possibility. For example, a record stating that the pelvis was found to be more than adequate by x-ray pelvimetry or that a suspected vertical incision was indeed transverse could help a physician support your decision. On the other hand, you could provide the physician with much of the information yourself. Many physicians will not believe their clients but use previous medical records as God's word: "Says here you have CPD. Sorry, in *your* case a VBAC is impossible." Your records may also be useful by providing information about the use of Pitocin, drugs, and medical interventions that may have led to your cesarean.

However, it is our experience that medical records are often misleading, inaccurate, illegible, and abbreviated. We have been told by hospital nurses and doctors alike that often the records are not filled out by the attending physician, nor are they always filled out at the time of birth. We have seen records with several handwritings and with numerous entries crossed out and rewritten. When there are three or four women in labor simultaneously, information is occasionally mixed.

Women often receive medical records with pages missing. Mary's records with her twins stopped after the birth of the first baby. When she called the hospital to receive the additional pages, she was told, "That's all there is." Joan's records stated, "The breech was delivered by cesarean section." Her baby had never been breech. Sue was sectioned "for fetal distress." Later the same record stated that fetal heart tones were strong throughout the entire labor and that the section was done for uterine inertia. Yet Sue had been six centimeters dilated when she arrived at the hospital and was recorded to be at nine centimeters an hour later, when the decision to perform the cesarean was made. Uterine inertia?? Donna was told that she needed a cesarean because her baby wouldn't "drop." She was told that her mid-pelvis was too small to accommodate her baby. Her medical records report that the baby was deeply engaged into the pelvis and that the cesarean was done for uterine fatigue. Scratch "uterine", pencil in "staff"? Her next baby, by the way, was a beautiful 9 pound VBAC after five hours of labor. Shelly was told that her baby was "under stress" and that she had to have an emergency c/section. Her medical report stated that the baby's heart beat was around 144 at all times. Mary, a nurse who had a section for CPD, read her report. "No evidence of CPD. Moulding compatible with this stage of labor." She says, "There is no need for me to re-read the report. The words have been etched in my memory since the day I first read them!"

Women whose records have doomed them to a lifetime of surgical births have gone on to deliver babies naturally. Nikki, Dee, and Bonnie all had completely contracted pelves, according to their medical records, but went on to have their babies naturally. The septum in Katie's uterus "precluded a vaginal delivery," yet she had a VBAC. Ginni, Jeanne, and Joanne had midline classical incisions. Their medical records forbade future vaginal delivery, yet they all had VBACs. Lynne and Eileen had fibroids. In spite of medical records that categorized these women as unfavorable or impossible VBACs, they all had their next babies without difficulty or complication.

We do not believe it is absolutely essential to have previous medical reports. Many previous reports arrived at the physician's office after a VBAC had been accomplished. Several doctors have said, "If I had read the records, I'd have done a repeat section." We know that the only way to determine if a VBAC is possible is to believe that it is and to give it your all.

On the other hand, if you want your medical records, you should be able to have them. Different states have different laws about medical records. To protect us, they say. No, to protect physicians and hospitals. Some hospitals deny us access to our medical records, information about our own bodies. That practice is an abridgement of human rights. In those states where consumers have legally challenged denial of "the right to access," courts have upheld that right. We cannot be denied access to our own records! As long as you permit your records to remain part of the medical domain, you won't own them. Although we would bet our money on your uterine incision itself, and on your own statements, over and above your medical records, those records are yours, inaccurate or not! Your right to them is as inalienable as your right to birth without interference.

Much in obstetrics is subjective. One doctor, upon examining a woman in labor, said, "She's already six centimeters dilated." The nurse, weary from a long day's work, wrote down, "Patient is only six cms." Another woman was making noises during labor. In her records it states that the "patient is loud and unmanageable."

There are doctors who keep meticulous records. We appreciate their thoroughness. But the majority of the records we have surveyed do a great disservice to the "patient" and do not accurately represent the obstetrical situation.

Reclaiming Responsibility

Of course, you know by now that we consider doctors to be superfluous at healthy, normal births. Approximately 80 percent of the babies in the world are delivered with midwives, not doctors, in attendance. This is common not only in underdeveloped countries, but in Sweden, Denmark, Finland, Holland and Japan—nations that have far lower infant-mortality rates than the United States. In fact, the United States is the only nation that has ever outlawed midwives. We are encouraged by "the return of the midwives" and pray that the art of midwifery is never lost. (As Lisa Frank remarks, "The grannies [granny midwives] are gaining!" However, in many states insurance companies will still not cover the cost of a midwife, let alone L.A. or cesarean prevention class.)

Childbirth educator Debra Evans writes:

> We will continue to experience a disparity between the management and the experience of childbirth *until women demand better treatment*. They are not likely to be served well by profit-motivated obstetricians subscribing to a paternalistic super-organization. The male bias, the economic system of health care in our country and the cultural definition of childbirth as a sickness requiring medical intervention prevent women from feeling whole as they give birth [emphasis added].

Marianne Brorup says, "It is a woman's right to birth with dignity and love. Why do we have to fight for that?"

In *Changing Childbirth*,[46] Diony Young reminds us that we cannot sit back and wait passively for change to occur. She makes suggestions for being an "active and informed initiator and participator" in the process of changing childbirth in our country. She remarks that "the most important strategy of all is to have the courage and determination to carry on the effort no matter what the obstacles may be." (Or, in the current phrase, "Don't let the turkeys get you down!")

In *Lying In: A History of Childbirth in America*, Dorothy Wertz remarks that women have set out to regain possession of their bodies and the life they have lost.[45]

Yes, we have.

We have also set out to regain possessions of our births. Recognizing our options and making well-informed, appropriate decisions is one step. Another step is letting those doctors, hospitals, and childbirth classes that we have eliminated from our list know why they were not chosen. Only when we begin to exert our influence as consumers will we be able to look forward to a time when all cesareans will once again be necessary cesareans.

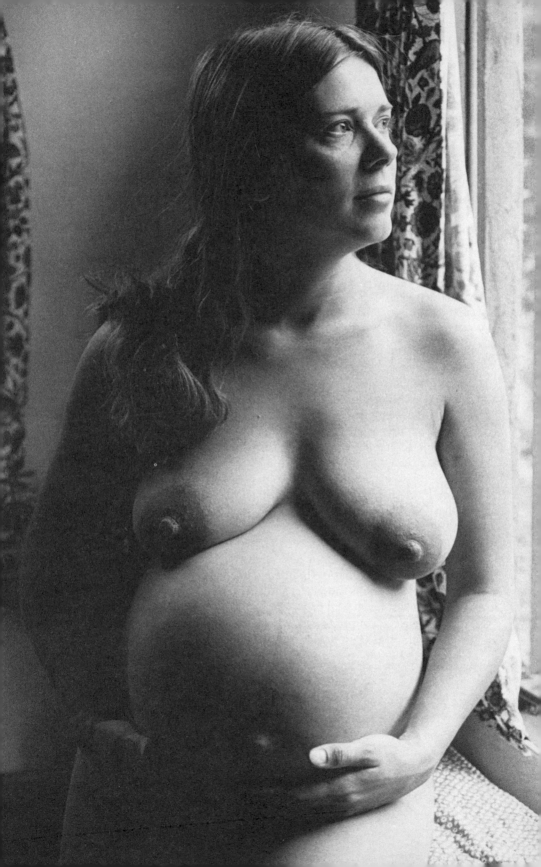

14 > In Case a Cesarean Is Necessary

Even though many of us would like to reduce the cesarean rate, we cannot eliminate *all* cesareans. If life deals you a cesarean, there's no need to throw down the rest of your cards. You can pick up your hand and play the remaining cards to win. Having a cesarean does not mean that every goal must be abandoned nor does it mean that you must relinquish all control over the experience. A cesarean can be a positive event for the whole family.

It is important to remain a conscious participant (both physically and mentally) throughout the pregnancy, delivery and postpartum period, even in the face of a serious medical situation. Maintaining understanding of oneself and of the event will result in feelings of satisfaction with the birth itself, whether the birth is vaginal or cesarean. At the point when a cesarean is suggested, the couple is often tired from long hours of labor, disoriented, and certainly vulnerable. In this weakened state, they will often agree to unwanted procedures and unnecessary policies just to "hurry and get the whole thing over with."

In order to be actively involved in your cesarean birth, you will need to do some homework during your pregnancy. Unless the reason for the cesarean is maternal disease or previously suspected placenta previa, there is rarely enough time to prepare for a necessary cesarean. It is, therefore, advisable to gather information ahead of time, and then tuck it away just in case a cesarean or a repeat cesarean becomes necessary.

Jini Duffy Fairley contributed this chapter. (See About the Contributors.)

Prenatal Planning

I suggest that you design a birth plan that describes the birth experience you desire. Learn your options through your reading as well as through discussions with other couples, with your medical team, and with the hospital. You may need to create some alternatives of your own. Focus on those options that are most important to you as a couple. Spell out your choices concisely, on one page for quick and easy reference. You may wish to obtain the signature of your primary physician to show that there has been discussion of and agreement with your plan. Ask that he respect your wishes as often as humanly possible. Do this early in your pregnancy. You may decide to change doctors or hospitals in order to achieve more of your goals for this birth. A birth plan, agreed upon by your physician, is one of the first steps toward a positive birth experience. Much of what follows will assist you in writing your plan.

There are several books on cesarean delivery that you may wish to add to your pregnancy reading list. None is complete unto itself, but each may offer information relevant to your own needs. For those few couples who must plan a cesarean, there are classes offered by community-based childbirth groups and hospitals. These classes offer information on nutrition and exercise during pregnancy, audio-visual aids to familiarize you with the operation, discussion of the procedures and policies available for the delivery, and suggestions to help you make postpartum adjustments. Choose a class taught by an instructor who does not "push" cesareans, one who explores with you the ways in which a cesarean could be avoided if at all possible. The classes, by the way, should not be an absolute prerequisite for the father's presence in the delivery room. After all, mothers are present for cesareans all the time without having taken any special classes. A father's "ticket" into the O.R. should not be a graduation certificate from cesarean classes, but his love for and interest in his mate and his infant.

Parent support groups for cesarean couples offer information and assistance. They can also offer emotional support. Again, beware of groups that accept the high rate of cesareans in your area as necessary and groups that do not advocate cesarean prevention and VBAC.

You should become well informed about your chosen physician's practices and about the hospital's policies regarding cesareans. A second opinion, if there is time, may help you to avoid an unnecessary cesarean. The second opinion should come from a physician who bears no allegiance to your particular doctor or hospital and who can therefore be more objective. Make certain that you discuss the following with your doctor and hospital in full detail: Their cesarean rate, their general attitude toward VBAC, recommended prenatal testing procedures, preferred preoperative medication (if any) and reasons for that preference, type of anesthesia perferred (and reasons), and types of incisions and stitches (sutures) preferred and why. Also determine if fathers and L.A.s are welcome at the cesarean. Find out the general management of the postpartum period, including pain medication options, and whether breastfeeding in the delivery and recovery room, and on demand, is encouraged. Determine when the I.V., catheter, and sutures will be removed, and when nutritious food will be offered. Make certain that sibling visitation in the mother's room (with baby present) is encouraged. Find out the average length of the hospital stay. During the discussion, let your needs be known. Ask for referrals of other women who had cesarean sections or VBACs with this physician or at the hospital and talk with them. If there is a long list of cesarean mothers readily available but few VBACs, it may make you think twice!

Often it is helpful and comforting for both you and your children, if you tour the hospital ahead of time. Include the cesarean facilities. Maternity units should provide a room where siblings can greet the newborn and parents shortly after the birth.

If you know you must have a cesarean, you can arrange to meet with the anesthesiologist ahead of time (although anesthesiologists are not used to dealing with fully conscious human patients). I encourage you to choose a regional anesthesia. This will allow you to be awake to welcome your baby; it is possible in most circumstances. Many women are told that a general anesthetic must be administered, even when there is no medical reason. You should find out which situations warrant general anesthesia. In the rare circumstances that general anesthesia is required, fathers should be permitted to be present. One woman who wrote to C/SEC remarked, "It was a great disappointment having to be knocked out. But when I woke up (still in the operating room), the first thing I saw was my husband holding our baby. Under the circumstances, that gave me the most amount of joy I could have felt." Cesareans have also been performed under hypnosis and with acupuncture.

Preoperative tests and blood work can be done on an outpatient basis the day before a scheduled cesarean in order to avoid spending a lonely night in the hospital.

Fortunately, more and more physicians are encouraging women to go into labor before the cesarean is performed. This helps to insure a full-term infant who is ready to be born. If this option is not available because of "inadequate staffing" or "unavailable operating rooms," you probably belong in another hospital. Most hospitals have plenty of practice in "emergency" cesareans—they deliver approximately 20 percent of their babies that way.

Delivery

During any childbirth experience, there are many choices to be made. You may be faced with the decision about a cesarean during the course of pregnancy, but more often it arises during labor. Your mate, your L.A., and the medical team should be involved with you in the decision-making process. You can certainly ask to be alone with your mate, or with your mate and advocate, to discuss your options. Dr. Murray Enkin[5] reminds us:

> The decision to *do* a cesarean is one which the doctor can make. The decision to *have* a cesarean is one which the parents should make. Parents must be given the information to make an informed decision, including what the operation entails, the indications, the risks, the benefits, the short and long term effects, what effects it may have on the baby and on the parent-child bond, on breast-feeding, and on subsequent pregnancies.

You should know whether your husband/mate will be welcomed at the delivery and in recovery. More and more, doctors and hospitals are responding to the parent's need to share the moments of birth. The NIH Cesarean Task Force[12] states, "Hospitals are encouraged to liberalize their policies concerning the option of having the father or surrogate attend the cesarean birth"(p. 20). Your L.A. should be allowed to accompany you to the O.R. and recovery, not in place of your mate, but in addition to him. She can continue to act as an advocate for both of you and provide you with emotional support during the procedure. She can answer your questions. She can also take pictures of you and your baby and tape-record the birth!

Only a small area on your back (for the regional anesthesia) and a small portion of the lower abdomen near the pubic hairline need to be shaved. It is very uncomfortable and completely unnecessary to be shaved from head to toe and back to front. One woman wrote to C/SEC, "I was shaved from top to bottom, belly and boob."

Most of the women C/SEC counsels refuse preoperative medications, which pass through the placenta to the baby and which often cause additional problems for both mother and baby.

The low transverse incision is the safest and strongest. Discuss with your physician the circumstances under which he would perform a low vertical or classical incision. On the abdomen, it is preferable cosmetically as well to have a low transverse incision.

Right from the preoperative prep to the end of your hospital stay, you have the right to know the available alternatives and to make plans and decisions. When and how you choose to exercise this right is up to you. Preparation during your pregnancy will allow you to be an active and knowledgeable participant, thereby enhancing your birth experience.

Both parents should have the option of viewing the birth, either without a screen or by mirror. If the hospital won't provide a mirror, bring your own. It can be sterilized if necessary! A running commentary about what is happening, what to expect, and when, is helpful and reassuring to both parents and should be provided by the physician or a staff member. The woman's arms need not be strapped down. During the birth or at any other time, the parents—or the mother—can restrict observers. Whenever possible, the baby should be delivered gently and slowly, allowing the cord to drain before it is cut.

Immediately after the birth, the baby should be given to the parents. It is vitally important that the healthy infant delivered by cesarean remain with the parents from birth. The parents and baby should have skin-to-skin contact, touching, stroking, and holding, while the incision is being repaired. (You may wish to arrange for a pediatrician of your choice to be present so as to avoid any unnecessary separation after assessment of the newborn.) Weighting and footprinting and other extraneous busywork can be done later. If the baby is in need of special attention, the father can accompany the baby while the L.A. remains with the mother.

Many cesarean couples refuse to allow silver nitrate to be put into their babies' eyes. You can save your newborn this unnecessary discomfort and interruption of the bonding process. Parents and baby should remain together in the recovery room, where breastfeeding can be initiated.

Postpartum Planning

Complete or modified rooming-in should be an option for all cesarean mothers! The mother should dictate when *she* wants the baby, whether or not this coincides with hospital policy. The first day or two can be difficult if you don't have the help of your mate or a friend or relative. The hospital should have 24-hour visiting privileges for your mate or a helping friend.

Even if you develop a fever, you and your baby should not be separated. You can be quarantined together!

A private room should be made available for you if you so desire. If not, a cesarean roommate would provide understanding company, and there are certainly enough cesarean roommates to go around. An electric bed is a must to facilitate changes in your position as easily and painlessly as possible. A wheelchair should be available if needed. You should be assigned a room near the nursery if you so desire. If your baby is in the special-care nursery, you should be assigned a room as near to your baby as possible.

It will be useful to know the hospital's transfer policy. If your baby requires intensive care at another hospital, are there provisions for you to be transferred as well? Most cesarean women are in no shape to check themselves out on the first day or so after the surgery to follow their babies.

Your older children will need to be with you. They should be given the opportunity to bond with their new sibling. Many hospitals understand the value of family visitation. The baby stays in mom's room so that the siblings meet him in person, rather than just looking at him through a glass wall. Your children need to be reassured of your love and well-being. Even if you are not quite up to par, what they imagine has happened to you when you are away is often far worse! Make certain your hospital is responsive in this area.

Remember that more and more women have the I.V. and catheter removed shortly after the birth. They also begin drinking water, light fruit juices, and broths, and eating yogurt and other nutritious foods within hours after the surgery. (One woman was told that she would be able to resume eating when she had her first bowel movement after surgery. "I kept wondering how I was going to have a bowel movement when I had had nothing to eat for three days," she remarked.)

Remember, too, that although the average length of stay after a cesarean is five to seven days, some women leave the hospital within 48 hours.

Your Newborn

It is important not to lose sight of the newborn and what he or she may need or be feeling. You can help to meet your baby's needs by lots of holding and cuddling and baby massage. Frederick Leboyer, author of *Loving Hands*, and cultural anthropologist Ashley Montagu, author of *Touching*, strongly suggest that babies born by cesarean be massaged soon after birth to release birth tensions and to provide tactile stimulation lost by not traveling through the birth canal. They recommend that this gentle massage should be continued through at least the first three to six months.[7,11]

In addition, the cesarean infant has the rights:

- To be delivered only when his/her lungs are mature and capable of functioning on their own
- To be born without extra or unnecessary medications, which cross the placenta and affect respiration
- To be greeted by both parents at birth
- To be greeted by the father if it is necessary that the mother have general anesthesia
- To receive immediate contact with mother and/or father, to experience feelings of love and security
- To receive the benefits of mother's milk
- To have his/her condition evaluated on an individual basis, without being isolated from parents as a matter of course

- To receive sufficient tactile stimulation the first days following birth, especially if birth was not preceded by labor
- To receive close, continued contact with parents during the hospital stay
- To meet siblings *soon* after birth*

The ideas, opinions, and suggestions presented here are given as food for thought in preparing for a cesarean delivery. Take great care in making each of your choices. Again, don't hesitate to seek a second (or third) opinion, or to change doctors and/or hospitals, if you have any doubts about the quality of care and sensitivity accorded you, or if the management policies are unacceptable to you. And make arrangements to have as much help as possible when you get home, so your energies can be directed to mothering and recovering.

For nine years I have been working with cesarean mothers, to guide them to VBAC or to help them make a necessary cesarean as positive and fulfilling as possible. My hope is to see the options of family-centered cesarean care exist everywhere for those who must birth surgically. However, my dream is to see the cesarean rate drop dramatically, since most cesareans performed in this country could be avoided.

---

*Adapted from an article by Linda Worzer, *C/SEC News*, Winter 1979.

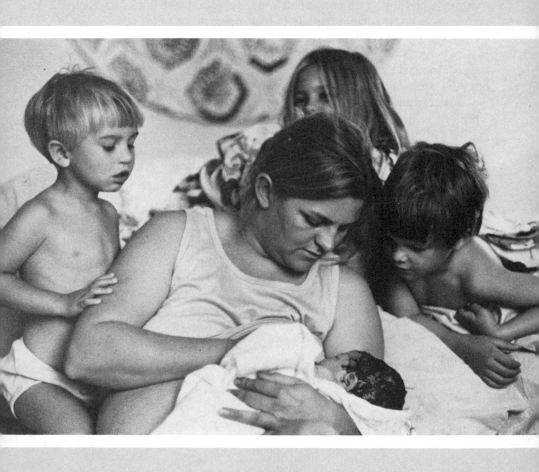

15 ❧ Voices of VBAC

The promise, the prophecy is within me.
That which I have waited for is now present;
No longer need I fear.
Within me shines
The first glimmering of the light,
And I am filled with the awareness
That the fulfilling of the prophecy
Is not a thing apart from me:
It is me.

—D. Parry

The letters that we shared with you earlier described the feelings of anger, disappointment, sadness, and depression that often follow a cesarean. Now we would like to share some of the exultation, joy, and love that come with the achievement of vaginal birth after cesarean.

The women who wrote of their VBACs in the letters presented in this chapter had been previously sectioned for many reasons. Some had been diagnosed as CPD, some had breech babies, others had long labors with many interventions and were accused of failure to progress. Some had had more than one cesarean, and some had had classical incisions. None of these things mattered at the moment that each gave birth, normally, to her very own VBAC baby. These letters permit us to relive those moments with VBAC mothers.

---

*From *Essence Book of Days for 1982*. Reprinted with the author's permission.

LETTERS FROM VBAC MOTHERS

The birth was what we wanted *though we had never dreamed it would all come off so well and with such positive feelings all around. The influence of the music on me and particularly the others around was special. It made so much difference to me and seemed to relax everyone around it. I found that relying on my own instincts was really the best way to go through the whole thing. Though loose-mouthed deep breathing helped, eventually I found I needed to make noise and did. I also found I got through the contractions well by smiling and thinking about that special baby that I'd be holding soon.*

—*Patsy* (Massachusetts)

The birth was all we had ever hoped it could be! We were both exhilarated by the birth and labor. The labor progressed well and I felt well supported by John and my L.A. I was terribly excited that labor had finally begun. I was also anxious initially, hoping I would be able to handle the stages of labor. It was strange though; once labor began I never doubted my ability to follow it through. The pushing stage was prolonged.

. . . It was very quiet and peaceful in each room. I was moved from labor to delivery and had to change tables. This was really the only aspect of the labor and birth not to my liking. I was aware before the labor that this would be done. The doctor had felt these moves would be necessary. . .

Since Aron was born an incredible feeling of accomplishment remains with me. The memories are priceless.

. . . During the labor I felt very much in tune with my body; to the point of withdrawal from those around me. I never talked through the labor and only asked if I was "getting anywhere" during the pushing stage. It was interesting to note, because I didn't speak neither did those around me. . . .

—*Judy* (Massachusetts)

Our first child was born by cesarean because my "pelvis was too small" and he weighed 8 lbs. 5½ oz. Our second child was born vaginally and he weighed 9 lbs. 2 oz. I had an easy birth but had a hard time convincing any doctor to allow me to try. In fact, no one in my area would agree so I simply stayed home until I was sure the baby would be born soon and Tommy was born about an hour after I arrived at the hospital. Most of the hour I spent listening to a doctor tell me I was attempting something dangerous and he would not be responsible if anything went wrong. Mostly it was a wonderful experience.

—*Dena* (Maine)

Our first baby was born by cesarean because of malposition and CPD. Our second birth experience: My daughter was born at 10:04 A.M. on July 18, 1980, vaginally. She was 8 lb. 8 oz., 21½", and a head circum. of 14½" (also after 2 hrs. of pushing). My original doctor had told me he would allow an attempted vaginal delivery; however, I was not completely satisfied with his enthusiasm. I chose to locate another doctor who had been wanting to further investigate the viability of VBAC. Together we researched it. Since my birth he has made this an integral part of his prenatal alternatives. He has been surprised at how few women wish to attempt it.—Anyhow, back to my birth. Labor began at 3:00 A.M. with a contraction which woke me from a sound sleep. I tried returning to sleep but found myself in the middle of another contraction 5 min. later. I was not having to use my Lamaze techniques for them but decided if I couldn't sleep I might as well time them. Mike and I left for the hospital just about 6:00 A.M. We arrived in Maternity at almost 6:30 A.M. I was checked by the nurse for progress and readied for the birth (blood work was done at this time "in case"). The results of my internal exam were 5 cm, 100% effaced and baby at least -5 in station. My doctor and I were concerned enough about the lack of engagement that a pelvimetry was done two days before to see if there was true CPD. At 7:00 A.M. I was between 5–6 cm so my doctor chose to rupture my membranes and insert an internal monitor. I was given the OK to push at 7:45 P.M. An hour and half later I was in the birthing chair watching our baby crown. Within another half hour she slid from me and was resting on my abdomen.

—Julie (California)

Anson was born half an hour after we got to the hospital. Hooray, Hooray! Dr. K. was totally non-interfering, kind, and caring. Our other son was present and both my husband and midwife stayed with me. I left the hospital two hours later. I didn't even check into the hospital. We all wonder if the struggle for a VBAC is worth it—well, it sure is!!!

—Cindy (New York)

My doctor told me that the next time I had a baby I'd "come in like a lady" (and have a repeat cesarean). Of course I switched doctors. I came in like a lady, all right—yelling and having a baby. The VBAC was wonderful.

—Sheryl (Massachusetts)

My only disappointment was my husband. He was so fascinated with it, he *could have been a male nurse watching his first birth. I had pictured us being very close and excited. When we discussed it later, he said he was very proud of me but he can't show emotions. Other than that, I'll take a VBAC over a cesarean any day. The difference in recovery time was incredible.*

—Betty (Massachusetts)

I am a registered nurse and I teach Lamaze. I have a low vertical incision. My first baby was born by c/section, deformed, and died almost immediately. My second baby was 9 lbs. 9 oz. girl, vaginally, no spinal, no forceps but a definite episiotomy. For myself, I can say that the ability to give birth to a healthy baby vaginally has given me a new sense of self-esteem, a new self-image, and a much closer bond between my husband and myself as well as between the baby and us. I have a great pride in my ability as a woman to utilize the body that God gave me and bear a child. I think much of these feelings are missing with a cesarean, no matter how lovely the cesarean experience is.

—Janice (Michigan)

"When is this nonsense going to end?" is what I kept saying to myself because for two weeks prior to the delivery I'd have contractions two minutes apart. One morning, I woke up with them one minute apart and I dilated to 2 cms. We thought I might be carrying twins so to be in labor early wasn't a surprise, but nothing ever happened. Anyway, here we are two weeks later and the "real thing" is upon us and I'm not so sure that what I've been so anxious to experience is as pleasant as I anticipated!

Thursday, Nov. 5, 1981. I had strong Braxton-Hicks type contractions all day. At 10 P.M. the contractions got strong enough to keep me awake and I started breathing thru them. Everyone was in bed but me. I was uncomfortable sitting so I walked around the house over and over until 2 A.M. and finally crashed on the couch on my side for 1½ hours and woke with another contraction. Richard, my husband, finally got up and hung out with me for an hour and we went back to bed at 5 A.M. and woke at 7:30 to the sound of the sweet voice of our three-year-old daughter, Carmen.

A bit disappointed to still be pregnant, I got up to begin my usual routine. Again around 9 A.M. the contractions started again three min. apart so I ate breakfast and went out for a walk. I had to stop walking during a contraction and sometimes bend over so pretended to be looking at something on the sidewalk so as not to alarm the neighbors!

My midwife arrived later that afternoon to tell me I was only three cms. I was discouraged so prepared myself for my labor to take a while longer than I imagined. The afternoon faded into evening and my contractions grew stronger and closer together. I was only comfortable on my knees on the couch during a contraction. We had a chiropractor come over to adjust my right hip because it felt out of place and I thought it would help progress. He adjusted my back, neck, hips and did some acupuncture and reflexology. When he was done I had dilated one more cm. I had pizza and salad for dinner, as I never lost my appetite! At 9 P.M. I decided to take a hot bath, and, while I was soaking, three midwives left and my main midwife went to sleep, leaving only my husband, his mother, and a friend up with me. At 11 P.M. we decided to wake my midwife to check dilation. She said, "Still 4 cms," which was no change for four hours!! I cried. I couldn't understand why such strong contractions weren't dilating my cervix! At midnite they tried to get me drunk so I could rest but it didn't work.

I walked, I squatted, I did pelvic rocks, I prayed, I drank herb teas, held combs, swore, cried, took tinctures—nothing helped.. Until 2 A.M. Sat., Nov. 7, we decided I was getting exhausted and Richard was getting worried that we should go to the hospital. That was the only time I got scared—when they were talking about taking me to the hospital! I said, "We still have one alternative! Break the water bag and see what happens!" So at 2 A.M., at 5 cms., we broke my water and ZAP—transition, here we come!

The contractions became incredibly strong. After each contraction I would think, "It can't get any stronger than that one!" But the next one would be even stronger! I wasn't quiet or laid back thru any of this process. I'm a nurse and have seen quite a few births and I kept wondering how anyone could lie still and keep their mouths shut thru a contraction! The next thing I knew, I was pushing. Someone got the birthing stool and here we go! Pushing was even more uncomfortable as I had hemorrhoids and they hurt like hell while I was pushing. Carmen got up just in time to see the last four pushes. Out popped the sweetest 7 lb. 14 oz. girl you ever saw. It took an hour to birth the 2 lb. placenta.

I was fortunate to have a group of people with enough confidence in me and the birth process to support us even after our previous cesarean experience. No M.D. in this area would help me.

—Dee (Colorado . . . Homebirth)

Three years ago, six months after my c/section, I took my records and x-rays to several doctors to obtain other opinions as to the necessity of my section. Several doctors thought I was a fanatic, some even recommended that I see a psychiatrist with my problem. Even my friends, husband, and mother initially thought I just couldn't accept the failing of my body and when I became pregnant they were fearful I would be risking my life and that of my unborn child if I pursued a VBAC. But I began receiving support from them. They even began cutting out articles on unnecessary cesareans.

My labor was 15½ hours . . . I ate during the labor—soup, toast, and applesauce . . . . When I pushed my baby's head out my first words were, "My baby!! I did it!"

*The birth has not only been a beautiful experience for myself and my husband,
but has confirmed the normalcy of my body, repaired my self-image, and detracted
from the negative memories surrounding my daughter's birth. My experience has
also been an incentive to a friend who is now planning a VBAC.*

—Fran (Connecticut)

*We have two daughters, both born by cesarean section [and now a VBAC son].
The first cesarean was supposedly due to cephalopelvic disproportion, complicated
by the baby presenting breech. The second section 13 months later was a repeat
elective cesarean. I was told I had a deformed pelvis and that my uterus would
rupture if I attempted a trial of labour. The following was written after my VBAC
labor:*

I feel good. Healthy, strong, full of love. Normal I birthed my own baby.

*They said I couldn't. They said, you're deformed, your babies will die, you can
get them in there, but we will have to cut them out for you. Why aren't you grateful:
we saved your life and your babies' lives, too. What kind of a person are you! Did
you have rickets, the obstetrician said, grinning. A five pounder couldn't maneuver
those bones. Can't you just accept that, you got your healthy babies, isn't that
enough?*

*NO. Not again. Three cesareans in three years? More morphine, Demerol, Syn-
tocinon, incisions, stitches, gas pains, catheters, nausea, infections, no energy?
Alan outside the O.R., congrats, we cut another healthy baby out of her?*

*Step no. one: another G.P. Then a look at the so-called facts. Two previous
cesareans due to an almost completely contracted pelvis. Two baby girls weighing
a whole 1½ pounds more than the magical five-pound limit. It looks hopeless.*

A little voice gaining strength: get another opinion.

*Our doctor agrees. We contact some midwives. Meanwhile, we negotiate for a
father-present cesarean that neither of us wants.*

*And then I sit in Dr. K.'s office, scared. I tell him I want a vaginal delivery,
a healthy baby. We look at the x-rays from Sarah. He agrees to a trial of labor.
I am stunned. Me, normal, you mean to tell me I might be able to do it? Maybe.*

*We turn our world upside down, borrow money, enlist the help of grandparents.
And read, exercise, relax, visualize, think positive, push away negative thoughts.
I hate every person who dares to mention cesareans.*

*July . . . we're in Vancouver. The waiting gets me down. Sarah was ten days
early, what's the matter with this kid? Five days before the due date we have thirteen
hours of labour. Everyone's dragged out of bed, a baby. Then, when we can't reach
the midwife, the contractions stop. Nothing. I want to cry, scream, sleep. I'll never
have this baby.*

*Due date comes. And goes. Our midwife is back in town. She says, anytime
now. Dr. K. says, any time now. Oh, sure, tell me another one.*

*Two days overdue. I have all the signs of labour, but am too depressed to
acknowledge them. Early evening, I casually ask Alan to time some contractions.*

*Sure, he says, and makes himself a nauseating chicken sandwich. I am mortified
and insulted. We start yelling at each other. Chicken vs contractions. This is
ridiculous. Let's phone somebody.*

*Just before ten, POP! Alan, quick, my water's broken, get me a towel, we have
to save Thomas's oatmeal sofa. Oh, dear God, I am not ready for this.*

*Margie comes and we drive to the midwife's house. Contractions are strong, two
minutes apart, I breathe. It hurts anyway.*

*The labour is unbelievable. Our midwife checks me. Rubs my belly, your body's
doing beautifully. She grins, we're having a baby!*

*I connect with someone for each contraction, grabbing whoever's closest. I need
everybody. I can feel the cervix stretching, the head heavy and powerful. I surrender,
think open. The power drags me thru contraction after contraction.*

*I am impatient and bitchy, but I don't care. I demand to know exactly how long
is this going to take.*

*3:30 A.M. I want to go the the hospital NOW. The van ride almost kills me.
Our midwife can't come up, she has her baby with her. She holds my face and tells
me I can do it.*

*Birthing suite, it's 4:00 A.M. Dr. F. comes in. He can't be serious, I'm only
four cm. We'll be here forever.*

*I squat on the toilet, I stand in the shower, I walk, sit, hang on Alan's shoulders.
I feel all wild inside. Baby rotates, I get onto my hands and knees. A cesarean
starts to look pretty good. My L.A. reads my mind. You're doing it. Yes, say yes,
I can do it, open up. Alan holds me, you can do it. The sun's come up.*

*It's 6:20 A.M. Someone's talking to me, Marianne, you have ten minutes to
pull yourself together. I want you up walking, talking when the doctor comes.
Okay, I say, and I feel better.*

I feel bossy, I'll show that doctor.

*6:35 A.M. Dr. F.'s in the doorway, rubbing his eyes like a sleepy bear. I grin
from my chair and take my time getting on the bed. He examines me carefully and
looks up, smiling: Everything's just fine. (That's nice.) If you feel any urge to
push . . . . (WHAT??? the whole room cheers.)*

*So I breathe and push—it's like being on a rollercoaster—and roar primevally;
the head's coming down, I can feel it, it's HUGE. I yell, "Out, baby!" It burns,
I feel myself tear.*

*Look, LOOK, Marianne, the head's out, another contraction and oh, what a
blessed relief as he (it's a BOY) slithers out like a greased seal. Only half an hour
to push him out. Oh, oh, he's perfect, Alan, it's a BOY.*

*I hear myself yelling, "I'm normal!" I love everyone in the room. I am holding
my baby, all gooey and warm and blue and pink. Margie comes in and we all
toast with semi-chilled champagne in styrofoam cups.*

*"I'm so grateful," Alan cries. I look around at everyone, I never want to let them
go. We did it together, what a team. Thank you, all of you.*

—Marianne (British Columbia)

. . . Max's birth will remain a peak experience in our lives. For me, it was the

culmination of twelve years of wondering about childbirth. I am hoping that my ability to overcome obstacles to a good birth will spread to other areas of my life and to other people . . .

—Katie (Massachusetts . . . Breech VBAC after two cesareans)

I pushed for six hours and finally, there he was, all 9+ pounds of him. It was incredible! Now that we have had a vaginal delivery, I feel much more strongly that cesareans are a brutal abuse of women in any case where one is not absolutely necessary. How shocking it is, that we have allowed such a practice to become so commonplace.

—Joanne (Connecticut . . . Classical incision)

I felt I had very good emotional and physical preparation. However, I still was amazed at the sheer amount of work that my body was doing. From early labor thru active labor and especially the pushing stage, it seemed like raw guts and stamina was what was required to continue!

I felt like sometimes I would miss the wave of an active labor contraction, then I would have to work it like crazy to get with it again.

. . . Sometimes I miss the beginning of a contraction and can't seem to ride the wave as long as I want to. At other times I can really feel the baby moving down inside me! It's wonderful! A little voice inside me is saying you're actually doing this—no medication! I can begin to feel a real burning sensation. . . . All of a sudden he pops out all at once all bloody, covered with vernix and beautiful! I first just stared, then I held him tightly. Phil cut the cord, no episiotomy, just a couple little tears. . . . Then push out the placenta all purple and full of blood. Everything is wonderful. I was in seventh heaven. My body was my own! I could move and be with my son and husband! Phil had tears in his eyes—we held one another— it was simply beautiful!

—Susan (Massachusetts)

I feel like I actually "missed" the birth in a way. I was so caught up in the painful sensations in my back that I didn't even want to watch the crowning and birth, although Jeff encouraged me to. I felt totally unaware of the purpose of it all. The baby wasn't a reality to me at all. It was all so different from what I'd anticipated. I guess because the heartbeat had fallen to 100 the doctor was anxious to have her be born. He encouraged me to push and put his fingers where he wanted me to direct the energy but I found it very difficult and felt like I wasn't performing very well. I had expected to be able to get myself together during second stage but it wasn't possible and so I'm disappointed that the baby was born before I could appreciate what was happening. It just wasn't the ecstatic, all-transcending experience I had looked forward to.

. . . Objectively there are so many good and positive aspects of the birth that I'm ashamed of my negative feelings. We have a sweet and beautiful new little girl to love. She is physically perfect although I had feared all sorts of deformities throughout my pregnancy. We had a vaginal delivery! That alone should satisfy me, it seems. I'm recovering quickly. Even the episiotomy doesn't seem very bothersome . . . . The hospital experience was by most standards fantastic. We gave birth in the birthing room and then stayed there four more hours enjoying the aftermath . . . . We had hoped that Aurora (our daughter) would attend the birth but the speed with which it all occurred as well as the hour made it impossible. . . . This brings me to my biggest problem with the experience. I just read an article and it perpetuates the idea that 2nd stage can be full of relaxation and a peaceful calm. Although I had anticipated at least a coherent 2nd stage, I experienced the very antithesis of what I had grown to expect through reading Kitzinger, Baldwin, Spiritual Midwifery, and Davis. I was insane—insane with the pain in my back, insane with the fear that I was dying, insane with the fear that the baby was dying, insane with the fear that I wasn't pushing right—it was horrible . . . . I feel so sad at the way this birth went. It was just so fast—1½ hours in all . . .

—Gretchen (New York)

I once ran the Boston Marathon. This was worse. Determination proved crucial, for my labor was long and difficult. I needed every ounce of will power to complete it. It was to last 27 hours, and by the 25th the doctor was posing grim alternatives. I decided I'd made a mistake. I should have had a cesarean right away. I not only wanted a cesarean, but I wanted general anesthesia as well. I wanted out—all the way.

And then a miracle. I felt the urge to push. But the pushing made the contractions seem mild by comparison . . . . and then I saw the birth begin. The head was a small darkness which, when I looked again, a few minutes later, had become a large ball with hair. "My God! There really is a baby inside of me," I thought. "It is not just pain." I felt a terrible burning sensation, but I knew I was making progress.

And then he was out. A whole body. A boy! Lying on the bed, between my legs. My husband and I looked at one another, awed. This was a phenomenon that surpassed anything we have ever witnessed or experienced. It was astounding. My child was born.

I nursed my son; the umbilical cord was cut, and he and I rested together for the next two hours. The exhaustion I felt during labor vanished. I was too excited to sleep that night. I had delivered a healthy eight pound, four ounce baby and the elation of his arrival lasted throughout my three-day hospital stay. (After the cesarean, I stayed eight.) Recovery from the delivery never felt like a recuperation. . .

At this moment, millions of women throughout the world are going through labor. It is an act of complete courage. That women get so little credit for it amazes me.

Both my daughter and son are beautiful. Each is a testimony to the wonder of creation. But the experience of giving birth is a life process so deep and so fundamental that to question the need or the wisdom of it, is to question the need for sleep, the need to eat, and the need to reproduce. I have done it and I feel whole.

—Wendy (Massachusetts)

I stayed at 7 cm. for three hours. My doctor broke the water and waited ½ hour. Not much progress so he decided to do a repeat cesarean. Anesthesiologist decided on a general. Had me prepped in the operation room. I had a contraction as I was moved to the table. The doctor checked me and I was fully dilated. I began pushing and delivered forty-five minutes later.

—Linda (Massachusetts)

As my first labor had been very long and erratic, I decided not to get too excited about this one, just to watch it come and go. Tried to rest, but couldn't, so I took a long walk to the lake, watched the sun coming up over the waters, the rippling of the spring, the fish and turtles, the chipmunks and squirrels, the fullness of the season, and felt at peace and unity with all creation.

Labor proceeded on and off throughout the afternoon, and I was able to doze a bit. My neighbor came by with some food and loving reassurance, and when the midwife came over in late afternoon I was 4 cm. dilated and almost fully effaced. I really enjoyed getting into my own inner space, my own rhythm and pattern of breathing, and getting very into Mary and Jesus and my teacher, Hazrat Inayat Khan. The light of their beings was a divine blessing. Took time as I could to give my little boy some loving energy (and occasionally yell at him) and appreciate my wonderful and supportive husband.

I think we all really knew I wasn't going to the hospital and in my heart had never really planned to, because by midnight the contractions were all-encompassing and we weren't going anywhere but onward.

. . . From that point on it just went fast and smooth, and at 1:45 Tara was born. A very ecstatic birth, the room and house full of heavenly beings. . . . As the sun came up our assistants drove away, leaving Aric and me still in bed with our new little girl . . .

P.S. Tara was ¾ lb. more than my first child, Gabriel, and the physician who did the c/sec for him said never even to attempt any but cesarean births because I was so small!

—Noor-Un-Nisa (New York . . . Homebirth)

Labor proceeded rapidly at home—from 2 A.M. to 6:30 A.M. I was at 8 centimeters—when we got to the hospital things slowed down—contractions got further apart—stayed strong but progress slowed—after about 1½-2 hours I decided to relax and not let the hospital "get to me"—in one more hour I was fully dilated and pushing. An excellent Bradley course and plenty of reading enabled me to consciously overcome the negative hospital vibrations and get on with my work. The birth went well and we were pleased with our care—and especially being able to come right home. We delivered in a labor bed in a birthing room—the baby never left us. We recovered in the same room and went home after 5 hours. Friends and neighbors and family are astounded (1) that a VBAC is even possible and (2) that we left the hospital immediately. My older son was spared any long-term separation and recuperating at home is wonderful.

Next time we plan a homebirth.

—Susan (New Jersey)

The coaching of staff nurse and Cameron really got me through the pain of pushing so long and hard. My bottom really hurt. It was all worth it when I saw my little boy! My husband has been on a cloud and he says that no man should deprive himself of the birth of his child. He was totally amazed even after knowing what was going to happen. Being there is really believing it!

—Bonnie (Connecticut)

It was harder than I expected. A cesarean birth in my opinion is easier! However, it was much more rewarding for me, and I would never opt for another cesarean. I had no I.V. or fetal monitor; and it was a beautiful, intimate, spiritual experience. I couldn't have asked for more.

—Cathy (New Jersey)

The birth was much better than we both expected! We did not have to "fight for our rights" as the hospital staff was very sensitive to our needs. Thanks to VBAC classes, we were well prepared. There were no complications. I took a shower about 1½ hours after the birth, and was so amazed at how good I did feel! The head nurse was especially supportive. She was all for our idea of leaving the hospital whenever we felt was right, and tried to get everything in order for us as soon as she could. The baby was never admitted to the nursery. He never left our sight. It was all such a great experience. Thank you again for helping make this possible for us. People still don't believe it can be done and no one can get over the fact that we were home all in the same day. But we're telling everyone we can in the hopes that we can let someone know who can benefit from it as we did.

—Marcy (Massachusetts)

The birth was everything that I had wanted it to be. I wanted to be relaxed and I was. I wanted to labor at home and I did. I feel one big beautiful experience in my life that my husband and I will never forget.

. . . There were no complications. I think the reason is because I had no interventions. I was able to walk and do what felt better to me. My mind was clear and I was not uptight. I never thought about my two previous sections. I relaxed when my contractions began. I was loose. Whenever a contraction came on I remembered to loosen up and relax.

Our birth of our 3rd son was beautiful. Everything went just as I expected it to.

—Debbie (Massachusetts)

First, how do I feel? Fantastic, great. I'd commute half way across the country for a vaginal delivery again. I feel a sense of accomplishment, joy, happiness that is difficult to describe. I went into Cate's birth with a lot of feelings that I would have difficulty coping with the pain. I'd been brought up to see myself as a coward. And I'd had memories of situations where there were powerful feelings and I was not in control of the situation. So I had tried to minimize the idea that there would be pain. However, the discomfort that I felt was not at all as I had imagined it would be. I would rather not have had to have an episiotomy; but I'd choose it any day if it was the price to avoid a cesarean.

. . . I wasn't prepared for the fame. Nurses on the postpatum floor were asking about me—how I was doing—before I went down to them. I asked my nurse how they even knew about me. Her reply, "Oh, everyone in this hospital knows about you." Another mother came up to me about three days after Cate was born asking how we'd decided to try for a vaginal delivery, how we'd gathered information, etc. I overheard a couple speak of me as they passed my room the first day or two. I was still having trouble voiding Tuesday. My nurse asked if I'd had the same problem with Seth. When I told her that he'd been a cesarean, she said, "Oh, you're the one . . ." I got the impression that everyone thought that I was terribly brave or gutsy or something; I really don't know why. I didn't do anything that they hadn't done.

. . . I could go on forever. But there is one last point. Jeff and I both feel that having two L.A.s with us made the difference. I'm not sure we'd have made it without them.

—Carol (Massachusetts)

Expectations—wonderful to start pushing and feel her crowning. Hard work, but pushing seemed effortless compared to contractions . . . Special care nurse—excellent choice—was able to work closely with us. She made a personal visit to our home—met us at door of hospital. My husband talked to resident, labor coach, anthesiology, doctor, and all insisted on a saddleblock because of uterine examination to take place after birth.

I hadn't thought that far and let him ask all questions. We were told exam was necessary and painful. Wonder why the saddleblock couldn't be administered after birth?

—*Francine* (Rhode Island)

I felt very well prepared—(and never worried re: my uterus rupturing!). The birth was as I expected—tho the in vivo experience was more painful than anything I could imagine. But the joy of not undergoing another cesarean cannot be descibed. And when all was said and done, I had (and still have) such a feeling of pride that my body worked as it was meant to, that I had the perserverance to pursue, and that my beautiful baby had no medication in her.

—*Berta* (Massachusetts)

At one point I wasn't making too much progress in dilating and the doctor mentioned I would have to progress in a couple of hours or a cesarean might be called for. He said it didn't have to be a lot of progress, but some would be necessary. He said all this in a very low-key manner; it really wasn't threatening (although I was a little concerned). So I tried different positions to encourage dilation and after a short time on my knees with head and arms resting on pillows on the raised bed, I made rapid progress from 7 to 10 cm. . . .

After two previous cesareans, it was wonderful going home several hours after giving birth and being able to fully care for my baby!

—*Martha* (Connecticut . . . VBAC after two cesareans)

. . . the doctor was getting discouraged and starting to wonder whether the baby was going to make it out that way. Our midwife said, "A baby's head just doesn't come that far and not get out!" and she suggested that he leave the room for a few minutes. She held the cervix back, the head turned on its own, and when the doctor returned the head was crowning. I hate to think what might have happened had she, and he, acted on his discouragement. . . .

We are very happy with the way the birth happened. I'm glad that we were home for most of the labor. The few hours in the hospital didn't detract too much. Nobody bothered us about interventions beyond an I.V., and everybody was very good to us. The birth was natural and beautiful. It took actually pushing this baby out, for me to really understand that my body could do that. Although we were prepared and determined, it was a very exciting surprise! I started laughing when her shoulders were out, and didn't stop for two days!

. . . The only trouble was about the silver nitrate. We were told that we couldn't take our baby home until we authorized the eye treatment, so we simply left through the nearest exist when we were left alone.

—Michelle (Massachusetts)

. . . I was very pleased with the delivery phase—I delivered in bed, was able to take my time, everyone was calm, patient and very interested, lights were dim, no one wore masks and I was encouraged to watch my baby being born, to feel her emerge. My husband was the first to speak to our baby before she was fully born. He cut the cord (and I nursed before the cord was cut). She was not washed and I held her for more than an hour before she was wiped off and diapered.

—Jeanne (Massachusetts . . . Classical incision)

I did not expect a ten-day (mostly "on") labor. I don't think anyone or anything could have prepared us for that. But our 10 lb. 6¾ oz. just needed to take her time.

After the birth the nurses tried to hold on to me. They wouldn't call the pediatrician—it was a holiday—besides, "you've been through so much, why don't you stay until tomorrow." "The baby is so big, Doctor will want her to stay anyway." My 4-hour discharge became 12 and then only because I got dressed and said, "I'm leaving!"

. . . All in all—it was a good experience. I did not see the birth—was flat; but we had a beautiful girl. The children didn't suffer any deprivation. We really birthed the baby together. It was beautiful to get home—the love my other children have is beautiful.

—Chris (Massachusetts . . . VBAC after two cesareans)

I feel totally positive about this birth. I had to have an external monitor and heparin lock, at the insistence of our ob. He was head of the department at the hospital and wanted to set protocol for future VBACs.

—Elizabeth (New York)

I feel very happy I was able to do it—complete it—and not be separated from my loved ones. I'm convinced that if I'd been in the hospital—they would never have let me push for five hours and would have sectioned me.

—Myla (Massachusetts . . . Homebirth)

Much more painful than I expected. Couldn't stand the pain. I wanted to get it over with, wanted medication and/or epidural—politely refused by coach and husband! I could have fought them by saying, "Look, this is my body!" but I didn't because I knew I'd be sorry later. Even had secret desire for c/sec.

. . . One nice thing the L.A. suggested was touching baby's head as I was crowning. I never really had sensation of baby moving down birth canal—only of discomfort of contractions. So when I felt the head, it brought a form of reality to me and I started to relate, "Come on, baby, move out . . ."

—Marion (Massachusetts)

The birth was much longer than I expected. My water broke 40 hours before delivery. My contractions progressed very slowly. I partially attribute this to some hidden apprehension about if I could really make it. The end result was super! When the baby finally entered the world, that slippery body was marvelous. It was indeed worth all the effort, and the joy of a vaginal delivery is irreplacable.

—Elaine (Massachusetts)

I was thrilled and exhaused when Jackie was born. The bonding between us all is so much greater than with our c/section baby. I never gave a thought to my incision, and thank goodness our doctor was not overly concerned either.

—Ginni (Massachusetts . . . Classical incision)

The birth was more than I had expected in some ways. Being at home during labor was unexpected, but pretty terrific.

. . . Feel pretty wonderful about seeing our daughter born. Held her on my abdomen until cord stopped pulsating; watched her color change from purple blue to more of a pink, and we bonded. One of the most amazing things was seeing her whole head outside of me, but the rest of her body inside.

—Joan (Maine)

We're sure the fact we were home enabled us to have our VBAC. If I was in the hospital when I got stuck at 8 cm., I would have been labeled a failure to progress again and pressured into another cesarean. . . . We called the doctor to cancel our appointment since we'd already had the baby! He was happy for us! We thank God for giving us our dream of a birth at home and for providing us with some of His infinite birthing knowledge.

—Kathy (New York . . . Homebirth)

I am very, very high—this is the most exciting, exhilarating thing I have ever done. The final stages of the labor were much faster and more intense than I expected, given my leisurely beginnings. It was very hard to leave my bedroom, panting through the urge to push, to go to the hospital, but once we arrived and established a rhythm again I was quite comfortable there. I just knew we'd succeed.

—Judith (Massachusetts)

As with the two previous labors, I could not deal with the pain from 4 cm. on. But the difference with this birth is that for some reason (good physical shape, good diet, knowledge, mental preparation, no intervention), the labor did make progress. And even though I "gave up" and begged for relief, my supporters (husband, labor coach, doctor, nurse) continued to provide positive support and would not let me give up. And I treated all of them so badly while I was in pain. I will be forever indebted to them for their persistance. In a way, by selecting these people and letting them know beforehand what I wanted and needed in labor to help me achieve a vaginal delivery, I suppose I set myself up to win even though I wanted to quit when the going got rough. The pushing stage was not as exciting as I imagined, but at least it was fast. When I finally squeezed the baby out, I could not believe my eyes. Only the umbilical cord which connected me to him assured me that he belonged to me. When the baby was born—my personality changed abruptly from total insanity to total peace! The pain was all gone! My recovery was perfectly wonderful. . . . I felt overwhelmingly happy and totally at peace. It was certainly hard work, but worth it. Finally, I must credit Michael with understanding my desires so well that he wouldn't let me give up, even though it was very difficult for him to "torture" (his words) me so. Baby Nathan is so happy, peaceful, and alert, and his brothers are enjoying him immensely (not to mention his proud parents).

—Janet (Massachusetts . . . VBAC after two cesareans)

. . . Finally we moved back to the bed and that was probably the hardest part,

the final descent of his head. I remember thinking it was too much . . . I even verbalized before he was born, out loud: "Whose idea was this, anyway?" Everyone but me got a chuckle. And I found that the last several pushes were very painful as they tried to manipulate the vaginal opening around his head. They showed me the head in a mirror. I was not impressed at this point. They all kept remarking during the crowning, "Look at the size of this head!"

His head was born as well as his body, and he was immediately put on my belly all creamy and smelling just wonderful. I was relieved and everyone was really happy. . . . Our friends came in. Everyone just milled around, we had a little champagne and a toast to the new baby. After the cord stopped pulsing, the doctor called Tom back in the room and handed him a pair of scissors and told him where to cut the cord. Tom didn't expect that, was a little taken aback but I think was pleased.

—*Donna* (Massachusetts)

Hospital policy didn't allow my L.A. to stay with me.

My doctor was busy "politicking"—trying to calm down nurses, anesthesiologist, etc.—he couldn't be a labor coach (if he had known how)—I had no real support to cope with negative thoughts. Pushing was very painful and I found I had doubts about my ability to "get the baby out."

Positive aspects—We had a VBAC! My husband (a very reserved person) said it was worth all the effort! Several days later he said now he feels we could do a homebirth "next time"! (Before, he didn't want a "next time"!) I feel the same way—I'd like to do it again, our way.

—*Colleen* (New York)

We did it! At the stroke of midnight Noah made his entrance. What an incredible experience—the long climb up the mountain is sure worth it! What a team David and I were. In 1½ hours in a nice hot tub I dilated from 5 cm. to 9 cm. and started to get pushing urges. . . . I got out of the tub, made myself beautiful, and moved into our set-up birthing room. I pushed for 45 minutes and that's it. That seemed so short to me . . . . we used affirmations . . . Noah was born while I was squatting on the floor massaging his head and perineal area with warm olive oil. He came out pink, wide-eyed and gorgeous. . . . I was quiet in early labor, but my heavens, the strength I seemed to derive from loud sounds during pushing! Visualization was very effective, too. It was a terrific experience.

—*Nan* (Ohio . . . Homebirth)

We have had a lot of people question us as to whether we had planned a homebirth

*or not. It was not exactly planned, although I might have been subconsciously
planning it. We refer to it as being allowed to happen. A lot of people have told
me how lucky I was that nothing went wrong. I don't feel it was just luck.*

—*Paula* (Rhode Island . . . Homebirth after four cesareans)

*It took us three years to build up the courage to try for another baby, naturally
assuming that another c/section was necessary, which neither of us wanted to face.
Fortunately, . . . I met VBAC women through my La Leche League group. They
put me in touch with a completely sympathetic doctor. My preparation was mainly
psychological—I made up my mind that I could do it—and I wouldn't listen to
the skeptics (all those raised eyebrows inquiring, "Aren't you endangering the life
of your unborn baby?"—statements that can only be attributed to a lack of knowledge, so I'd consider the source and ignore the comments). Every time I would get
doubtful or worried I'd talk to one of the two women living in my town or to my
doctor. They were always reassuring and understanding.*

*One week before my due date my water broke, but this time I was given the
chance to go into labor. My labor was erratic, but my doctor told me about a
woman who went five days after her water broke before delivering—he even offered
to put me on antibiotics if I went beyond 24–48 hours—so I was encouraged. I lay
down as little as possible during labor. I sat in a rocking chair or walked down the
halls of the maternity ward. After sixteen hours, my labor began in earnest, and
three hours later I was on the delivery table and pushing and watching my husband
assist in the delivery of our baby boy. I'll never forget my elation at being able to
experience this, just to see my husband's face so full of complete wonder and joy,
and to hold my son immediately after birth. He was totally alert, calm, and his
eyes never left my face. The whole experience was wonderful for us all, and to think
we could have missed out on this all!!! Of course, afterward, many people were
amazed at our success and even congratulated us on our "courage" (if they only
knew how much more frightened we were about the prospect of another cesarean).
How proud and fortunate we are to be part of the VBAC revolution. You
see . . . it can and is being done!*

—*Shirley* (Massachusetts)

*I really never believed it was possible. I was sure my section wasn't necessary
when it was done, but not that a better trial of labor might not have ultimately
led to the same thing. This time I had 24 hours of the kind of labor they did a
section for after 7 hours last time!*

*I was delighted, my doctors amazed, only now I feel like I have to live down a
"Superwoman" image. It may not be major surgery but it's no piece of cake either.
I think my husband expects me to scale the Prudential Building tomorrow!. . .*

*Everyone seems to think my success was due to a determination I never felt.
"VBAC" scared me because I didn't feel a "religious" commitment to it—I was
strong enough without it, with the right support people. Also, my "mindset" never*

thought of medication—there's labor or there's surgery, and I probably spent the morning yelling, "Get the knife!"—fortunately, no one listened.

—Barbara (Massachusetts)

. . . When the monitor began to disturb me late in labor it was removed. That obstacle hurdled, the nurse then brought in the I.V. and again we told her no.

. . . Our physician arrived around 4:30 A.M. He came into the room, asked how I was doing, and said, "Well, I'm here, I hope I don't see you again." I was happy to see that he was secure enough with himself and VBAC that he didn't feel he had to check up on us. I saw my labor "team" as myself, my husband, our midwife (and baby, of course!), and I was grateful for the doctor's passive support. (I never did see him again during the entire labor and delivery) . . .

. . . The baby had been posterior through the labor and finally he turned. With that came incredible pain and pressure and within one or two contractions his head was born. His cord was tight around his shoulder so I needed to continue to push him out without contractions. That really was difficult, but was accomplished in a short time. He arrived at 9:30 A.M. and was fine and healthy and I was so glad he was out! The pediatrician suctioned him and then brought him over to me. Anna unwrapped him and laid him right on my chest and then turned down the lights. I did not have an episiotomy (also no shaving) . . . Ben stayed at my breast until shortly before 11:00 A.M., when the pediatrician returned to do the exam. I got washed and dressed and then got Ben ready, and at 11:30 A.M. Ben, Dennis, and I joined Nathan and Hannah—and home we went!

. . . More thoughts . . .

Ben was born on my birthday!

"The squeaky wheel gets the oil"—I made myself a pain in the neck with the hospital during the pregnancy with requests, meetings, negotiations. But we got excellent service from them for our efforts.

This whole experience has been an incredible affirmation to me of my belief in God's grand design.

—June (Rhode Island)

I had labored before, so I knew somewhat of what happens. This time I rather enjoyed the intensity of labor—that feeling of timelessness and intense focus on one's own body.

My labor started very slow—we stayed home for the first 28 hours as it didn't become active until about 20–22 hours after the mucous plug popped. We arrived at 6 or 7 A.M. Saturday at 7 cm. Even though I had done much preparing, I still had a hard time walking into that cold, sterile labor room. Luckily we had a nice view out the window and the sky was so blue. We were soon in transition. Beth massaged my legs and abdomen and Andy massaged my shoulders. We did most of transition in the bathroom where I could stand during contractions and sit in between them.

We moved to the delivery room as pushing started. I had not been ready for the bad memories the delivery room evoked. But I felt prepared enough to say to myself— "O.K. there's nothing else you can do but get on with the task at hand."

This stage of labor was the hardest for me. After pushing for what seemed like a long time, I began to feel I was making no progress. This is where we had failed before, and I began to feel the same was happening again. Everyone was encouraging, but I hadn't left the last labor totally behind. I wish I had brought a mirror. Beth finally told me to put my hands in my vagina to feel the head—That certainly helped . . . I made a lot of noise this time, and it felt good! Interestingly, the fear of scar rupture never once entered my mind. I thought it would be a big problem.

Lindsey was born and put on my abdomen—a feeling I will never forget. It's one of those experiences that will stay clear in my memory, probably forever. Andy and I have felt a closeness we never knew before.

I'm grateful to all those who helped us achieve this goal. They all have a special place in our hearts.

—*Deborah* (Massachusetts)

I feel very good about the birth. As the time approached I realized my two "firsts" were (1) I didn't want to have to pee in a bedpan or pot and (2) I was self-conscious about making noise. I was able to walk to the bathroom until 2 P.M. and didn't need to pee after that, and when the time came, I didn't care one whit about moaning and then hollering!

If I had ordered this labor and delivery it couldn't have been better. Progress was steady and I didn't ever feel all the work was getting nowhere. It was during the day, I was surrounded by family and friends, etc., etc. I was a bit confused by the feel of the pushing contractions but I was able to say so and was coached well. Finn was great. He really came through as promised; we couldn't have been closer. By the time I even thought about transition it was over. I have no complaints, and I'm sitting, sore-bottomed, on top of the world!

—*Nora* (Vermont . . . Homebirth)

The birth was nothing like I had anticipated. I was looking forward to a long labor with lots of loving touching, slowly building to a crescendo. It all happened too quickly for me to integrate it. When we arrived at the hospital and I was examined, I was 7 cm. When the doctor arrived 15 minutes later and examined me I was fully dilated. I had constant back labor and invented a new type of breathing that went, "ha, ha, ha, PUSH!". . . .I think the biggest problem was *having no relief at all between contractions. I kept feeling like I wasn't handling any of it very well. Joe was wonderfully encouraging and the doctor kept saying that the baby would be born soon but I didn't even care. I was in too much pain to experience what was actually happening. When I was proclaimed fully dilated, I thought something was going to change. I had expected the contractions to be different and further apart. Instead they just kept on coming as before, with intense back pain. I had no real urge to push. I sort of wanted to just stop everything at that point, having lost sight of the ultimate goal. But the doctor insisted that I push, and with a lot of very loud grunting and groaning I pushed her out in 15 minutes, feeling all the while that I wasn't pushing very effectively. Because of the baby's lowered heart rate there was an air of urgency that I found it hard to meet. Mostly I'm disappointed that I didn't act at all like the ladies in the childbirth movies. I think if it had been slower I could have handled it better. But the second that she was out, I felt WONDERFUL. I couldn't believe I could have felt so awful such a short time before. I took a shower two hours after the birth and went home less than 36 hours later. I am so* grateful not to have had another cesarean.

—Mary Jo (New York)

I tried not to have too many expectations, but rather to consider this a first-time labor and delivery. I was prepared for a long labor and pushing stage (and both were long!) and if necessary, for a c/section (as there were signs of fetal distress at the beginning). However, I was confident throughout that this would be a vaginal delivery.

Both Peter and I felt that this was a totally different—totally opposite!—experience from Ian's birth (our first child, by c/section, after 18 hours of labor), in terms of medical intervention, the hospital atmosphere, our doctor, and overall psychological support. Our labor coach was invaluable; in fact, she made all the difference. Whereas during Ian's birth the nurses kept saying, "Oh, just another hour" (which wasn't true), Vickie, our coach during Derek's birth, would say, "It's going slow, but you're making progress." Her presence took a good deal of the burden away from Peter.

. . . Peter assisted during the birth: he delivered Derek's head and I lifted Derek out. It was really an incredible experience. We felt, when it was over, that it had been a triumph.

—Christine (Massachusettes)

I was told my tailbone was crooked. He said it protruded too far and wouldn't let a baby pass. Well, it must have unprotruded because I did it with room to spare.

—Coreen (California)

A *10 lb. 11 oz.* baby. I can't believe I birthed all that baby! Completely natural!! The scar was checked. It was perfect. I squatted to deliver and picked her up and walked down the corridor with her.

—*Helen* (Canada)

I want to report a tremendous birth experience. I had as close to a homebirth as possible with my husband, our children, and two close friends—and no interventions. Had very little contact with the staff. No episiotomy or tearing. The doctor arrived at the same time as Davy's head.

—*Coleen* (Pennsylvania)

After four years of research and hard work the birth was surprisingly fast and simple, but also awe-inspiring. We had no medication or intervention of any kind.

—*Mary* (Oregon)

About two weeks before Mike was born, my doctor in Toledo told me that he couldn't deliver me naturally, as much as he wanted to. He had consulted a doctor whose specialty is vaginal births after cesarean. He told my doctor that without having anesthesia on 24-hour call, it was too risky for me to deliver in any of the hospitals in my area. We were referred to another doctor who gave us the pros and cons of trial labor and told us to discuss it and let him know. Of course, our minds were already made up.

We left for the hospital about 2:15 (it's a 45-minute drive), and when we got there I was examined and found to be completely dilated. We went straight to delivery and Mike was born a few minutes later. We were flying high!!

—*Ann* (Michigan)

My first child was a cesarean for all the wrong reasons. This time, I resolved to have a homebirth provided there were no complications prenatally. I did not inform the hospital of my intent but rather made arrangements with two excellent midwives to deliver at home.

During my first pregnancy, I was classified as a class A gestational diabetic, so my doctors were pressuring me to agree to a repeat c/section at the 40th week on my due date. I refused to agree to this, stating I would hold out to 42 weeks, provided I didn't spill sugar in my urine and the nonstress tests they were conducting stayed good.

Three days before my due date, I began experiencing contractions of sufficient severity to prohibit me from sleeping. One day after my due date, I delivered Angela Maria at home into loving hands. Her father cut the cord, and she stayed with me constantly. It was one of the greatest experiences of my life.

—Mary Jo (Ohio . . . Homebirth)

I DID IT!!
The birth went well—just as we had hoped, although the baby came three weeks early (one week before we were to leave for Atlanta to have him there). I was totally prepared—Rob did a fantastic job coaching and I did a fantastic job coping!!
. . . I could see the baby's head coming, and I could see myself making it all happen—FANTASTIC—God knows how many women I have watched pushing in childbirth films, but this time I was watching ME do it and it was the thrill of my life!! I Gave Birth to my baby on my own—without any medical interference or intervention—I knew *I could do it!* . . . I'm *terrific!!*

—Cyndie (Florida . . . VBAC after 2 cesareans)

. . . Being an obstetrician, and my baby being three weeks late, posterior, and floating, I was hung up for hours at four cm. (when the membranes finally ruptured, there was thick meconium and audible decelerations) . . . The end result was a spontaneous vaginal delivery of a healthy 8 lb. 4 oz. son—there was plenty of room! I was so happy—I'm still grinning. He was 9 oz. heavier than the CPD baby. He was the same length. I had an easy recovery from the c/sec, but there was no comparison. When I went home the next day, I picked number-one son up and gave him a huge hug. You can't do that with a fresh incision. Also, I was only away from home for 36 hours the whole time. Everything is going well. I have enough milk to drown twins.

—Caroline (Pennsylvania)

Ten years ago I had to have an emergency c/section and the baby died. I grieved for years. This summer I had a beautiful baby girl vaginally, without drugs or complications. It was wonderful and the most thrilling experience of my life, and my daughter, Elizabeth, is so healthy.
I wanted to write to support your work and tell you how glad I am that you are helping people understand that it is O.K. to have a vaginal birth after a cesarean birth.

—Cathy (Colorado)

I was subjected to a cesarean operation for my first child. When I became pregnant with my second daughter, my husband and I began asking some very important questions, i.e.: Why a repeat? How safe are they? What about the dangers of major surgery? What is high risk? I became disgusted with the medical profession in general, obstetrical routine, hospital policies, and the final straw was finding out that my previous c/sec was unnecessary. At that point we chose homebirth as our SAFEST alternative, found a competent lay midwife, and proceeded to enjoy the loving, gentle, 5½ hour, uncomplicated birth of our second daughter, in the privacy and dignity of our own home.

—Laurie (Colorado . . . Homebirth)

I am a doctor's wife. I am personally involved in his practice as an office worker, but, more importantly to me, as a prenatal and birth attendant. My first baby was delivered via c/section and my second delivered by my husband at home with no problems . . . . We just had a woman deliver an 8 lb. boy vaginally, who had had a 6 lb. girl taken by c/section. We are working with another cesarean woman and are hopeful. We feel that whatever the outcome, she will have a positive birth experience, which will help boost her sagging self-image.

—Addie (Idaho . . . Homebirth)

My VBAC was wonderful. My husband was very anxious that it be a VBAC, because he would not be allowed in for a repeat cesarean. (He was told that fathers are not prepared for surgery—neither are mothers, but we are expected to be there.) At the birth, he was so excited, he fainted and hit his head on a table. He required 3 stitches and a 24-hour hospital stay. I left the hospital (with the baby) 8 hours after the birth, to be home with our 4-year-old.

—Laura (Vermont)

Well, we did it—a beautiful normal delivery (after our previous c/sec with the twins). It all went so fast, they didn't have a chance to use an internal monitor, catheter, I.V., shave, episiotomy, or anything! At 3 centimeters my water broke, and exactly ½ hr. later I pushed Jonathan out myself—no one helped me. What happened was, I told them I had to push about 25 min. or so after the water broke. They didn't believe me—told me to pant and not push—I said, "Forget it—the kid is on its way out." So I pushed once, and he came out, completely (in bed). It was super! It's great not having an epis.—I was never sore—and I feel wonderful after this labor and delivery.

—Ann (Arizona)

I dilated to 10 cm. in 3 hrs. of active labor (vs 5 cm. in 72 hrs. last time) and then took 4 hrs. to push Joshua out! I had a wonderful midwife, incredibly supportive and intuitive, and excellent labor coaching as well as moral support from my husband. I did not lie down at all but either stood up or was on all fours throughout. I birthed my baby while standing (slightly squatting) and sipped a lot of orange juice and honey throughout labor.

—Anne (Arizona)

They're identical and were born VBAC! It was the grandest thing I've ever done. When I had a contraction I kneeled on my stairs and rested on another stair. I didn't do any "method" of breathing and it was so much better. My blood pressure was high at the end of the labor and Rita kept telling me to just visualize it coming down. My own doctor wasn't there and the doctor was awful. He told me I could die in labor and if I didn't hurry I'd have to have them by 8:15 "one way or the other." He did an episiotomy without telling me and told the midwife afterwards not to meddle.

I showered and walked, although he wanted me in bed. The girls were 6–5 and 6–9. I am really proud.

—Julie (Massachusetts . . . VBAC twins)

If you recall, I spoke to you last year and told you that I was pregnant but my doctor was very pessimistic about the size of my pelvis. He agreed to a trial of labor. I swam a lot during this pregnancy and felt very strong. I also arranged to have a midwife come to our home and then to the hospital with us.

Labor began at 2 A.M. By 5 P.M. I hadn't even begun to dilate, despite walks, baths, etc. If it hadn't been for the midwife's encouragement, we would have believed it couldn't work. I took blue and black cohash tincture and a hot bath. By 8:00 I was 4 cm. We stupidly called the doctor then, who demanded that we be in the hospital by 9:00.

I was checked in by 9:30 and feeling great and relaxed. I was 5 cm. At 12:30 A.M. (I'd been feeling like I was in transition for quite a while) I was at 6 cm., and the baby was posterior and the head unengaged. The doctor became very insistent on doing a cesarean. He said that getting hung up in dilation with the head unengaged was a classic rupture situation. I didn't buy that and neither did the midwife. I refused the c/sec. The doctor threatened to go off the case and called in the cesarean team. I demanded a second opinion and refused to sign the consent forms.

I got a second opinion from one of the other doctors who would have assisted in a cesarean. He broke my waters and told my doctor to let me labor some more if I wanted to. After that the two doctors kept coming in and pushing back my cervix—painful! An hour and a half later they let me get in the birthing chair, and at 4:26 A.M. our daughter was born! What a high experience. I birthed her without even any tears, and she weighed almost 8 lbs.! One highlight was when they brought in the cesarean consent forms: I told them I wouldn't sign any God-damned papers. I'll never think of myself as a weak person again.

—Susan (Massachusetts)

I am now the proud mother of a baby daughter that I delivered naturally.

—Janis (California)

My daughter was born very naturally and quite easily in fact, on New Year's eve! There aren't any words to describe the experience.

—Eva (California . . . Homebirth)

After two cesareans, our daughter wangled her way into the world before a section could be done. I'm an instructor in Fertility Awareness, so I knew she was conceived late in the "cycle" and due before the ob-gyn calculated—thus I was able to schedule the operation for after *her due date.*

—Judith (California . . . VBAC after two cesareans)

I was told I had an absolutely contracted pelvis, so I had a section. The next time around, my absolutely contracted pelvis delivered an 8½ lb. baby!

—Nikki (Massachusetts)

The thing that upset me most about my cesarean was that the doctor greeted my hope for future vaginal births with the emphatic statement that he was sure that I could never have . . . a vaginal birth because of my small structure. This statement grated on my brain for the next year and a quarter. With a family history of two sisters and their 5 cesarean births behind me, along with the doctor's fore-

boding statement, what I really needed was some good strong encouragement that my body could achieve a vaginal birth. I got much of this from VBAC classes.

My object was to convince myself that my body could do it. *For my own peace of mind, I had to make sure nothing in my surrounding environment during pregnancy or delivery could interfere with that goal. I also wanted to work on finding processes that could help achieve that goal. I spent countless energy and hours on all of this . . . I also worked on convincing my husband that my first cesarean was indeed a negative experience, which I didn't want to repeat, regardless of the fact that a healthy daughter resulted from it.*

. . . During my pregnancy, and continuing through labor, I tried to find techniques that would help me "open up." One such technique was that besides addressing personal prayers to G-d, I repeatedly recited a blessing that thanks G-d for creating humans with all the proper orifices (which I not only said fervently but also calligraphed many times during labor) . . . and meditated on my vaginal area opening properly to birth the baby . . . . I also learned a Hebrew song that translates, "Open for me the gates of righteousness that I may enter them and praise G-d." I borrowed an artpiece inspired by that same verse on which to meditate, both at home and in the hospital. Finally, I wrote up positive affirmations that my body would work and in detail described how my body had worked for me in the past . . . I also hashed out my concerns about the birth with my friend and she gave me such emotional support and spiritual uplifting, as well as being at my side during labor and delivery. . . .

With all this preparation, I delightfully accomplished birthing Este Rachel Emunah. *When I went into labor, I was very calm. I ate to my heart's desire (in fact, even more than usual!) I called on my husband for assistance in relaxing and focusing . . . During labor this time, he also gave me spiritual support by studying a certain Chasidic text with me, which was related to the labor process. I did a lot of laboring in the comfort of my own home and fortunately only ended up spending 3 hours in the hospital. The only way I survived the intense contractions of transition was by singing the "Opening of the Gates" song enthusiastically while my husband soothed me even more by harmonizing . . . At the hospital, my wishes were met, and I emerged victorious from my internal struggle with the ever-so-special reward of my second precious daughter, Este Rachel Emunah. Her third name means "faith." We gave that name to her to signify that I had the faith in G-d that my body could work, and it certainly did just that!*

—*Laurie* (Massachusetts)

. . . At 2:30 P.M. Tuesday (after 3 days of strong, albeit intermittent contractions) I thought for sure my uterus was in trouble. Nancy said I must have been feeling the cervix opening, because the uterine scar would not be anywhere near that point. I realized that she was right *and my contractions went to just under 2 min. apart. We called the midwife (who had been at anoother birth that morning) and Nancy again around 3:30. The midwife arrived at 4:30 and about 5:15 we*

went upstairs to do an internal exam. I was 5–6½ cm.! Very stretchy, and the waters were bulging and stretching me to 7 + cm. with each contraction!!! I was going to do it! I was going to have this baby the way nature intended for babies to be born! . . .

When we got to the hospital at 7 P.M. the doctor, who had been out with his son, and our friends were waiting for us. The doctor checked me and I was now 7 + cm. He went to take his son home. I did a lot of squatting (I couldn't get low enough to the floor for my body!) and sitting on the toilet and commode. I drank juice. I talked to my son and husband between contractions, made jokes, and asked to take a nap. The baby and my body said, "NO!" and I had another contraction. Ben (our other child) went home at about 9:30 P.M. Some time after that my waters broke or were broken by the doctor who checked me during a contraction. It wasn't important to me at that point, because they would have broken on their own. After a 5-day labor . . . . I pushed for less than a hour, squatting on the floor. We had lots of hot compresses and vitamin E oil and perineal massages. Andy held me and breathed with me and was totally there for me as I/we birthed our baby. I lifted her from my body and brought her right to my breast. The doctor watched and took pictures. Arayel Rohana was born at 10:28 P.M. At 2 A.M. we were on our way home.

At 7 on Wednesday morning Ben came into our room, as he does each morning. We were all in bed, right where we were supposed to be, and there was his sister. They spent the better part of the next hour looking at each other, bonding and smiling.

—Jami (Massachusetts)

My water broke and for two days I had intermittent contractions. About 7:00 P.M. they finally began to get more regular. At 1:00 A.M. I called our midwife and when she arrived I was only 2 cm. dilated, although the contractions were very strong. She told me to slowly inhale through my nose and exhale through my mouth in 3 short breaths. She told me to visualize my cervix opening. I fell asleep imagining a donut with its hole getting bigger and bigger. I woke up at 4:00 A.M. fully dilated and ready to push!! At 6:15 our son was born. It was the most wonderful experience of my life.

—Judy (Massachusetts . . . Homebirth after two cesareans)

Our first daughter was delivered by cesarean section when my induced labor "failed to progress." Our second daughter was delivered by elective c/section because we were not educated.

. . . Planning for our 3rd child was emotionally draining. I found it exhausting to interview and choose obstetricians (a first choice and back-up), pediatricians, *and hospitals that would support us in the natural process of birth. There is no doubt it would have been easier to have major surgery. I admire the obstetrician we chose for his progressive views in a very conservative medical community. Although he may not have truly understood the reasons for our choosing a VBAC, he was willing to support our decision while providing excellent medical back-up if it should have been needed.*

We chose to have a midwife with us at home to monitor our labor and to act as our advocate once we entered the hospital. Her presence and encouragement enhanced our experience tremendously. We planned to stay at home as long as possible during labor. I was most comfortable at home, and we felt this would decrease the likelihood of medical intervention.

My labor was hard work but a part of the birth experience I treasure. I spent two nights and two days in my rocking chair breathing during contractions and watching our children play or talking to Ray or our midwives between them. At home there was no I.V.—I had food and fluids as I needed them. There was no fetal monitor— a fetal scope was used to listen to our baby's heartbeat and I was able to walk about in our house and outdoors between contractions. There was no medication— there was understanding and patient encouragement from those around me. Drugs were never an issue. And there was no mention of surgery. My body was designed to deliver our baby and, of course, I could do it. I was under no pressure to perform. We were all working and waiting together for our child to be born.

The hospital cooperated in honoring the requests we had outlined in a letter. However, we found hospital personnel generally unaccustomed to assisting in natural childbirth. Hospital policies and procedures were distracting. I found myself trying to listen only to Ray and our midwife—to their reassurance, suggestions, and encouragement. And I depended upon them to also reassure hospital personnel and our obstetrician that I was doing fine.

I have never worked so hard as I did during the second stage of labor. All the fears and questions I had during transition vanished as I realized my body really did know how to have our baby. Ray and our midwife were a tremendous help. Time lost meaning and I lost perspective that our labor would soon come to an end. I was surprised when a nurse, seeing that our child's birth was imminent, initiated our flight to the delivery room. And, although I had felt our baby's head numerous times, I was amazed when I saw a baby's head—our baby's head—in the mirror.

No words can describe the joy and love we felt as our hands lifted our baby into the world. We had done it—and we had done it our way! We had delivered our baby—a big (9 lbs. 10½ oz.), healthy baby boy. We had dared to dream, and that impossible dream had come true.

It wasn't until our son was lying on my abdomen that I was really ready to say good-bye to our pregnancy. Then I was anxious for the umbilical cord to be severed so I could hold him in my arms, stroke him, nurse him, and welcome him into the world. He was beautiful!

We left the hospital later that same morning. We wanted to reunite our family and introduce our son to his sisters. There were lots of kisses and hugs waiting at home.

Postscript: After nine months of educating ourselves and working so hard to avoid unnecessary surgery, we found it impossible to subject our son to unnecessary surgery. He was not circumcised.

—Karen (Massachusetts . . . VBAC after two cesareans)

The doctor was waiting for the placenta and out popped two more little feet. I knew it all the time. My labor took four days after the water broke. The neonatologist said all that time really helped their lungs to develop because they were early.

—Mary (Massachusetts . . . VBAC twins after two cesareans)

For some mothers, cesarean birth is a normal and pleasant way to have a baby. Not for me. I was in a car accident, which caused a placental abruption, and my first baby, which was born by cesarean, was stillborn. I associated all my sorrow with cesarean section. I didn't ever want another cesarean.

During my next pregnancy I asked about a natural birth. My physician was too scared. I was also afraid of having another stillbirth. So I had a cesarean 10 days prior to my due date. Mark was the first husband allowed in for a cesarean. We were thrilled to share the birth and have a healthy daughter.

When I became pregnant with our next child, I wanted to have it naturally. The people in this area were so terrified, that I was sectioned. I was in labor, but it was going too slowly for them.

With my fourth pregnancy I labored and thought I'd deliver vaginally. One nurse came in and said I was trying to murder my baby by going into labor. I knew I didn't need the operation. I was more scared of what was going to be done to me than delivering naturally. There was no support. I was 2 cm. when I went to the hospital. They would have sent anyone else home. Another cesarean.

Finally, when I got to Esther's birth I had her vaginally. I never had one pain I didn't love. I had a very long labor from beginning to end. It was an incredibly joyous experience. I experienced the pushing phase in both an orgasmic and holy way.

After the second cesarean, I was very depressed. I sought psychiatric help. But my natural birth cleared the coast. I had been so preoccupied with the cesareans that I could hardly think of anything else. People would say, "What beautiful children," and I'd say, "Yes, but they had to be born by cesarean." I kept on having babies close together (5 in 7 years) because I had to do it. I am no longer preoccupied with childbearing. It is all worked through now, and it is all HEALED.

—Marie (Connecticut . . . VBAC after four cesareans)

My labor was long and it was hard. It was pacing the hospital floors for almost a day, hot showers, cold showers, back rubs, muscle relaxers, which I asked for because I thought I was too uptight. It virtually caused my labor to stop, so Pitocin was used. It was all very hard. But, I endured it. When I thought to myself, "Why am I doing this? Why did I want to experience all this pain?" I remembered all the women before me who had had their babies naturally spanning all the centuries from the corners of the globe. Despite our differences in customs, I knew we were the same women. I also thought about women in this country today and tomorrow who, because of my having a vaginal birth after a c/sec, would know that it can be done. I could reassure myself by knowing they would be given the confidence to try it themselves when they heard it was possible. And I thought of all the women who in this past century had been robbed of experiencing their own child's birth because of recommended medication.

After it was over I reflected on the difference between my first child's birth, by c/sec, and my second, natural, birth experience. I couldn't explain it. Why had the passage down the birth canal made such a tremendous difference? It was as if I had never given birth to my first child, he had been plucked from me. The second I had pushed from my body and she felt so much more a part of me.

Not any less important was the physical difference. The moment she slipped out of my body the pain was over. If I had had another c/sec the pain of contractions would only have been replaced by the pain of the incision. That pain would have lasted for weeks with no rests in between. The physical contrast was remarkable. This affected the way I felt mentally and my ability to cope with my new responsibility.

—Carol (Massachusetts)

Changing my thoughts about my previous birthings opened a path for Benjamin's natural delivery. The cesarean birth of my twin boys had left me feeling depressed about my failure to push them out of me and I suffered deeply because of the violation to my body through surgery. I then attempted to have a VBAC with my next hospital birth. Again medical technology intervened and with negativity all around (except from my husband), I had another cesarean. At least this time I was awake and "allowed" to bond with my daughter. Only eight months later I was pregnant again and more determined than ever NOT to repeat my cesareans.

With a trained counselor I learned of my own traumatic birth through recall, processing my mother's pregnancy, labor, and delivery. I also experienced the physical sensations of pain, felt the fear and violence of my birth through months of rebirthing (a technique of circular breathing with eyes closed in a prone position). I began doing affirmations such as, "It is now safe and pleasant for my baby to come out vaginally." I forgave myself for creating the cesarean births to protect my babies from the birth trauma I had experienced, and I thanked myself for loving my babies so much that I underwent surgery so that their births would be gentle. My husband and I took VBAC classes to learn all we could.

Benjamin!!

Eleven hours of labor seemed long to me at the time but I had been waiting seven years to push a baby into the world! And I had spent a total of seventy-two hours laboring during the three attempts to birth my four children vaginally.

Benjamin's labor was considered an "average" labor. Average?? How can such an experience be classified as average? It is the single most spectacular event in my life. The most creative, rewarding, intensely loving act I ever experienced. The climax of my husband's and my relationship.

The labor began in a very peace-filled manner on my due date. That evening, as usual, I was lying down to nurse my sixteen-month-old daughter Heidi to sleep on her bed. She shared the room with Justin and Nathan, who would be seven years old in a week. The children were quietly listening to me talking to the baby inside me. "I know it is time for you to come out, baby. My body feels tired from carrying you inside me so long. Now it is time for you to come out." Justin asked, "Can the baby hear you?" "Not very well, but it understands me. Shall we all ask it to come out?" I replied. "Baby . . . come out, come out, we want to see you," both boys softly spoke. Then I said, "Let's sing, 'Like a Leaf or a Feather in the windy windy weather, We will whirl around and twirl around and all fall down together.'" We sang the song together three times and the next moment my labor began with a contraction that lasted about a minute. This is it! My opportunity to experience my power as a woman, to achieve mastery over the past failures to birth my babies out of my body. My chance to push a child into the world as nature intended. Oh how exciting it was and how sure of myself I felt! This time I would be in my own safe home with my family and self-chosen attendants . . . . From that first contraction they were coming every five minutes and lasting a minute. This was the true progress of a working labor. (The true work of a labor in progress?) I had this kind of labor before but there was no dilation in my cervix. This time I could visualize opening with each contraction.

I phoned the Department of Environmental Affairs radio room to get ahold of the boat Eric was on. He was 100 miles away by land and it was his first day at his new job. I could hear the radio operator say, "Labor, labor," and I knew that this brief message would be understood. Eric told me later that in his haste to get off the boat he nearly leaped into the ocean instead of onto the dock. I was in the tub when he arrived. His face radiated so much love and excitement it was dazzling to look at him!

. . . If I had been in the hospital I would have been frightened by the insistence of the doctors to perform a cesarean. After two cesareans, they would have insisted on a cesarean due to meconium and a period of time with little progress. Thank GOD we were at home with competent and patient attendants. Looking into their eyes was like gazing into pools of calm water. It was wonderful.

—Heather (Massachusetts . . . Homebirth after two cesareans)

I loved labor and delivery—all of it. The birth was twice as good as I had hoped for in my dreams.

—Ruth (Massachusetts)

Katie's Poem

We did it!
I yelled
We did it!

Because we knew
It was right.
You won't cut me
Not again, ever!

My baby knew.
My husband knew.
My heart knew.
Now the whole world can know.

They didn't fool me
With their jargon.
They didn't fool us
With their threats.

It was *my* responsibility.
It was *my* baby's birth.
Now, it's my joyous memory
And a part of who I am.
                    —*Esther B. Zorn*

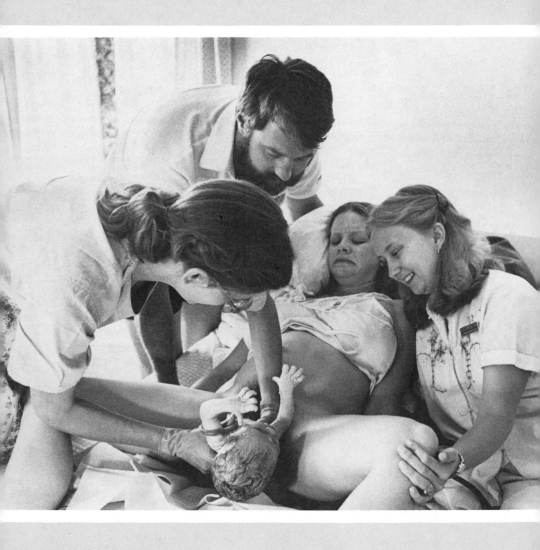

16 ❧ Cesarean Deliverance

The future does not belong to those who are content with today . . . . It will belong to those who can blend passion, reason and courage in a personal commitment.

—Robert Kennedy

During the time it took you to read this book, several thousand American women were strapped to operating tables and delivered of their babies by cesarean section. In most situations, both mother and baby would have been safer if the knife had never been raised.

During the time it took you to read this book, other women were giving birth to their babies purely and joyfully. They had carefully chosen those who would attend them and had prepared their bodies well for their labors of love. These women refused invasive and interfering techniques that would confuse their bodies and increase their chances for problems during labor and delivery. They refused to be cut unnecessarily. Some had had previous cesareans, but they did not allow their prior experience to rob themselves and their new babies of the right to a normal, healthy birth. In reclaiming our rights as women, and in *giving birth*, there is deliverance.

The desire to birth normally and purely connects all women to one another. The experience of birthing bonds us to those who have come before: our mothers, our grandmothers, our great-grandmothers. It joins us to all our sisters who share this Earth with us. We are a part of a universe that works. What better legacy—what better gift—to leave our children than the belief that this is so.

In *A Woman in Residence*, Dr. Michelle Harrison presents a powerful vision. "I have fantasies in which women stand up in the thousands and thousands and say they are going to deliver their babies without having them cut out of their bellies."

We, too, have a vision. We dream of the time when the birthing room will once more be the domain of those who rule it best: mothers and their babies.

381

We dream of a time when every pregnant woman can birth her baby in an atmosphere of total love and support. We dream of the time when doctors will once again be free to do what they do best: heal the sick. Ours is not an impossible dream.

Some will never allow themselves to share our visions and to hear what we have to say. The truth is often painful—no less sharp than knives, thousands of them, cutting into women's bellies and their bottoms. But the truth is that the time has come for women to acknowledge their strength. The time has come for us to regain trust in our bodies and pride in the process of birth. The time has come for us to respect our own ability to make responsible choices about childbearing.

It is time to turn frustration into energy, confusion into clarity, anger into action. It is time for us to tap our self-respect, our spirit, and our power. Only then will we emerge from birth intact. Only then will the cesarean epidemic be brought under control. Only then will we be delivered.

The future of childbirth in America does not belong to those who are content with the medical and technocratic practices of today. It belongs instead to those who are willing to speak in defense of the original plan. It belongs to those of us who can look beyond the tools, tubes, chemicals, and machines and see the safety and joy inherent in nature's design. WE ARE THE PRESERVERS OF THE BLUEPRINTS. The knife, not our voices, will be silent.

---

*New York: Random House, 1982.

APPENDICES

Appendix A

REMEMBER . . . EVERY LABOR IS **UNIQUE!**

Phase of Labor	What You Might Feel
Stage I Effacement and Dilatation A. Early phase: 0–2 fingers or 0–4 cm. Contractions: 30–60 seconds; 5 minutes or more apart (from start to start)	Increased vaginal discharge Diarrhea or constipation Light cramping or tightening "Show" Ruptured membranes (this can happen at any time right up to baby's birth)
B. Mid-phase: 2–4 fingers or 4–8 cm. Contractions: 45–60 seconds; 3–5 minutes apart	Stronger, more frequent contractions More serious concentration Preoccupation Dependence on companionship Restlessness
C. Latter phase: 4–5 fingers or 8–10 cm. Contractions: 60–90 seconds; 2–3 minutes apart (or back to back)	Total involvement and detachment Apprehension "Sleeping" between contractions Increased pressure Heavy show Desire to push Some women feel: shaky, leg cramps, hot, perspiration, cold, nausea, vomiting
Stage II Birthing of Baby: 10 min–4 + hours Contractions: 45–90 seconds; 2–5 minutes apart	Contractions may slow down and change character Urge to push Pressure to rectum and perineum Total involvement Stretching (burning) sensation Feel head moving down
Stage III Expulsion of placenta	Contraction: Some women are so involved with baby, they don't feel it!!

Remember: Waves come to shore, noisy trucks do finally pass by, and the view from the mountain *you've climbed* somehow is more breathtaking, exhilarating, majestic!

Labor Chart

What You Can Do	What To Remember
Light foods and tea (or juices or broth) Time a few contractions Call midwife or labor attendant Slow, relaxed breathing Relaxation exercises Urinate frequently Rest!! (or take a nice walk outside) Take some pictures, get things ready	Many women feel energetic, excited, impatient, talkative— *SAVE YOUR ENERGY!!* If it is nighttime, try to fall back to sleep for a while Hot water trickled over abdomen usually feels good during early phase
Continue concentrated breathing (lighten up if necessary) Effleurage (cornstarch) Tea, juices, water for thirst Broth, yogurt, toast, etc., for hunger Release all body parts Vary position (sitting, standing, etc.) Pillows to support all body parts	Concentrate on *one* contraction at a time A back rub or thigh massage might feel great You can continue taking a walk Continue to relax On "hands – knees" for back labor may help
Breathing—light, using partner for eye contact and rhythm Feel your spouse's touch and love Wake up in time for contraction Stay in the present time Make sure room is tranquil and full of confident support and caring Change positions if necessary Thigh massage between contractions	These contractions may be no stronger than previous ones—only longer, perhaps (some may have double peaks) The people around you are there to help and support you Reassure her gently and lovingly: "Stay with it"; "You're terrific"; "Open . . ."; "You *can* do it" Your baby is coming soon! (If she asks for medication, she needs more support)
Relax perineal muscle Physical support to woman Push gently—let body rhythms determine length and intensity Push with vagina (loosen mouth!) Be ready to stop pushing when head crowns	Get mirror (and eye glasses!!) ready *Hot* compresses and vitamin E oil feel great and HELP on perineum Squatting encourages rotation of baby's head (posterior) and increases pelvic diameter Reach down and touch your baby's head
Love your baby! Gently push with contraction	Your placenta has helped to give life to your baby—you might want to take a close look at it.

Remember: VBAC labors rarely need any medical interventions (and, in fact, interventions often adversely affect the outcome).

Appendix B ❧ Preventing Unnecessary Cesareans

by E. L. Shearer

Reason for C/Sec	Avoidable Factors	Alternatives
I. Dystocia— CPD Failure to progress Prolonged labor Arrest of labor Uterine inertia Failed induction Failed forceps	1. Lack of patience with normal labor process; misinterpretation of Friedman labor curve. (it's a *mean*, not a *norm*; there is a normal human variation in length and pattern of labor.)	1. Trust a woman's body unless clear clinical signs of fetal or maternal distress; stay at home until 5 cms.; go home if arrive at hospital and less than 3–4 cms.
	2. Recumbent position; lack of mobility in first stage. (When woman is upright and ambulatory, first stage is shorter, contractions stronger and more efficient, gravity helps, baby enters pelvis at a better angle, mother is more comfortable and feels less pain. Supine position leads to maternal hypotension and reduced uterine blood flow.)	2. Stay out of bed and *WALK!* Avoid semireclining position; no I.V. unless specifically indicated, then on mobile stand; monitor by auscultation unless electronic fetal monitoring specifically indicated, then alternate fetal monitoring with periods of walking.
	3. Exaggerated pushing with prolonged breath-holding in semireclining or reclining position. (Squatting increases pelvic diameters, can increase available area 20–30%; gravity helps; baby descends at better angle. Hard, lengthy pushes result in ineffective pushing out-of-sync with uterus's own bearing-down efforts, as well as maternal exhaustion. Pushing with closed glottis,	3. Avoid semireclining or reclining position for second stage; squat, kneel, stand, or sit on toilet, especially if second stage long or uncomfortable; use these or side-lying position to rotate posterior or transverse head. Push only with body's own rhythm;

Reprinted by permission of the author.

holding legs up, pushing with heels result in tense, tight legs, buttocks, pelvic floor, and vagina, delaying baby's descent and causing more stress on baby's head and mother's soft tissues.)

4. Too hasty use of Pitocin after premature rupture of membranes or after due-date; elective induction; artificial rupture of membranes early in labor. (If cervix unready for labor, induction will be ineffective or labor prolonged. Pit can result in contractions too strong, long, and close together, increasing likelihood of use of analgesics or anesthesia, and of fetal distress, discussed later in this appendix. Pit associated with excessive third-stage bleeding and neonatal jaundice. With precautions, risk of infection after ruptured membranes very small in healthy, well-nourished women. Induction solely on the basis of dates runs risk of premature baby if dates wrong; there is a normal variation in length of gestation.

Artificial rupture of membranes removes protection for baby's head, can lead to excessive molding; increases likelihood of infection with internal exams, leads to concern over length of labor because of fear of infection.)

5. Fasting in labor. (Labor is hard physical work and requires lots of calories to burn. Digestion slows down in active labor, but continues slowly. A 5% glucose solution insufficient to supply energy needs. Times when inhalation anesthesia required are rare; fasting

mother avoid holding legs up, pushing with heels, or closing glottis; mother emphasize opening up and tuning into body's signals, not technique.

4. No Pitocin after ruptured membranes unless signs of infection; wait at home for labor (risk of infection and anxiety both lower there); eat at will and drink lots.
No post-dates induction unless signs of placental deterioration.
NO elective induction (banned by FDA).
No artificial rupture of membranes except in late labor in a few selected cases.

5. Eat at will in labor; drink lots.

does not eliminate risk of acid aspiration; effects on maternal and fetal metabolism and uterine functioning of prolonged fasting not clearly known.)

6. Narcotics in first stage. (Central nervous system depressants can slow uterine functioning, especially if given in latent phase or if labor progressing slowly already.)
   Epidurals in first or second stage. (Slow first stage by withdrawing blood from uterus and retarding uterine functioning; slow second stage by eliminating urge to push, weakening abdominal muscles; higher incidence of failure of baby's head to rotate.)

7. Maternal anxiety and fear. (Cause release of catacholamines, which withdraw blood from internal organs and relax smooth muscle, thus slowing labor down. Release of oxytocin also inhibited by fear, anxiety, and tension.)

II. Fetal distress

1. Misinterpretation of electronic fetal monitoring tracings. (Tracings are difficult to interpret, as some variations are normal; electronic monitoring produces many false

6. No narcotics or epidurals. Walking or other positions, relaxation, massage, shower or bath, breathing patterns, loving support, and encouragement instead.

7. Increase mother's self-confidence by emphasizing birth as *normal physiological function*, not only in childbirth classes and during pregnancy, but from childhood; give extra support in labor; stay home in early labor; improve community options for safe out-of-hospital births and alternative in-hospital births.

1. Monitor by auscultation unless electronic monitoring specifically indicated (according to NIH, no benefit

positives.) Reliance on electronic fetal monitoring for diagnosis. (According to NIH, this is a *screening*, not a *diagnostic*, tool.)	of EFM over auscultation demonstrated, except in high-risk cases). Confirm diagnosis with fetal scalp sampling before intervening.
2. Reclining position. (Supine position can cause maternal hypotension, reduce blood flow to uterus; labor less efficient and prolonged.)	2. Stay upright, out of bed, or on side.
3. Narcotics. (Central nervous system depressants can depress maternal respiration; cross placenta quickly and can depress fetus, especially if already stressed.) Epidurals. (Can lead to maternal hypotension, withdraw blood from uterus, as well as prolong labor.)	3. No narcotics or epidurals.
4. Pitocin. (Can cause contractions too long, strong, and close together for baby to recover oxygen supply in between, especially if already stressed; increases maternal discomfort and anxiety, raises likelihood of use of narcotics or epidurals.)	4. Use Pitocin rarely and sparingly; turn down or off once labor established. Stimulate labor by giving mother a rest, getting her up to walk, helping her relax, or stimulating nipples, instead of Pitocin.
5. Exaggerated pushing with prolonged breath-holding (Valsalva maneuver). (Can reduce oxygen to baby by retarding blood return through extreme intrathoracic pressure, and by using up oxygen with mother's own efforts; supine position leads to maternal hypotension and reduced uterine blood flow.)	5. Push physiologically with body's own rhythms, in upright or side-lying position hold breath no longer than 6-7 seconds.
6. Hyperventilation. (By several mechanisms, reduces oxygen available to baby.)	6. Help mother relax upper body, avoid rapid breathing.

	7. Maternal anxiety. (Reduces blood flow to uterus and oxygen available to baby.)	7. Help mother relax; see earlier paragraphs of alternatives.
III. Breech presentation	Automatic, blanket rules about how to deliver breech babies.	Prenatal exercise to turn baby; external version; x-ray at labor onset and trial of labor; skilled, confident midwife or obstetrician.
IV. Toxemia Hypertension Placental abruption Placental insufficiency Premature birth Low birthweight	Inadequate nutrition, during intrauterine life, childhood, adolescence, and pregnancy. Use of drugs in pregnancy—prescription, over the counter, and recreational, including alcohol and especially smoking. Restriction of blood volume and placental size by restricting salt intake or using diuretics.	Education about nutrition and use of drugs in pregnancy—before pregnancy begins, in early pregnancy, and in childbirth classes. *Avoid ALL drugs* if possible. Avoid use of diuretics, salt to taste; increase protein intake, maintain fluid and salt intake, if fluid retention and high blood pressure become problems. Feed low income pregnant women and growing girls. (Most low birth weight, premature births, perinatal and infant mortality in US occur to poor and minority women.)
V. Previous cesarean	Automatic, once-a-C/S-always-a-C/S policies. NIH and	Labor and vaginal birth unless

ACOG have both stated that vaginal birth is a safe option in most cases after a prior cesarean.

2–4 times greater risk of maternal mortality, increased risk of maternal morbidity and neonatal respiratory disease with elective repeat cesarean. Increased maternal-infant separation, stress on attachment process, decreased maternal self-esteem all may follow C/S. Risk of dehiscence (separation) of lower segment (horizontal) scar about 0.5%, with risk of serious rupture much less. Risk of maternal or fetal death little or no higher than without previous C/S.

i) classical uterine scar (skin doesn't matter)*

ii) new indication for C/S in this pregnancy.

*Parents may choose to take 1–3% risk of serious rupture with classical scar. If so, may want to go to hospital as soon as labor begins, have IV in place, blood ready, OR and anesthesia alerted, constant labor nursing supervision. With horizontal lower segment scar, same labor supervision and management as for any other labor.

Appendix C 🐦 VBAC Classes: Questions for Private Discussion

What do I want from this birth?

What do I need from you during this pregnancy?

What are my strongest feelings about our last birth?

What was it like for me when the decision was made to have a cesarean?

What feelings did I have during the surgery?

What feelings surface when I think about another cesarean birth?

What were those first weeks at home like?

How do I imagine this time will be different?

What can we do to make it different?

What will I need from you if this is a cesarean birth?

What will I need from you if this is a vaginal birth?

What feelings do I have now about this pregnancy?

What are we like sexually during this pregnancy?

What are my fantasies about this birth?

What would I settle for?

How do I feel about all the preparation that is necessary for this birth?

How do I want to be during labor?

How do I want us to be during labor?

What are my greatest fears about this pregnancy/birth?

What are my greatest joys?

What do I want for this baby?

How can we work to be the best team, the strongest unit, we can possibly be, during the next months?

What if labor takes a very long time?

List ten things that relax you that could help during labor.

List ten things you could do for someone in labor.

List ten things you want done for you during labor.

Tell me places you like to be touched.

Appendix D ❧ VBAC Classes: Questions for Open Discussion

How do I feel about our chances for a VBAC? What have we done to enhance our chances for the kind of birth we'd like?

How do I think I'll feel if a cesarean becomes necessary? What have we done to insure it will be the best possible experience?

How do I feel about my (your) incision?

What can we do to "pave the way" for other couples wishing a VBAC?

What beliefs/attitudes have I uncovered that may have influenced the last birth? What new beliefs/attitudes are present that will help?

What do I think it will be like having another addition to our family? What concerns do I have?

What is the single most important thing I learned through my childbirth classes?

How do I feel knowing labor is painful? What techniques/ideas/people can I call upon during that time for help?

In what ways does my relationship with my spouse (partner) affect how I feel about the birth?

Do I feel comfortable about where the birth will take place? About the people we have chosen to be there?

How do I feel about my (partner's) pregnant body? How does being pregnant affect our sexuality/sexual life?

Comparing this pregnancy to the last, these are the things that are different:

What frightens me most is:

What makes me feel most excited and happy about this coming birth is:

What I regret most about my cesarean is:

What I am most angry about is:

What I am most excited about is:

What our baby most wants me to know today is:

How does this statement make you feel? There is no perfect birth.

Do you feel your previous birth had any effect on your relationship with your baby?

What do you want/need most from your doctor and midwife/LA? Have you communicated these wishes to them?

Appendix E ❧ Resource Groups

Alternative Birth Crisis Coalition
Box 48371
Chicago, Ill. 60648

American Academy of Husband
  Coached Childbirth
Box 5224
Sherman Oaks, Cal. 91413

American College of Home Obstetrics
664 North Michigan Ave., Suite 600
Chicago, Ill. 60611

American Foundation for Maternal
  and Child Health
30 Beekman Place
New York, N.Y. 10022

American Society for
  Psychoprophylaxis in Obstetrics
  (ASPO)
1411 K St. N.W.
Washington, D.C. 20005

Association for Childbirth at Home,
  International
Box 1219
Cerritos, Cal. 90701

Cesarean Connection
c/o Cynthia Duffy
Box 11
Westmont, Ill. 60559

The Cesarean Prevention Movement
Box 152
University Station
Syracuse, N.Y. 13210

Conscious Childbirth (formerly
  Cesarean Birth Alliance)
c/o Barbara Brown Hill & Lynn
  Richards
39 Denton Avenue
E. Rockaway, N.Y. 11518

Council for Cesarean Awareness
5520 S.W. 92nd Avenue
Miami, Fla. 33165

C/SEC, Inc. (Cesareans/Support,
  Education & Concern)
22 Forest Road
Framingham, Mass. 01701

C-Section Experience of Northern
  Illinois
1220 Gentry Road
Hoffman Estates, Ill. 60195

The Farm
156 Drakes Lane
Summerstown, Tenn. 39483

HOME
511 New York Avenue
Takoma Park
Washington, D.C. 20010

Informed Homebirth
Box 788
Boulder, Colo. 80306

International Childbirth Education
  Association (ICEA)
Box 20048
Minneapolis, Minn. 55420

International Women's Council on
  Obstetrical Practices
149 Pratts Mill Road
Sudbury, Mass. 01776

La Leche League, International
9616 Minneapolis Avenue
Franklin Park, Ill. 60631

Maryland Cesarean Section
  Association
Box 10431
Baltimore, Md. 21209

National Association of Parents and
  Professionals for Safe Alternative in
  Childbirth (NAPSAC) (has directory)
Box 267
Marble Hill, Mo. 63764

Nutrition Action Group (NAG)
Box 124
Bedford Hills, N.Y. 10507

Offspring
1465 Mass. Ave.
Arlington, Mass. 02102

Psychophysiological Associates
1749 Vine Street
Berkeley, Cal. 94703

Appendix F ❧ Sample Affirmations

Woman:

I am a strong and capable woman.

I am creating a totally positive and new birth experience.

My pelvis is releasing and opening (as have those of countless women before me).

I am accepting my labor and believe that it is the right labor for *me,* and for *my baby.*

I now feel the love that others have for me during the birth.

I am treating my mate lovingly during the birth.

I have a "success consciousness."

I have a beautiful body. My body is my friend.

I now see my last birth as a learning experience, from which I am growing and changing.

I embrace the concept of healthy pain.

I am welcoming my contractions.

I have enough love to go around.

There is always enough love for me.

I am strong, confident, assured, and assertive and still feminine!

I am helping my baby feel safe so that she can be born.

Man:

I am taking care of myself during this pregnancy.

I see my wife as a strong and capable woman, and this does not threaten me.

I am supporting her during her labor, even when she is in pain.

I am expressing my love to my wife easily and frequently.

I am accepting the labor that is meant for us.

I am accepting feelings of helplessness.

I am sensitive, tender, open, and trusting.

I am feeling the love that others have for me when I need support.

Put stars by the affirmations that feel right for you. Write the affirmations many times furing the course of a week. Say them aloud, and use your name in the sentences. Then use the second and third persons. *Example:* "I, Susan, am a strong and capable woman. You, Susan, are a strong and capable woman. She, Susan, is a strong and capable woman." Add other affirmations that would be helpful to you personally.

·→ *References*

Chapter 2 • The Knife Unsheathed

1. "Actual Maternal Deaths in U.S. as Much as Double Rates Reported," NAPSAC *News*, 6 (Winter 1981), no. 4.
2. Arms, Suzanne, *Immaculate Deception* (New York: Houghton Mifflin/Bantam, 1975).
3. Avery, Mary Ellen, "Does Delivery by Section Matter to the Infant?" *New England J. Med.*, 285 (1971):917.
4. Bampton, Betsy A., & Joan M. Mancini, "The Cesarean Section Patient Is a New Mother, Too," *J. Ob. Gyn. Nursing*, 2 (July-Aug. 1973).
5. Boston Women's Health Book Collective, *Our Bodies, Ourselves* (New York: Simon & Schuster, 1971).
6. Browne, Lynn (Richards), "What Every Pregnant Woman Should Know about Cesareans," in Stewart & Stewart, *Compulsory Hospitalization* (n. 48, this chapter), 1:153–59.
7. Collins, Chase, "Random Voodoo," *Ms.* (Aug. 1977).
8. Committee on Obstetrics, Maternal and Fetal Medicine, American College of Obstetricians and Gynecologists, "Guidelines for Vaginal Delivery after a Cesarean Childbirth" (Washington, D.C.: ACOG, 7 Jan. 1982).
9. Corea, Gena, "The Cesarean Epidemic," *Mother Jones* (July 1980).
10. "Delivery after Cesarean Section," *British Med. J.* (5 July 1969).
11. Doering, Susan G., "Unnecessary Cesareans: Doctor's Choice, Parent's Dilemma," in *Compulsory Hospitalization* (n. 48, ch. 2), 1:145–52.
12. Evrard, John R., & Edwin M. Gold, "Cesarean Section and Maternal Mortality in Rhode Island: Incidence and Risk Factors 1965–1975," *Ob. Gyn.*, 50 (Nov. 1977), no. 5.
13. Gaskin, Ina May, *Spiritual Midwifery* (Summertown, Tenn.: Book Pub. Co., 1977).
14. Haire, Doris, *The Cultural Warping of Childbirth* (Milwaukee: ICEA, 1972).

15. Harrison, Michelle, A *Woman in Residence* (New York: Random House, 1982).
16. Hauskenecht, Richard, & Joan Rattner Heilman, *Having a Cesarean Baby* (New York: Dutton, 1978).
17. Hazell, Lester D., *Commonsense Childbirth* (New York: Berkeley, 1969).
18. Kitzinger, Sheila, *The Experience of Childbirth* (New York: Penguin, 1962).
19. Klaus, Marshall, et al., "Maternal Attachment: Importance of the First Post-Partum Days," *New England J. Med.* (2 Mar. 1972).
21. Knox, Richard A., "Report Urges Caesarean Policy Change," *Boston Globe* (25 Sept. 1980).
22. Knox, Richard A., "Frequency of Cesarean Birth Brings a Warning from Baird," *Boston Globe* (31 Dec. 1981).
23. Marieskind, Helen, *An Evaluation of Cesarean Section in the United States* (Washington, D.C.: Dept. of HEW, 1979).
24. McClellan, Muriel S., & William A. Cabianca, "Effects of Early Mother-Infant Contact following Cesarean Birth," *Ob. Gyn.*, 56 (July 1980), no. 1.
25. McGaughey, Harry S., Jr., Robert C. Brames, Guy M. Harbert, Jr., & W. Norman Thornton, Jr., "Pregnancy and Labor following Cesarean Section," in *Controversy in Obstetrics and Gynecology*, ed. Duncan E. Reid and T. C. Barton (Philadelphia: Saunders, 1969). Douglas, R.G., is also in Reid and Barton.
26. *Medications Used during Labor and Birth* (Milwaukee: ICEA, 1978).
27. Meyer, Linda D., *The Cesarean (R)Evolution* (Edmonds, Wash.: Charles Franklin, 1979).
28. Milinaire, Caterine, *Birth* (New York: Harmony, 1974).
29. Minkoff, Howard, & Richard H. Schwarz, "The Rising Cesarean Section Rate: Can It Be Safely Reversed?" *Ob. Gyn.*, 56 (Aug. 1980).
30. Mitchell, Kathleen, & Marty Nason, *Cesarean Birth: A Couple's Guide for Decision and Preparation* (San Francisco: Harbor, 1981).
31. Montagu, Ashley, *Touching: The Human Significance of the Skin* (New York: Harper & Row, 1978).
32. Norwood, G.A., et al., "Vaginal Delivery after Cesarean Section," *Ob. Gyn.*, 42 (1973):589.
33. National Institutes of Child Health and Human Development, *Draft Report of the Task Force on Cesarean Childbirth* (Bethesda, Md.: NIH, Sept. 1980).
34. National Institutes of Child Health and Human Development, *Cesarean Childbirth (NIH Consensus Development Conference Summary)*, vol. 3, no. 6 (Bethesda, Md.: NIH, May 1981).
35. National Institutes of Child Health and Human Development, *Cesarean Childbirth (NIH Final Report)*, (Bethesda, Md.: NIH, Oct. 1981).
36. O'Connell, W.I., "Vaginal Delivery following Cesarean Section," *Pacific Med. Surg.* (1966):343.
37. Peterson, Gayle H., *Birthing Normally* (Berkeley: Mindbody Press, 1981).
38. Pettiti, Diana, "Have Increased Cesarean Delivery Rates Resulted in Lower Neonatal Mortality Rates?" paper presented at *Birth & Family J.* Conference, San Francisco, 16 & 17 Oct. 1981.
39. Pettiti, Diana B., et al., "In-Hospital Maternal Mortality in the U.S.: Time Trends and Relation to Method of Delivery," *Ob. Gyn.*, 59 (Jan. 1982), no. 1.

40. Pfeuffer, Robbi, "The Hazards of Hospital Childbirth," *Women's Yellow Pages (New England)* (Boston: Public Works, Inc., 1978).
41. Pritchard, Jack A., & Paul C. MacDonald, *Williams Obstetrics*, 16th ed. (New York: Appleton-Century-Crofts, 1980).
42. Saldana, Louis R., "Management of Pregnancy after Cesarean Section," *Am. J. Ob. Gyn.*, 135 (1 Nov. 1979):555.
43. Salk, Lee, "The Critical Nature of the Postpartum Period in the Human for the Establishment of the Mother Infant Bond: A Controlled Study," *Diseases Nervous System*, 31 (Nov. 1970).
44. Shearer, Madeleine, "Complications of Cesarean to Mother and Infant," *Birth & Family J.*, 4 (Fall 1977), no. 3.
45. Shulman, Norma, *Labor and Vaginal Delivery after Cesarean Birth: A Survey of Contemporary Opinion* (Framingham, Mass.: C/SEC, 1979).
46. Shy, Kirkwood, James P. Longerfo, and Lawrence E. Karp, "An Evaluation of Elective Repeat Cesarean Section as a Standard of Care: An Application of Decision Analysis," *Am. J. Ob. Gyn.*, 139 (15 Jan. 1981).
47. Sokol, R., et al., "Risks Preceding Increased Primary Cesarean Birth Rates," *Ob. Gyn.*, 59 (1982):340.
48. Stewart, David, & Lee Stewart, *Compulsory Hospitalization or Freedom of Choice in Childbirth?* (Chapel Hill, N.C.: NAPSAC, 1976).
49. Stewart, David, & Lee Stewart, *Safe Alternatives in Childbirth* (Chapel Hill, N.C.: NAPSAC, 1976).
50. Stewart, David, & Lee Stewart, *21st Century Obstetrics NOW!* (Marble Hill, Mo.: NAPSAC, 1977).
51. Tilden, Virginia Peterson, & Julien G. Lipson, "Caesarean Childbirth: Variables Affecting Psychological Impact," *Western J. Nursing Research*, 3 (1981), no. 2.
52. "Vaginal Birth following Cesarean Section," *ICEA Review*, 3 (Dec. 1979).
53. Young, Diony, *Bonding* (Minneapolis: ICEA, 1978).
54. Young, Diony, "Cesareans in the U.S.: A Sobering Situation," *ICEA News*, 18 (1979), no. 4.
55. Young, Diony, & Charles Mahan, *Unnecessary Cesareans: Ways To Avoid Them* (Minneapolis: ICEA, 1970).

Chapter 4 • Grieving and Healing

1. Bampton & Mancini (n. 4, ch. 2).
2. Borg, Susan, & Judith Lasker, *When Pregnancy Fails: Families Coping with Miscarriage, Stillbirth, and Infant Death* (Boston: Beacon, 1981).
3. Cohen, Nancy Wainer, "Minimizing Sequelae of Cesarean Childbirth," *Birth & Family J.* (Fall 1977).
4. Cohen, Marion, "Cesarean Poems," *Mothering* (Summer 1980).
5. Cohen, Marion, "This Is What I Do with Kerin," *Mothering* (Fall 1980).
6. de Jim, Strange, *Visioning* (San Francisco: Ash Kar Press, 1979).

7. Deutsch, H., *Motherhood*, vol. 2 of *The Psychology of Women* (New York: Grune & Stratton, 1945).
8. Drucker, Cindie Van Hook, & Arlene Hoogerwerf, "Emotional Aspects of Cesarean Childbirth," in *Compulsory Hospitalization* (n. 48, ch. 2), vol. 3.
9. Gawain, Shakti, *Creative Visualization* (Mill Valley, Cal.: Whatever Pub., 1978).
10. Hall, Carol, "It's All Right To Cry," from the album *Free To Be . . . You and Me* (New York: Bell Records, Stereo ARIII 34408, 1972).
11. Hallet, Elizabeth, "Birth and Grief," *Birth & Family J.* (1974), no. 4.
12. Hartman, Rhondda Evans, "A Study of Factors Affecting Satisfaction with the Birth Experience," in *Compulsory Hospitalization* (n. 48, ch. 2), vol. 3.
13. Hazell (n. 17, ch. 2).
14. Klaus, Marshall H., & John H. Kennell, *Maternal Infant Bonding* (St. Louis: Mosby, 1976).
15. Kubler-Ross, Elizabeth, *On Death and Dying* (Toronto: Macmillan, 1970).
16. Kushner, Harold, *When Bad Things Happen to Good People* (New York: Schocken, 1981).
17. McClellan & Cabianca, (n. 24, ch. 2).
18. Murphy, Joseph, *The Power of Your Subconscious Mind* (Englewood, N.J.: Prentice-Hall, Reward, 1981).
19. Panuthos, Claudia, & Barbara Bierkoe-Peer, *The Emotional Ups and Downs of Childbirth* (Boston: People Place, 1981).
20. Panuthos, Claudia, and Joanne Silva, *Positive Birthing* (Boston: People Place, 1982).
21. Peterson (n. 37, ch. 2).
22. Pizer, Hank, & Christine Garfink, *Coping with a Miscarriage* (New York: Dial, 1980).
23. Ponder, Catherine, *The Dynamic Laws of Healing* (Marina del Ray, Cal.: DeVorss, 1980).
24. Robinson, Bonnie, "Facilitating Attachment following Disturbed Birth Experiences," unpublished ms., Aug. 1981.
25. Shives, Vicki, "Coping with a Miscarriage," *Parents'* (Nov. 1980).
26. Simonton, Carl, & C. Simonton, *Getting Well Again* (New York: Bantam, 1978).
27. Tilden & Lipson (n. 51, ch. 2).
28. Willmuth, L.R., "Prepared Childbirth and the Concept of Control," *J. Ob. Gyn. Nursing* (Sept.-Oct. 1975), no. 4, p. 38.

Chapter 5 • *Of Sound Mind and Belly*

1. Adair, F., "Premature Rupture of Membranes," *Am. J. Ob. Gyn.*, 44 (1942):99.
2. Adair, F., & I. Brown, "Puerperal Sterilization," *Am. J. Ob. Gyn.*, 37 (1939):472.
3. Allahbadia, N.K., "Vaginal Delivery following Cesarean Section," *Am. J. Ob. Gyn.*, 85 (15 Jan. 1963), no. 2
4. Armon, P.J., "The Management of Patients Previously Delivered by Cesarean Section," *Central African J. Med.*, 17 (Aug. 1971):170.
5. Avery (n. 3, ch. 2).

6. Berman, V.M., "Cesarean Sections" (unpublished ms., references 1963-1972).
7. Bhattacharya, A.K., and G.P. Dutta, "A Study on Rupture of the Gravid Uterus," *J. Indian Med. Assn.*, 65 (16 Oct. 1975):221.
8. Birnbaum, S.J., "Postcesarean Obstetrics," *Ob. Gyn.*, 7 (1956), no. 6.
9. Borenstein, R., et al., "External Rupture of the Uterus," *Ob. Gyn.*, 40 (Aug. 1972):211.
10. Bottoms, Sidney, et al., "The Increase in the Cesarean Birth Rate," *New England J. Med.*, 302 (6 Mar. 1980):559.
11. Bright, M.V., "Abdominal Wound Healing following Cesarean Section," *J. Royal College Surg. Edinborough*, 19 (Sept. 1974):297.
12. *British Med. J.*, "Editorial: Delivery after Cesarean Section" (5 July 1969).
13. Browne, Alan D.H., & James McGrath, "Vaginal Delivery after Previous Cesarean Section," *J. Ob. Gyn. British Commonwealth*, 72 (1965):557.
14. Browne (n. 6, ch. 2).
15. Burkons, H.F., "Ruptured Uterus," *Am. J. Ob. Gyn.*, 42 (1941):75.
16. Camillieri, A.P., & T. Busittil, "Twice a Cesarean...," *J. Ob. Gyn. British Commonwealth*, 75 (Dec. 1968):1305.
17. Carswell, William, "The Current Status of Classical Cesarean Section," *Scottish Med. J.*, 18 (1973):106.
18. Case, B.D., et al., "Cesarean Section and Its Place in Modern Obstetric Practice," *J. Ob. Gyn. British Commonwealth*, 78 (March 1971):203.
19. "Cesarean Controversy update," *Upjohn Newsletter*, Dec. 1981.
20. Cohen, Nancy Wainer, *Vaginal Birth after Cesarean* (Framingham, Mass.: C/SEC, 1974; rev. ed. 1981).
21. Corcoran, R., et al., "Letter: Uterine Scar," *Lancet* (20 Mar. 1976).
22. Cosgrove, S.A., "Cesarean Section Surgery," *Ob. Gyn.* (May 1965):616.
23. Craigin, E.B., "Conservatism in Obstetrics," *New York Med. J.*, 104 (1 July 1916), no. 1.
24. Danforth, David N., *Textbook of Obstetrics and Gynecology* (New York: Harper & Row, 1966).
25. Davydov, S.N., et al., "Cineroentgenological Study of Uterine Function and the Scar after Cesarean Section," *Vopr. Okhr. Materin. Det.*, 20 (Feb. 1975):67.
26. Dewhurst, C.J., "The Ruptured Cesarean Section Scar," *J. Ob. Gyn. British Commonwealth*, 74 (1957):113.
27. Donald, I., *Practical Obstetric Problems* (London: Lloyd Luke, 1966).
28. Donnelly, M., "Cesarean Sections: A Five-Year Survey," *Ob. Gyn.*, 7 (1956):412.
29. Donnelly, M.P., and K.T. Franzoni, "Vaginal Delivery following Cesarean Section," *Ob. Gyn.*, 29 (June 1967):871.
30. Douglas, C.P., "Rupture of the Uterus," *Nursing Times* (17 Feb. 1977).
31. Douglas, R.G., S.J. Birnbaum, & F.A. MacDonald, "Pregnancy and Labor following Cesarean Section," *Am. J. Ob. Gyn.*, 86 (Aug. 1963):961.
32. Drew-Smythe, H.J., *Modern Trends in Obstetrics and Gynecology*, ed. K. Bowes (London: Butterworth, 1950).
33. Duckering, F.A., "Delivery after C/Section," *Am. J. Ob. Gyn.*, 51 (1946):621.
34. Eames, D.M., "Management of Pregnancies Subsequent to C/Section," *Am. J. Ob. Gyn.*, 65 (1953):944.

35. Eastman, N.S., ed., *Williams Obstetrics*, 11th ed. (New York: Appleton-Century-Crofts, 1956).
36. Evrard & Gold (n. 12, ch. 2).
37. Erhardt, C.L., & E.M. Gold, "C/Section in New York City:1954–55," *Ob. Gyn.*, 11 (1958):241.
38. Ferguson, Robert K., & Duncan E. Reid, "Rupture of the Uterus: A Twenty Year Report from the Boston Lying-In Hospital," *Am. J. Ob. Gyn.*, 76 (July 1958):172.
39. Gaskin (n. 13, ch. 2).
40. Golan, A., et al., "Rupture of the Pregnant Uterus," *Ob. Gyn.*, 56 (Nov. 1980):549.
41. Granat, M., "Oxytocin Contraindicated in Presence of Uterine Scar," *Lancet* (25 Dec. 1976):1411.
42. Greenhill, J.P., "Editorial: Vaginal Delivery after Cesarean Section: Morbidity," and "Management of Delivery after Previous Cesarean Section," *Yearbook of Obstetrics and Gynecology* (Chicago: Yearbook Pub., 1975), 162.
43. Greenhill, Jacob P., *Obstetrics and Gynecology* (Chicago: Yearbook Pub., 1975).
44. Gun, K.M., "Editorial: Rupture of the Uterus," *J. Indian Med. Assn.*, 65 (1 Dec. 1975):314.
45. Guttmacher, Alan, *Pregnancy and Birth* (New York: Viking, 1962).
46. Haeri, A.D., "Comparison of Transverse and Vertical Skin Incisions for Cesarean Section," *South African Med. J.*, 50 (10 Jan. 1976):33.
47. Hawrylshyn, P., et al., "Risk Factors Associated with Infection following Cesarean Section," *Am. J. Ob. Gyn.*, 139 (1981):294.
48. Harris, J.R., "Vaginal Delivery following Cesarean Section," *Am. J. Ob. Gyn.*, 66 (Dec. 1953):1191.
49. Hills, E.R., et al., "Rupture of the Pregnant Uterus," *J. National Med. Assn.*, 66 (Jan. 1974):66.
50. Hindman, D.H., "Pelvic Delivery after C/Section," *Am. J. Ob. Gyn.*, 55 (1948):273.
51. Horowitz, B.J., et al., "Once a Cesarean Always a Cesarean?" *Ob. Gyn. Survey (supp.)*, 36 (1981):592.
52. Jerusun, M.M., and S.W. Simpson, "Vaginal Delivery following C/Section," *Am. J. Ob. Gyn.*, 75 (1958):401.
53. Jordan, Brigette, "Studying Childbirth: The Experience and Methods of a Woman Anthropologist," in *Childbirth: Alternatives to Medical Control*, ed. Shelly Romalis (Austin: Univ. of Texas, 1981).
54. Kaltreider, D.F., and W.F. Krone, "Delivery following Cesarean Section," *Clinical Ob. Gyn.*, 2 (1959):1029.
55. Keefer, F.J., et al., "Successful Pregnancy following Repair of a Ruptured Uterus," *W. Va. Med. J.*, 71 (1975):316.
56. Kerr, J.M.M., "C/Section with Special Reference to the Lower Uterine Segment," *Am. J. Ob. Gyn.* 12 (1926):729.
57. Klein, Joseph, "Perinatal Morbidity and Mortality Associated with Cesarean Sections," *Ob. Gyn.*, 16 (1960), no. 5.
58. Klein, T., et al., "Rupture of the Gravid Uterus," *J. Reproductive Med.*, 6 (May 1971):218.

59. Kessler, I., et al., "Etiological and Diagnostic Problems in Rupture of the Uterus," study done by Dept. Ob. Gyn. Hebrew Univ. Med. School, Jerusalem, 1976.

60. Klufio, C.A., et al., "The Outcome of Pregnancy and Labor following Previous Cesarean Section at the Korle Bu Teaching Hospital," *Ghana Med. J.* (June 1973):150.

61. Krone, H.A., "Maternal Mortality in Cesarean Section as Compared to Vaginal Delivery," *Fortschrift Med.*, 93 (25 Sept. 1975): 1266.

62. Kleible, H.P., et al., "Abstract: Report on 21 Uterine Ruptures and the Influence of Single Row Uterotomy Stitching on Rupture Prevention," *Geburtshilfe Frauenheilkd*, 35 (July 1975):533.

63. Lane, F.R., & D.E. Reid, "Dehiscence at Repeat C/Section," *Ob. Gyn.*, 2 (1953):54.

64. Lavin, et al., "Vaginal Delivery in Patients with a Prior Cesarean Section," *Ob. Gyn.*, 59 (Feb. 1982):135.

65. Lawler, P.E., et al., "A Review of Vaginal Delivery following Cesarean Section, from Private Practice," *Am. J. Ob. Gyn.*, 72 (Aug. 1956):252.

66. Lawrence, R.R., *J. Ob. Gyn. British Empire*, 60 (1953):237.

67. Lull, C., & J. Ullery, "Continuous Spinal Anesthesia in C/Section," *Am. J. Ob. Gyn.*, 57 (1949):1199.

68. Mason, N.R., & J.T. William, "The Strength of the Uterine Scar after Cesarean Section," *Boston Med. Soc. J.*, 162 (1910):65.

69. Macafee, C.H.G., *Irish J. Med. Science*, 38 (1958):81.

70. McGarry, J.A., "The Management of Patients Previously Delivered by Cesarean Section," *J. Ob. Gyn. British Commonwealth*, 76 (Feb. 1969):137.

71. McLane, C.M., *Am. J. Ob. Gyn.*, 20 (1930):650.

72. McTammany, J.R., "Vaginal Birth after Cesarean," in *Compulsory Hospitalization* (n. 48, ch. 2), vol. 1.

73. Meehan, F.P., et al., "Vaginal Delivery with Caudal Anesthesia after Cesarean Section," *British Med. J.*, 2 (1972):740.

74. Mendelsohn, Robert, *Mal(e) Practice* (Chicago: Contemporary, 1981).

75. Meier, Paul, "Trial of Labor after Cesarean Section," paper presented at *Birth & Family J.* Conference, San Francisco, 16 & 17 Oct. 1981.

76. Merrill, Berkeley S., & C.E. Gibbs, "Planned Vaginal Delivery following Cesarean Section," *Ob. Gyn.*, 52 (July 1978):40.

77. Minkoff & Schwarz (n. 29, ch. 2).

78. Mokgokong, E., & E. Marivate, "Treatment of the Ruptured Uterus," *South African Med. J.* (Sept. 1976).

79. Norwood, et al. (n. 32, ch. 2).

80. Morley, G.W., "Once a Cesarean, Always a Cesarean?" *J. Am. Med. Assn.*, 178 (1961):1128.

81. Mowat, James, "Abdominal Wound Dehiscence after Cesarean Section," *British Med. J.* (May 1971).

82. Mphahlel, M., "The Outcome of Labour following Previous Cesarean Section," *South African Med. J.*, 46 (1972):1851.

83. Murphy, Harry, "Delivery following Cesarean Section: Ten Years Experience at the Rotunda Hospital, Dublin," *Irish Med. J.*, 69 (1976):533.
84. Mussenden-Jackson, C., "Once a Cesarean, Always a Cesarean Not Always True," *Ob. Gyn. News* (1 Oct. 1981).
85. National Institutes of Child Health (n. 34, ch. 2).
86. Notelovitz, M., & D. Chrichton, *South African Med. J.*, 41 (1967):323.
87. "Never on a Sunday or Holiday," *Alive Magazine*, no. 36 (June 1981).
88. O'Connell (n. 36, ch. 2).
89. O'Driscoll, K., "Rupture of the Uterus," *Royal Soc. Med. Proc.*, 59 (1966):65.
90. Oxorn-Foote, *Human Labor and Birth*, 4th ed. (New York: Appleton-Century-Crofts, 1980).
91. Palerme, G.R., and E.A. Friedman, "Rupture of the Gravid Uterus in the Third Trimester," *Am. J. Ob. Gyn.*, 94 (1966):571.
92. Pauerstein, Carl, "Once a Section, Always a Trial of Labor? *Ob. Gyn.* 28 (Aug. 1966), no. 2.
93. Pauerstein, Carl, et al., "Trial of Labor after Low Segment Cesarean Section," *Southern Med. J.* (Aug. 1969).
94. Pearce, D.J., et al., "Letter: Rupture of Uterine Scar in a Patient Given Epidural Analgesia," *Lancet*, 1 (29 May 1976): 1177.
95. Peel, J., *J. Ob. Gyn. British Cwlth*, 75 (1968):1282.
96. Pettiti, Diana, et al., "Cesarean Sections in California: 1960–1975," *Am. J. Ob. Gyn.*, 133 (1979), no. 4.
97. Poidevin, L., *Cesarean Section Scars* (Springfield, Ill.: Thomas, 1965).
98. Pritchard & MacDonald (n. 41, ch. 2).
99. Rehns, Marsha, "Debate: Are Repeat Cesareans Necessary?" *Childbirth Educator*, 1 (Oct. 1981).
100. Reid and Barton, *Controversy in Obstetrics* (Philadelphia: Saunders, 1969).
101. Research Resource Reporter, "Number of Cesarean Deliveries Can Be Reduced," 5 (Oct. 1981), U.S. Dept. Health & Human Services, P.H.S., NIH Bldg. 31, Rm. 5B13, Bethesda, Md. 20205.
102. Richards, Lynn, & Barbara Brown-Hill, VBAC *Workbook: A Self-Help Guide for Parents and Professionals in Preparation for the* VBAC *Experience* (S. Hadley, Mass.: J.F. Bergin Publishers, Inc.), 1983.
103. Riva, H., & J. Breen, "Analysis of 100 Consecutive Vaginal Deliveries following Cesarean Section," *Am. J. Ob. Gyn.*, 76 (1958):192.
104. Riva, H., & J. Teich, "Vaginal Delivery after Cesarean Section," *Am. J. Ob. Gyn.*, 81 (1961):501.
105. Rubin, L.L., et al., "Maternal Death after Cesarean Section in Georgia," *Am. J. Ob. Gyn.*, 139 (15 Mar. 1981).
106. Ruiz-Velasco, V., et al., *J. Gyn. Ob. Biol. Reprod.* (Paris, Sept. 1973): 673.
107. Saldana (n. 42, ch. 2).
108. Salzmann, B., "Rupture of Low-Segment Cesarean Section Scars," *Ob. Gyn.* 23 (1964):460.
109. Schmitz, H.E., & G.R. Baba, "Vaginal Delivery following C/Section," *Am. J. Ob. Gyn.*, 57 (1949):669.
110. Schmitz, H.E., & G.J. Gajewski, *Am. J. Ob. Gyn.*, 61 (1951):1232–41.

111. Schwartz, O.H., "The Cesarean Scar," *Am. J. Ob. Gyn.*, 36 (1938):962.
112. Shearer, Elizabeth, "NIH Consensus Development Task Force on Cesarean Childbirth: The Process and the Result," *Birth & Family J.*, 8 (Spring 1981):1.
113. Shearer, Elizabeth, "Education for VBAC," *Birth & Family J.*, 9 (Spring 1982):1.
114. Shy et al. (n. 46, ch. 2).
115. Silfen, S., & R. Wilf, "Summary on Booth Maternity Hospital's Services of VBACs," paper presented to the *Birth & Family J.* Conference, San Francisco, 16 & 17 Oct. 1981).
116. Skelly, H.R., et al., "Rupture of the Uterus: The Preventable Factors," *South African Med. J.*, 50 (24 Mar. 1976):505.
117. Smith, A.M., "Letter: Rupture of the Gravid Uterus," *Lancet*, 1 (22 Jan. 1977):195.
118. Smith, A.M., "Letter: Uterine Rupture in Labor," *British Med. J.* (24 May 1976):446.
119. Sokol et al. (n. 47, ch. 2).
120. Sorokin, Yoram, "Should All Previous Cesarean Sections Be Sectioned Again?" (unpublished manuscript, 1979).
121. Stone, Martin, ed., "Changing Indications for Cesarean Section," *ACOG Update*, 4 (1981), no. 11.
122. Timonen, S., et al., *Ann. Chir. Gyn.*, 59 (1970):173.
123. Waniorek, A., "Hysterography after C/Section," *Ob. Gyn.*, 29 (1967):192.
124. Waters, E.G., "Use and Abuse of C/Section," *Am. J. Surg.*, 69 (1945):208.
125. Wilson, A., "Labor and Delivery after C/Section," *Am. J. Ob. Gyn.*, 62 (1951):125.
126. Wilson, St. George, *J. Ob. Gyn. British Empire*, 38 (1931):504.
127. Wolfson, A., & M. Lancet, "Management of Postcesarean Deliveries," *Ob. Gyn.*, 6 (1955):625.
128. Young (n. 54, ch. 2).
129. Zarou, E.S., "Analysis of 400 Consecutive C/Sections," *Am. J. Ob. Gyn.*, 63 (1952):122.

Chapter 6 • The Fallacy of Natural Childbirth

1. Arms (n. 2, ch. 2).
2. Bean, Constance, *Labor and Delivery: An Observer's Diary* (New York: Doubleday, 1977).
3. Berezin, Nancy, *The Gentle Birth Book* (New York: Pocket Books, 1951).
4. Browne, Lynn (Richards) (n. 6, ch. 2).
5. Davis, Elizabeth, "Energy Cycles in Pregnancy and Childbirth," *Yoga* (May-June 1980), no. 32.
6. Dick-Read, Grantly, *Childbirth without Fear* (New York: Harper, 1944).
7. Doering, Susan G. (n. 11, ch. 2).
8. Frank, Lawrence, *On The Importance of Infancy* (New York: Random House, 1969).
9. Gaskin (n. 13, ch. 2).
10. Hazell (n. 17, ch. 2).
11. Milinaire (n. 28, ch. 2).

12. Montague (n. 31, ch. 2).

13. Peterson (n. 37, ch. 2).

14. Pfeuffer (n. 40, ch. 2).

15. Rosen, M., & L. Rosen, *In the Beginning: Your Baby's Brain before Birth* (New York: Plume, 1975).

16. Schwartz, Leni, *The World of the Unborn* (New York: Richard Marek, 1980).

17. Speir, Bonnie, *Birth Whole for Optimal Health* (Open Eden, 1231A Oxford St., Berkeley, Cal. 94709, 1980).

18. Stewart & Stewart (n. 49, ch. 2).

19. Stewart & Stewart (n. 48, ch. 2).

20. Stewart & Stewart (n. 50, ch. 2).

21. Tanzer, Deborah, *Why Natural Childbirth?* (New York: Schocken, 1976).

22. Verny, Thomas, & John Kelly, *The Secret Life of the Unborn Child* (New York: Summit, 1981).

23. Young (n. 53 ch. 2).

Chapter 7 • Increasing Your Potential for Normal Birth

1. Bing, Elisabeth, *Moving through Pregnancy* (New York: Bantam, 1980).

2. Breams, Marianne, *Swim for Fitness* (San Francisco: Chronicle, 1979).

3. Brewer, Gail, *What Every Pregnant Woman Should Know: The Truth about Diet and Drugs in Pregnancy* (New York: Random House, 1977).

4. Brewer, Thomas, *Metabolic Toxemia of Late Pregnancy: A Disease of Malnutrition* (New Canaan, Conn.: Keats, 1982).

5. Clark, James W., *Clinical Dentistry*, vol. 1: *Local Anesthesia* (New York: Harper & Row, 1980).

6. Coffin, Lewis A., *The Grandmother Conspiracy Exposed* (Santa Barbara, Cal.: Capra, 1974).

7. Committee on Public Information, *Diet and Hyperactivity: Any Connection?* (Chicago: Institute of Food Technologists, 1976).

8. Dilfer, Carol, *Your Baby, Your Body* (New York: Crown, 1977).

9. Dufty, William, *Sugar Blues* (New York: Warner, 1976).

10. Ewald, Ellen Buchman, *Recipes for a Small Planet* (New York: Ballantine, 1973).

11. *The Farm Vegetarian Cookbook* (Summertown, Tenn.: Book Pub. Co., 1975).

12. *FDA Drug Bulletin*, "Surgeon General's Advisory on Alcohol and Pregnancy," 1 (July 1981), no. 2.

13. Gardner, Joy, *Healing the Family: Pregnancy, Birth and Children's Ailments* (New York: Bantam, 1982).

14. Gaskin (n. 13, ch. 2).

15. Gawain, Chi-uh, *Yoga with the Unborn* (Mill Valley, O.: Whatever Pub., 1980).

16. Glasser, Ronald, *The Greatest Battle* (New York: Random House, 1976).

17. Goldbeck, Nikki, & David Goldbeck, *The Supermarket Handbook* (New York: New American Library, Signet, 1976).

18. Hyland, Jackie, "The Sugar Pushers" (source unknown).

19. Jelliffe, D.B., & E.F.P. Jelliffe, "The Uniqueness of Human Milk," *Am. J. Clinical Nutrition*, 24 (Aug. 1971).
20. Johnson, Roberta B., ed., *Whole Foods for the Whole Family* (Franklin Park, Ill.: La Leche League, 1981).
21. Jones, Lyn, & Pam England, "Herbs for Pregnancy and Birth," *Mothering* (Spring 1982).
22. Katzen, Mollie, ed., *The Enchanted Broccoli Forest* (Berkeley: Ten Speed, 1982).
23. Katzen, Mollie, ed., *The Moosewood Cookbook* (Berkeley: Ten Speed, 1977).
24. Kimball, Charles, "Commentary: Endorphins and Analgesia," *ICEA Review*, 4 (Dec. 1980), no. 3.
25. Kinderlehren, Jane, *Confessions of a Sneaky Organic Cook* (Emmaus, Pa.: Rodale/New American Library, 1971).
26. Kramer, H.S., & V.A. Milton, "Complications of Local Anesthetics," in *Dental Clinics of North America*, ed. C.C. Alling, 17 (July 1973):443.
27. La Leche League, *Whole Foods for the Whole Family* (Franklin Park, Ill.: La Leche League, 1981).
28. La Leche League, *The Womanly Art of Breastfeeding* (Franklin Park, Ill.: La Leche League, 1981).
29. Lance, Kathryn, *Running for Health and Beauty* (New York: Bantam, 1978).
30. Lansky, Vicki, *Feed Me I'm Yours* (Wayzata, Minn.: Meadowbrook, 1978).
31. Lappé, Frances Moore, *Diet for a Small Planet* (New York: Ballantine, 1975).
32. Montague, Ashley, *Life before Birth* (New York: New American Library, Signet, 1978).
33. Naeye, R.I., "Update on Maternal Weight Gain and Pregnancy Outcome," *Modern Med.* (30 Jan.–15 Feb. 1980).
34. Noble, Elizabeth, *Essential Exercises for the Childbearing Year* (Boston: Houghton Mifflin, 1976).
35. Nofziger, Margaret, *A Healthy Pregnancy on a Vegetarian Diet* (Summertown, Tenn.: The Farm, 1975).
36. Null, Gary, & Steve Null, *The Complete Handbook of Nutrition* (New York: Dell, 1972).
37. *Nutrition in Pregnancy: An Annotated Bibliography of Scientific Studies* (Chicago: Society for the Protection of the Unborn through Nutrition, 1981).
38. Odent, Michel, "The Evolution of Obstetrics at Pithiviers," *Birth & Family J.*, 8 (Spring 1981), no. 2.
39. Parvati, Jeanine, *Hygieia: A Woman's Herbal* (Berkeley: Freestone, 1979).
40. Pirani, et al., "Smoking during Pregnancy: Its Effects on Maternal Metabolism and Fetoplacental Functioning," *J. Ob. Gyn.*, 52 (Sept. 1978), no. 3.
41. Pryor, Karen, *Nursing Your Baby* (New York: Pocketbooks, 1973).
42. Ray, Sondra, *The Only Diet There Is* (Millbrae, Cal.: Celestial Arts, 1981).
43. Ribble, Margaret, *The Rights of Infants* (New York: Signet, 1973).
44. Robertson, Laurel, et al., *Laurel's Kitchen* (Petaluma, Cal.: Nilgiri, Bantam, 1976).
45. Rodale Press Editors, *Be a Healthy Mother, Have a Healthy Baby* (Emmaus, Pa.: Rodale, 1973).
46. Rosen, Mortimer, & Lynne Rosen, *Your Baby's Brain before Birth* (New York: New American Library, 1975).

47. Shute, Wilfred, "Recent Vitamin E Research," *C/SEC Newsletter*, 1 (Spring-Summer 1976), no. 2.
48. Smith, Lendon, *Feed Your Kids Right* (New York: Delta, 1979).
49. Smith, Lendon, *Improving Your Child's Behavior Chemistry: A New Way to Raise Happier Children into Healthier Adults* (Englewood Cliffs, N.J.: Prentice-Hall, 1976).
50. "Smoking: The Truth No One Else Will Print," *Mother Jones* (Jan. 1979).
51. Taub, Harold, ed., *Natural Health and Pregnancy* (New York: Pyramid, 1968).
52. Urbanowski, F., *Yoga for New Parents* (New York: Harper & Row, 1975).
53. Weathersbee, Paul, & Robert Lodge, "Alcohol, Caffeine and Nicotine Usage in Pregnancy," *U.S. Pharmacist* (Mar. 1981).
54. Williams, Phyllis, *Nourishing Your Unborn Child* (New York: Avon, 1975).
55. Wynne, Margaret, & Arthur Wynne, "The Importance of Maternal Nutrition in the Weeks before and after Conception," *Birth*, 9 (Spring 1982), no. 1.
56. Yamamoto, Koji, and Joanna Yamamoto, "Exercising for Easy Childbirth," *East/West J.* (April 1980):76.
57. Zucker, Martin, "Childbirth Made Easier with Vitamin C," *Let's Live*, 47 (Oct. 1979), no. 10.

Chapter 8 • Diagnostic Time Bombs?

INFORMED CONSENT?

1. American College of Obstetricians and Gynecologists, *Standards for Obstetric-Gynecologic Services*, 5th ed. (Washington, D.C.: ACOG, 1982), p. 108.
2. Annas, George, *The Rights of Hospital Patients* (New York: Avon, 1975).
3. Elkins, Valma, *Rights of the Pregnant Parent* (New York: Shocken, 1976).
4. Stewart, David, "Informed Consent," *ICEA News*, 17 (1978), no. 1.
5. Stimeling, Gary, "Will Common Delivery Techniques Soon Become Malpractice?" *J. Legal Med.* (May 1975).
6. *Patient's Bill of Rights* (Boston: Blue Cross Blue Shield of Mass, 1979).
7. *The Pregnant Patient's Bill of Rights and Responsibilities* (Minneapolis: ICEA, n.d.).
8. Young, Diony, "Ethical Considerations for American Obstetricians Approved," *ICEA News*, 21 (Aug. 1982), no. 3.

WOMEN AS LAB RATS

9. Corea, Gena, *Hidden Malpractice: How American Medicine Mistreats Women* (New York: JOVE, 1977).
10. Daly, Mary, *Gyn/Ecology* (Boston: Beacon, 1978).
11. Dworkin, Andrea, *Our Blood* (New York: Perigree, 1981).
12. "Human Milk, Nutrition, and the World Resource Crisis," *Science*, 1975.
13. *ICEA Sharing*, "New Device Tested—A New Intra-Penal Contraceptive," vol. 3 (1975), no. 3.

14. Larned, Deborah, "The Epidemic of Unnecessary Hysterectomy," in *Seizing our Bodies*, ed. Claudia Dreifus (New York: Vintage, 1978).
15. Ratner, Herbert, ed., "Medical Hazards of the Birth Control Pill," *Child & Family* (Dec. 1969).
16. Seaman, Barbara, "The Dangers of Oral Contraception," in Dreifus (n. 14, this chapter).
17. Schorr, Daniel, *Don't Get Sick in America* (Nashville: Aurora, 1970).
18. Weiss, Kay, "What Medical Students Learn about Women," in Dreifus (n. 14, this chapter).

ULTRASOUND

19. Abdulla, Usama, et al., "Effects of Diagnostic Ultrasound on Maternal and Fetal Chromosomes," *Lancet* (16 Oct. 1971).
20. Bichler, Joyce, *DES Daughter* (New York: Avon, 1981).
21. Bolsen, Barbara, "Question of Risk Still Hovers over Routine Prenatal Use of Ultrasound," *JAMA Med. News*, 247 (23 Apr. 1982).
22. "Diagnostic Ultrasound Equipment," *Federal Register*, 44 (13 Feb. 1979), no. 31.
23. Dilanni, Denisce, "Ultrasound," *Mothering* (Summer 1982).
24. Liebeskind, D., "Diagnostic Ultrasound: Effects on the DNA Growth Patterns of Animal Cells," *Radiology*, 131 (April 1979):177.
25. *Microwaves and Radiowaves*, CIP Bulletin, Center for the Biology of Natural Systems (St. Louis: Washington Univ. 1980).
26. Shearer, M., ed., "The Risks of Diagnostic Ultrasound—a Literature Survey and a Response," *Birth & Family J.*, 4 (Fall 1977).
27. Shearer, M., "The Risks of Fetal Monitoring from the Consumer's Point of View," lecture given at Newton Wellesley Hospital, Boston, in 1978.
28. Sherman, Carl, "Biological Effects of Ultrasound on Mother, Fetus Are Considered," *Ob. Gyn. News* (15 May 1982).
29. Stewart & Stewart (n. 48, ch. 2).
30. Stratmeyer, M.E., "Research in Ultrasound Bioeffects: A Public Health View," *Birth & Family J.*, 7 (Summer 1980).
31. Sweet, Gail Grenier, "Diagnostic Ultrasound," *Mothering* (Spring 1981).
32. Transcript of Cable News Network Program on Ultrasound, New York (May 1982).
33. Wright, Margaret, "How To Avoid an Ultrasound Scan," AIMS (Assn. for Improvements in Maternity Services), 21 Franklin Gardens, Hitchin, Hertshire, England (1982).

AMNIOCENTESIS, OCTS, NON-STRESS TESTS

34. Brewer, Gail, & Janice Presser Greene, *Right from the Start* (Emmaus, Pa.: Rodale, 1981).
35. Chayen, S., ed., "An Assessment of the Hazards of Amniocentesis," *British J. Ob. Gyn.*, 85 (Supp. 2, 1978).
36. Edwards, M., & Penny Simkin, *Obstetric Tests & Technology: A Consumer Guide* (Seattle: Pennypress, 1980).

37. Ettner, Frederick, "Hospital Technology Breeds Pathology," *Women & Health*, 2 (Oct. 1977).
38. Evarts, Lucy, "Amniocentesis Benefits and Risks," *Childbirth Alternatives Quarterly*, 3 (Fall 1981).
39. Freeman, R., "An Evaluation of the Significance of a Positive Oxytocin Challenge Test," *Ob. Gyn.*, 47 (1976): 1.
40. Gluck, L., "Iatrogenic RDS and Amniocentesis," *Hospital Practice*, 12 (17 Mar. 1977): 11.
41. King, James F., "More Muddy Water: Antepartum Fetal Assessment Techniques," *ICEA News*, 20 (Nov. 1981).
42. "The Obstetrician's Dilemma," *Med. J. Australia* (4 Dec. 1976).
43. Patrick, John, ed., *Seminars in Perinatology*, 4 (Oct 1980).
44. Teramo, K., & S. Sipinen, "Spontaneous Rupture of Fetal Membranes after Amniocentesis, *Am. J. Ob. Gyn.*, 52 (Sept 1978).

X-RAYS

45. Bottoms et al. (n. 10, ch. 5).
46. Caldicott, Helen, *New Directions for Women*, 9 (Jan.-Feb. 1980).
47. Campbell, J. A., "X-Ray Pelvimetry: Useful Procedure or Medical Nonsense?" *J. National Med. Assn.*, 68 (1976):514.
48. *FDA Drug Bulletin*, "Statement on Use of Pelvimetry X-Ray Examination" (Nov. 1981).
49. Fine, E., et al., "An Evaluation of the Usefulness of X-Ray Pelvimetry: Comparison of the Thoms and Modified Balls Methods with Manual Pelvimetry," *Ob. Gyn.*, 137 (1980):15.
50. Gaskin (n. 13, ch. 2).
51. Hannah, Walter, "X-Ray Pelvimetry: A Critical Appraisal," *Am. J. Ob. Gyn.*, 91 (1965), no. 3.
52. Jagani, N., et al., "The Predictability of Labor Outcome from a Comparison of Birth Weight and X-Ray Pelvimetry," *Am. J. Ob. Gyn.* (1 Mar. 1981).
53. Joyce, D., et al., "Role of Pelvimetry in Active Management of Labor," *British Med. J.*, 4 (1975):505.
54. Kelly, K., et al., "The Utilization and Efficacy of Pelvimetry," *Am. J. Roentgenology*, 125 (1975):66.
55. Laube, D.W., et al., "A Prospective Evaluation of X-Ray Pelvimetry," *J. Am. Med. Assn.*, 246 (1981):2187.
56. Macht, S., & P. Lawrence, "Congenital Malformations from Exposure to Roentgen Radiation," *Am. J. Roentgenology*, 73 (1955):442.
57. Marieskind, Helen, *An Evaluation of Caesarean Section in the United States* (Seattle: U.S. Dept. HEW, 1979).
58. Mendelsohn (n. 74, ch. 5)
59. Meyer, M., et al., "Long Term Effects of Prenatal X-Ray on Development and Fertility of Human Females," *Biological & Environmental Effects of Low Level Radiation*, vol. 2 (Vienna: International Atomic Energy Commission, 1976).

60. Miller, R., & W.J. Blot, "Small Head Size after In-Utero Exposure to Atomic Radiation," *Lancet* (14 Oct. 1972).
61. Stewart, A.J., et al., "A Survey of Childhood Malignancies," *British Med. J.*, 1 (1958):1495.
62. U.S. Department of Health and Human Services, *The Selection of Patients for X-Ray Examinations: The Pelvimetry Examination* (Rockville, Md.: Bureau of Radiological Health, 1980).
63. Varner , M., et al., "X-Ray Pelvimetry in Clinical Obstetrics," *Ob. Gyn.*, 56 (Sept. 1980).

Chapter 9 • Birth Interventions

LABOR BEGINS

1. Akil, H., et al., "Antagonism of Stimulation: Produced Analgesia by Naloxone, a Narcotic Antagonist," *Science*, 191 (1976):961.
2. Arnold, Linda, *Nine Months: Songs of Pregnancy and Birth* (Santa Cruz: Ariel Records, Arnold, 1979).
3. Bean (n. 2, ch. 6).
4. Bombeck, Erma, "Giving Birth to Immodesty," *Boston Globe* (28 Feb. 1978).
5. Brewer & Greene (n. 34, ch. 8).
6. Cogan, R., ed., "Endorphins and Analgesia," *ICEA Review*, 4 (Dec. 1980).
7. Davis, Elizabeth, *Guide to Midwifery: Heart and Hands* (Santa Fe, N.M.: John Muir, 1981).
8. Gaskin (n. 13, ch. 2).
9. Gintzler, Alan, "Endorphin-Mediated Increases in Pain Threshold during Pregnancy," *Science*, 210 (1980):192.
10. Haire (n. 14, ch. 2).
11. Kloosterman, G.J., *MAMA [Mid-Hudson Area Maternity Alternatives] News*, 2 (Nov.-Dec. 1979).
12. Kimball, Charles, "Commentary," *ICEA Review*, 4 (Dec. 1980).
13. Korte, Diana, & Roberta Scaer, "A Survey of Maternal Preferences: What Mothers Want—Not What They Have," in *Compulsory Hospitalization* (n. 48, ch. 2), vol. 3.
14. Luce, Judith, "Childbirth without Mothers: More Violence against Women," *Sister Courage* (Apr. 1976).
15. "Maternal Stress and Pregnancy Outcome," ed. S. MacKay, *ICEA Review*, 4 (Apr. 1980).
16. Mendelsohn, (n. 74, ch. 5).
17. Montague, Ashley, "Social Impacts of Unnecessary Intervention and Unnatural Surroundings in Childbirth," in *21st Century Obstetrics Now!* (n. 50, ch. 2).
18. Odent, Michel, "The Evolution of Obstetrics at Pithiviers," *Birth & Family J.*, 8 (Spring 1981).

19. Phillips, E., *Obstetrics and Gynecology Combined for Students* (London: Lewis, 1962).
20. Shearer, Elizabeth, "The Art of Labor Support," *Childbirth Educator* (Fall 1981).
21. Sobel, D., "The Hospital Fever," *Harvard* (May-June 1978).

MATERNAL POSITION IN LABOR

22. Andrews, Claire M., "Changing Fetal Position," *J. Nurse Midwifery*, 25 (Jan.-Feb. 1980).
23. Caldeyro-Barcia, R., "Some Consequences of Obstetrical Interferences," *Birth & Family J.*, 2 (1977):34, 73.
24. Caldeyro-Barcia, R., "The Influence of Maternal Position on Time of Spontaneous Rupture of the Membranes, Progress of Labor, and Fetal Head Compression," *Birth & Family J.*, 6 (Spring 1979).
25. Carr, Katherine Camacho, "Obstetric Practices Which Protect against Neonatal Morbidity: Focus on Maternal Position in Labor and Birth," *Birth & Family J.*, 7 (1980):249.
26. Flynn A., & J. Kelly, "Ambulation in Labour," *British Med. J.*, 2 (1976):842.
27. Huch, A., & R. Huch, "Transcutaneous, Noninvasive Monitoring of PO_2," *Hospital Practices*, 11 (June 1970):6.
28. Kitzinger, Sheila, *Women as Mothers* (Glascow: Fontana, 1978).
29. Mackay, Susan, ed., "Maternal Position during Labor and Birth," *ICEA Review*, 2 (Summer 1978).
30. Mendez-Bauer, C., et al., "Effects of Standing Position on Spontaneous Uterine Contractility and Other Aspects of Labor," *J. Perinatal Med.*, 3 (1975):89.
31. Miller, Frank C., "Ambulation and Measurement of Uterine Efficiency," *Birth & Family J.*, 8 (Fall 1981).
32. Read, J.A., F.C. Miller, & R.H. Paul, "A Randomized Trial of Ambulation versus Oxytocin for Labor Enhancement," *Am. J. Ob. Gyn.*, 139 (15 Mar. 1981).
33. Roberts, J.E., "Alternative Positions for Labor," *J. Nurse Midwifery*, 25(4) (1980):11.
34. Roberts, J.E., & C. Mendez-Bauer, "A Perspective on Maternal Position during Labor, *J. Perinatal Med.*, 8 (1980):255.
35. Roberts, Joyce, "Which Position for First Stage?" *Childbirth Educator* (Summer 1982).
36. "Supine Called Worst Position during Labor and Delivery," *Ob. Gyn. News* (1 June, 1975).

THE "PREP," I.V.S, EATING DURING LABOR

37. Birnbaum, D.A., "The Iatrogenesis of Damaged Mothers and Newborns," in *21st Century Obstetrics Now!* (n. 50, ch. 2).
38. Brewer (n. 34, ch. 8).
39. Haire (n. 14, ch. 2).
40. Kenepp, N., et al., "Effects on Newborn of Hydration with Glucose in Patients Undergoing Ceserean Section with Regional Anesthesia," *Lancet* (22 Mar. 1980).

41. Kitzinger, Sheila, "Second Stage," lecture given at Boston College, Boston, in November 1981.
42. Mendelsohn (n. 74, ch. 5).
43. Nimmo W., et al., "Narcotic Analgesics and Delayed Gastric Emptying during Labor," *Lancet* (19 Apr. 1975).
44. Phillips (n. 19, this chapter).

AMNIOTOMY . . . AND INFECTION

45. Abramovici, H., et al., "Meconium during Delivery: A Sign of Compensated Fetal Distress," *Am. J. Ob. Gyn.*, 118 (1974):251.
46. Althabe, O., "Influence of the Rupture of Membranes on Compression of the Fetal Head during Labor," paper presented at Pan American Health Organization's Conference on Perinatal Factors Affecting Human Development, Washington, D.C., 1969.
47. "Amniocentesis May Increase Fetal Loss, Morbidity," *Ob. Gyn. News*, 14 (1 Apr. 1979).
48. Brewer (n. 34, ch. 8).
49. Brotanek, V., & J. Hodr, "Fetal Distress after Artificial Rupture of Membrane," *Am. J. Ob. Gyn.*, 101 (1968):542.
50. Caldeyro-Barcia, R., et al., "Adverse Perinatal Effects of Early Amniotomy during Labor," in *Modern Perinatal Medicine*, ed. L. Gluck (Chicago: Year Book Medical, 1974).
51. Caldeyro-Barcia, R., et al., "Effects of Rupture of Membranes on Fetal Heart Rate Pattern," *International Gyn. Ob.*, 10 (1972):169.
52. Caldeyro-Barcia, R. (n. 23, this chapter).
53. Ettner, Frederick, "Hospital Technology Breeds Pathology," *Women & Health*, 2 (Oct. 1979).
54. Gabbe, S.G., et al., "Umbilical Cord Compression Associated with Amniotomy: Laboratory Observations," *Am. J. Ob. Gyn.*, 126 (1976):353.
55. Granat, M., "Oxytocin Contraindicated in Presence of Uterine Scar," *Lancet* (25 Dec. 1976):1411.
56. Holland, E., "Cranial Stress in the Fetus during Labor," *J. Ob. Gyn. British Empire*, 19 (1922):549.
57. *Lancet*, "Oxytocic Drugs Associated with Uterine Rupture," (Dec. 1976).
58. McKay, S., ed., "Amniotomy," *ICEA Review*, 3 (Summer 1979).
59. Meis, Paul, et al. "Late Meconium Passage in Labor: A Sign of Fetal Distress," *Ob. Gyn.*, 59 (1982):332.
60. Mendelsohn (n. 74, ch. 5).
61. Ment, L., et al., "Neonates with Seizures Attributable to Perinatal Complications," *Am. J. Diseases of Children*, 136 (1982):548.
62. Miller, F., et al., "Significance of Meconium during Labor," *Am. J. Ob. Gyn.*, 122 (1975):573.
63. Muller, P.F., et al. "Perinatal Factors and Their Relationship to Mental Retardation and Other Parameters of Development," *Am. J. Ob. Gyn.*, 109 (1971):1205.
64. Peterson (n. 37, ch. 2).

65. Saldana (n. 42, ch. 2).

66–67. Schwartz, et al., "Fetal Heart Rate Patterns in Labors with Intact and with Ruptured Membranes," *J. Perinatal Med.*, 1 (1973):153.

68. Schwarcz, R., et al., "Influence of Amniotomy and Maternal Position on Labor," *Proceedings*, 8th World Congress on Gynecology and Obstetrics, Mexico, 1976, p. 377.

69. Zalen, Richard, & Edward Quilligan, "The Influence of Scalp Sampling in the Cesarean Section Rate for Fetal Distress," *Am. J. Ob. Gyn.* 135 (1979):239.

FETAL MONITORING

70. Banta, D., & S. Thacker, "Electronic Fetal Monitoring: Is It of Benefit?" *Birth & Family J.*, 6 (Winter 1979).

71. Chard, Tim, & Martin Richards, ed., *Benefits and Hazards of the New Obstetrics* (Philadelphia: Lippincott, 1977).

72. Ettner, Frederick, "Hospital Technology Breeds Pathology," *Women & Health*, 2 (Sept.-Oct. 1977).

73. Feminist Health Works, reprint on Internal Fetal Heart Monitoring, 231 Centre St., New York, N.Y. 10013.

74. "Fetal Monitoring: For Better or Worse?" *Harvard University Focus* (10 Dec. 1981).

75. Fernandez-Rocher, L., and H. Oulette, "Fetal Bleeding: An Unusual Complication of Fetal Monitoring," *Am. J. Ob. Gyn.*, 125 (1976):1153.

76. Gassner, C.B., and W.J. Ledger, "The Relationship of Hospital-Acquired Maternal Infection to Invasive Intrapartum Monitoring Techniques," *Am. J. Gyn.*, 126 (1976):33.

77. Haverkamp, Albert, "Does Anyone Need Fetal Monitors?" in *Compulsory Hospitalization* (n. 48, ch. 2), vol. 1.

78. Haverkamp, A.D., et al., "The Evaluation of Continuous Heart Rate Monitoring in High Risk Pregnancy," *Am. J. Ob. Gyn.*, 125 (1976):310.

79. Hughey, M., et al., "The Effect of Monitoring on the Incidence of Cesarean Section," *Ob. Gyn.*, 49 (May 1977).

80. Jarzembski, W.B., "Benefits, Limitations, Fallacies, and Hazards of Electronic Monitoring of the Human Body," in *Compulsory Hospitalization* (n. 48, ch. 2), vol. 1.

81. Katz, Barbara, "Electronic Fetal Monitoring and the Law," *Birth & Family J.*, 6 (1979):251.

82. Kitzinger (n. 41, this chapter).

83. Low, et al., "Prediction of Intrapartum Fetal Acidosis by Fetal Heart Rate Monitoring," *Am. J. Ob. Gyn.*, 139 (1981):299.

84. Low, J., et al., *"The Prediction of Intrapartum Fetal Metabolic Acidosis by Fetal Heart Rate Monitoring,"* *Am. J. Ob. Gyn.*, 139 (1981): 299.

85. Marieskind (n. 57, ch. 8).

86. Mendelsohn (n. 74, ch. 5).

87. Murphy, J.R., et al., "The Relation of Electronic Fetal Monitoring Patterns to Infant Outcomes," *Am. J. Epidemiology*, 114 (1981):539.

88. *NAPSAC News*, "Fetal Monitors Spread Infectious Germs—NIH," 5 (1980), no. 2.

89. Oestreicher, Annette, "ACOG Backs Fetal Monitoring Despite Tie to More Cesareans," *Med. Tribune* (18 June 1980).

90. Paul, R.H., & E.H. Hon, "Clinical Fetal Monitoring," *Am. J. Ob. Gyn.*, 118 (1974), no. 4.

91. Sarah, Becky, "Electronic Fetal Monitoring—How Safe Is It?" *Family J.*, 2 (July-Aug. 1982).

92. Shearer, Madeleine, "Electronic Fetal Monitoring from a Consumer's Point of View," from a lecture given in Boston in 1978.

93. Shearer, Madeleine, "Fetal Monitoring: For Better or for Worse?" in *Compulsory Hospitalization* (n. 48, ch. 2).

94. Shearer, M.T., "Some Deterrents to Objective Evaluation of Fetal Monitors," *Birth & Family J.*, 2 (Spring 1975):58.

95. Siddiqi, Shameen, et al., "Necrotizing Fasciitis of the Scalp: A Complication of Fetal Monitoring," *Am. J. Diseases of Children*, 136 (Mar. 1982).

96. Thompson, M., & A. Cohen, "Fetal Monitoring: For Better or Worse," *Harvard Focus* (10 Dec. 1981).

97. Timor-Tritsch, I., et al., "Electronic Monitoring of the Fetal Heart Rate and Uterine Contractions during Cesarean Section under Balanced Anesthesia, *Ob. Gyn.*, 48 (Sept. 1976).

DRUGS

98. Arms, Suzanne, *Immaculate Deception* (n. 2, ch. 2).

99. Bond, Virgina, et al., "Pulmonary Aspiration Syndrome after Inhalation of Gastric Fluid Containing Antacid," *Anesthesiology*, 51 (1979):452.

100. Brackbill, Yvonne, et al., "Informed Consent and Obstetric Drugs: An Ethical Hiatus," transcript of testimony given before the Subcommittee on Science and Technology, Washington, D.C., 30 July 1981; reprinted in *NAPSAC News*, 7 (Fall 1982).

101. Brackbill, Yvonne, "Lasting Behavior Effects of Obstetric Drugs," in *Compulsory Hospitalization* (n. 48, ch. 2).

102. Brackbill, Y., "Obstetrical Medication and Infant Development," in *Handbook of Infant Development*, ed. Joy Osofsky (New York: Wiley, 1978).

103. Brewer (n. 34, ch. 8).

104. Cohen, Sheila, "Aspiration Syndromes in Pregnancy," *J. Anesthesiology*, 51 (Nov. 1979).

105. Dowie, M., & C. Marshall, "The Benedectin Cover-Up" *Mother Jones* (Nov. 1980).

106. Elkins, Valma Howe, *The Rights of the Pregnant Parent* (New York: Shocken, 1976).

107. Ericson, Avis J., *Medications Used during Labor and Birth* (Milwaukee: ICEA, 1978).

108. *FDA Drug Bulletin*, "Pregnancy Labeling," 9 (Sept. 1979).

109. Glasser, Ronald, *The Greatest Battle* (New York: Random House, 1976).

110. Goodlin, Robert, "Naloxone and Its Possible Relationship to Fetal Endorphin Levels and Fetal Distress," *Am. J. Ob. Gyn.*, 139 (1981):16.
111. Haire (n. 14, ch. 2).
112. Haire, Doris, *How the FDA Determines the "Safety" of Drugs—Just How Safe Is "Safe"?* (Washington, D.C.: National Women's Health Network, 1980).
113. Haire, Doris, "Research in Drugs Used in Pregnancy and Obstetrics," testimony presented to the Subcommittee on Investigation and Oversight of the House Committee on Science and Technology, Washington, D.C., 30 July 1981.
114. Kenepp (n. 40, this chapter).
115. Kron, R., et al., "Newborn Sucking Behavior Affected by Obstetrical Sedation," *Pediatrics*, 37 (1966):1012.
116. Lowbin, Abraham, "Organic Causes of Minimal Brain Dysfunction," *J. Am. Med. Assn.* (30 Aug. 1971).
117. Meyers, R., & S. Meyers, "Use of Sedative, Analgesic and Anesthetic Drugs during Labor and Delivery: Bane or Boon? *Am. J. Ob. Gyn.*, 133 (1979):83.
118. O'Brien, T.E., & J.A. Bulmer, "Drugs and the Human Fetus," *U.S. Pharmacist* (Mar. 1981):44.
119. Ostler, Carol Wood, "Obstetrical Premedication and Infant Outcome," *Consumers for Choices in Childbirth*, 5 (Apr. 1980).
120. Peterson (n. 37, ch. 2).
121. Petrie, Roy, et al., "The Effect of Drugs on Fetal Heart Rate Variability," *Am. J. Ob. Gyn.*, 130 (1978):294.
122. Ritchie, Susan, "Risks and Benefits of Some Common Labor Medications," *LICA [Long Island Childbirth Alternatives] Quarterly* (Fall 1979).

SECOND STAGE

123. Baldwin, Rahima, *Special Delivery*. Millbrae, Cal.: Les Femmes, 1977.
124. Banta, D., & S. Thacker, "Risks and Benefits of Episiotomy: A Review," *Birth*, 9 (Spring 1982):1.
125. "Brain Damage by Asphyxia at Birth," *Scientific American* (1969).
126. Brendsel, C., G. Peterson & L. Mehl, "Episiotomy: Facts, Figures and Alternatives," in *Compulsory Hospitalization* (n. 48, ch. 2).
127. Brewer & Greene (n. 34, ch. 8).
128. Caldeyro-Barcia, R., "The Influence of Maternal Bearing Down Efforts during Second Stage on Fetal Well-Being," *Birth & Family J.*, 6 (1979):17.
129. Cogan, R., & E. Edmonds, "The Unkindest Cut?" *Contemporary Ob. Gyn.*, 9 (1977):55; *J. of Nurse Midwifery*, 23 (1978):17.
130. Cohen, Wayne R., "Influence of Duration of Second Stage on Perinatal Outcome and Puerperal Morbidity," *Ob. Gyn.*, 49 (1977):266.
131. Daly (n. 10, ch. 8).
132. "Epidural Analgesia," *ICEA Review*, 5 (Aug. 1981).
133. Erickson, Avis, *Medications Used during Labor and Birth* (Seattle: ICEA, 1978).
134. Frankfort, Ellen, "Vaginal Politics," in Dreifus (n. 14, ch. 8).
135. Gaskin, (n. 13, ch. 2).

136. Harris, Carol, "On Avoiding Episiotomies," *H.O.M.E. Newsletter*, 4 (Summer 1979), no. 2.

137. Kitzinger, Sheila, *Some Women's Experiences of Episiotomy* (London: National Childbirth Trust).

138. Kitzinger, Sheila, *The Complete Book of Pregnancy and Childbirth* (New York: Knopf, 1980).

139. Kitzinger, Sheila, "The Rhythmic Second Stage," *Birth Center Newsletter* (Summer 1978).

140. Kloosterman (n. 11, ch. 9).

141. Maltau, J.M. & H.T. Anderson, "Epidural Anaesthesia as an Alternative to Caesarean Section in Prolonged, Exhaustive Labour," *Acta Anaesth. Scand.* (Denmark), 19 (1975):349.

142. McNeal, C., & R. McNeal, "The Neurophysiology of Letting Go," *Special Delivery Newsletter*, 3 (Spring 1980).

143. Mead, Margaret, & Niles Newton, "Cultural Patterning and Perinatal Behavior in Modern Perspectives," in *Psycho-Obstetrics*, ed. J. Howells (New York: Brunner-Mazel, 1972).

144. Mendelsohn (n. 74, ch. 5).

145. Miller, Frank, et al., "Effects of Paracervical Block on Uterine activity and Beat to Beat Variability of the Fetal Heart Rate," *Am. J. Ob. Gyn.*, 130 (1978):284.

146. Noble, Elizabeth, "Controversies in Maternal Effort during Labor and Delivery," *J. Nurse Midwifery*, 26 (Mar.-Apr. 1981):18.

147. Noble (n. 34, ch. 7).

148. Stevens, Richard, "Psychological Strategies of Pain Management in Prepared Childbirth: A Review of the Literature," *Birth & Family J.*, 3 (1977), no. 4.

149. Stewart & Stewart (n. 49, ch. 2).

150. Stewart & Stewart (n. 50, ch. 2), vol. 2.

151. Stewart, David, & Lee Stewart, eds., "Warning, Episiotomy Can Be Lethal," *NAPSAC News*, 5 (Summer 1980).

152. Sweet, Gail Grenier, "Exhale Pushing," *Mothering* (Spring 1982).

BABY'S VERY OWN INTERVENTIONS

153. Baker, Sue, "Persistent Couple Change Silver Nitrate Law," *ICEA News*, 19 (May 1980).

154. Bard, J., "Newborn Jaundice," *Childbirth Courier* (Oct.-Nov. 1972).

155. Brewer & Greene (n. 34, ch. 8).

156. Carter, N., *Routine Circumcision: The Tragic Myth* (Cal.: Noontide, 1980).

157. Cogan, R., ed., "Circumcision," *ICEA Review*, 5 (Apr. 1981).

158. Countryman, Betty Ann, *Breastfeeding and Jaundice* (Franklin Park, Ill.: La Leche League, 1978).

159. Gartner, L.M., "Jaundice and Liver Disease in the Newborn," in *Neonatal-Perinatal Medicine*, ed. Behrman (St. Louis: Mosby, 1977).

160. Gerrold, David, *Moonstar Odyssey* (New York: New American Library, 1977).

161. Graham, K., "Physiological Jaundice: What Is It?" *ICEA Sharing*, 4 (Winter 1977).

162. "Human Milk, Nutrition, and the World Resource Crisis," *Science* (May 1975).

163. Jelliffe & Jelliffe (n. 19, ch. 7).
164. McKay, S., ed., "Physiologic Jaundice of the Newborn," *ICEA*, 3 (Spring 1979).
165. Mendelsohn (n. 74, ch. 5).
166. Preston, N., "Whither the Foreskin? A Consideration of Routine Neonatal Circumcision," *J. Am. Med. Assn.*, 213 (14 Sept. 1970).
167. Pryor, Karen, *Nursing Your Baby* (New York: Pocket Books, 1973).
168. Reeder, Sharon, et al., *Maternity Nursing*, 13th ed. (Philadelphia: Lippincott; Oxford & Edinburgh: Blackwell Scientific Pubs., 1976).
169. Samuels, Mike, & Nancy Samuels, "Circumcision," *Family J.*, 2 (1982), no. 5.
170. Shulman, J., et al., "Surgical Complications of Circumcision," *Am. J. Diseases Children*, 107 (Feb. 1964).
171. "Silver Nitrate," *Federal Monitor*, 4, no. 2, p. 7.
172. Simkin, P., & M. Edwards, *When Your Baby Has Jaundice* (Seattle: Pennypress, 1979).
173. Speir, Bonnie, *Birth Whole for Optimum Health* (Berkeley: Open Eden, 1982).
174. Spezzano, Charles & Jill Waterman, "The First Day of Life," *Psychology Today* (Dec. 1977).
175. Stewart & Stewart (n. 48, ch. 2), vol. 1.
176. Stewart, D., & L. Stewart, eds., "Jaundice," *NAPSAC News*, 7 (Spring 1982).
177. *The Womanly Art of Breastfeeding* (Franklin Park, Ill.: La Leche League, 1981).
178. Topp, Sylvia, "Why Not to Circumcise Your Baby Boy," *Mothering*, 6 (1977).
179. Wallerstein, E., *Circumcision: An American Health Fallacy* (New York: Springer, 1980).
180. Whittaker, Nancy, & Judy Strasser, "The Silver Nitrate Challenge," *Mothering* (Spring 1981).
181. Whittaker, Nancy, "Neonatal Jaundice," *Mothering* (Summer 1982).
182. Wood, J., *The Circumcision Controversy* (Intact Educational Foundation, 1980).
183. *Circumcision* (a book of reprints from *Mothering*, available for $3.50 from Box 2046, Albuquerque, N.M. 87103).

AFTER THE BIRTH

184. Caplan, Frank, *The First Twelve Months of Life* (New York: Bantam, 1978).
185. Committee on Environmental Hazards, American Academy of Pediatrics, "Infant Radiant Warmers," *Pediatrics*, 61 (1978):113.
186. Fraiberg, Selma, "How a Baby Learns To Love," La Leche League Reprint no. 122 (1979).
187. Fraiberg, Selma, *Every Child's Birthright: In Defense of Mothering* (New York: Bantam, 1977).
188. Francis, Babette, "Successful Lactation and Women's Sexuality," La Leche League Reprint no. 148 (1978).
189. Jelliffe (n. 19, ch. 7).
190. Jones, Sandy, *To Love a Baby* (Boston: Houghton Mifflin, 1981).
191. Kitzinger, Sheila, "How Hospitals Disrupt Family Bonding" in *Compulsory Hospitalization* (n. 48, ch. 2), vol. 1.

192. Klaus, M., et al., "Maternal Attachment: Importance of the First Postpartum Days," *New England J. Med.*, 286 (1972):460.
193. La Leche League, *Womanly Art of Breastfeeding* (Franklin Park, Ill.: La Leche League, 1981).
194. Peterson, G., & L. Mehl, "Some Determinants of Maternal Attachment," *Am. J. Psychiatry*, 135 (Oct. 1978).
195. Pryor (n. 167, this chapter).
196. Raphael, Dana, *The Tender Gift: Breastfeeding* (Englewood, N.J.: Prentice-Hall, 1973).
197. Thevenin, Tine, *The Family Bed: An Age Old Concept in Child Bearing* (Minneapolis: Tine Thevenin, P.O. Box 16004, 1976).
198. White, Mary, & M.C. Thornton, "Together, and Nursing, from Birth," La Leche League Reprint no. 20 (1978).
199. *White Paper on Infant Feeding Practices* (Washington, D.C.: Center for Science in the Public Interest, 1974).
200. Young (n. 53, ch. 2).
201. Young, Diony, *Changing Childbirth: Family Birth in the Hospital* (Rochester, N.Y.: Childbirth Graphics, 1982).

JUDICIOUS USE OF MEDICAL INTERVENTIONS

202. Birnbaum, David, "The Iatrogenesis of Damaged Mothers and Newborns," in *21st Century Obstetrics Now!* (n. 50, ch. 2), vol. 1.
203. Ehrenreich, B., & D. English, *For Her Own Good: 150 Years of the Experts' Advice to Women* (Garden City, N.Y.: Anchor Press/Doubleday, 1979).
204. Exacto, Dr., "Memoirs of A Surgeon," *National Lampoon* (Nov. 1978).
205. Hazell (n. 17, ch. 2).
206. Kloosterman, G.J., quoted in Arms (n. 2, ch. 2).
207. Lamaze, F., quoted in Arms (n. 2, ch. 2).
208. Pfeuffer, Robbi, "The Hazards of Hospital Childbirth," *Women's Yellow Pages (New England)* (Boston: Public Works, 1978).
209. Rich, Adrienne, *Of Women Born* (New York: Norton, 1976).
210. Shaw, Nancy Stoller, *Forced Labor: Maternity Care in the United States* (New York: Pergamon, 1974).
211. Shearer, Elizabeth Connor, "Education for VBAC," *Birth & Family J.*, 9 (Spring 1982).
212. Stewart & Stewart (n. 49, ch. 2).
213. Wertz, D., & R. Wertz, *Lying In: A History of Childbirth in America* (New York: Random House, 1975).

Chapter 11 • *Labor Support*

1. Baldwin, Rahima, *Special Delivery* (Millbrae, Cal.: Les Femmes, 1977).
2. Barna, Ed, "Chant for Transition," *Mothering*, 15 (Spring 1980).

3. Bergman, Steve, "Suite Baby Dreams." Cassette tape, P.O. Box 481, Carmel Valley, Cal. 93924.
4. Bing, Elisabeth, and Libby Colman, *Making Love during Pregnancy* (New York: Bantam, 1977).
5. Davis (n. 7, ch. 9).
6. Gaskin (n. 13, ch. 2).
7. Gass, Robbie, "Welcome to the World." *Trust in Love* (Ashby, Mass.: Spring Hill Records).
8. Gawain, Shakti, *Creative Visualization* (Mill Valley, Cal.: Whatever Pub., 1978).
9. Goodman, Ellen, "Stop the Press! A Breakthrough Medical Discovery," *Boston Globe* (16 Sept. 1980).
10. Jordan, Brigette, "Studying Childbirth: The Experience and Methods of a Woman Anthropologist," in Shelly Romalis (n. 21, this chapter).
11. Kitzinger, Sheila, from her lectures on labor support, 1975–1982.
12. Korte, D., & R. Scaer, "A Survey of Maternal Preferences: What Mothers Want— Not What They Have," in *Compulsory Hospitalization* (n. 48, ch. 2), vol. 3.
13. Lederman, R., et al., "The Relationship between Psychological Variables and Specific Complications of Pregnancy, Labor, and Delivery," *J. Psychosomatic Research*, 20 (1976): 207–10.
14. Lederman, R., et al., "The Relationship of Maternal Anxiety, Plasma Cate Cholomines and Plasma Cortisol to Progress in Labor," *Am. J. Ob. Gyn.* (Nov. 1978):495–99.
15. Leigh, Janet, from her lectures on the art of labor support, 1972–82.
16. Mehl, Lewis, *Mind and Matter: Foundations for Holistic Health* (Berkeley, Cal.: Mindbody Press, 1981).
17. Peterson (n. 37, ch. 2)
18. Peterson, G., et al., "The Role of Some Birth-Related Variables in Father Attachment," *Am. J. Orthopsychiatry* (1979).
19. Peterson, G., & L. Mehl, "Some Determinants of Maternal Attachment," *Am. J. Orthopsychiatry*, 135 (Oct. 1978), no. 1.
20. Rich, Adrienne, "The Theft of Childbirth," in Dreifus (n. 14. ch. 8).
21. Romalis, Coleman, "Taking Care of the Little Woman: Father-Physician Relationships during Pregnancy and Birth," in *Childbirth: Alternatives to Medical Control*, ed. Shelly Romalis (Austin: University of Texas Press, 1981).
22. Shearer, Elizabeth, "Labor Support," *Childbirth Educator* (Fall 1981).
23. Sosa, R., J. Kennell, M. Klaus, et al., "The Effect of a Supportive Companion on Perinatal Problems, Length of Labor, and Mother-Infant Interaction," *New England J. Med.* (11 Sept. 1980):597.
24. Young & Mahan (n. 55, ch. 2).

CHILDREN AT BIRTH

25. Anderson, Sandra Van Dam, and Penny Simkin, *Birth: Through Children's Eyes* (Seattle: Pennypress, 1981).
26. Bernstein, Anne, *The Flight of the Stork* (New York: Dell, 1978).
27. Farrell, Sherrie, *Gabriel's Very First Birthday* (Seattle: Pipeline, 1976).

28. Gordon, Sol, & Judith Gordon, *Did the Sun Shine before You Were Born?* (New York: Okpaku, 1974).
29. Hathaway, Marjie, & Jay Hathaway, *Children at Birth* (Sherman Oaks, Cal.: Academy, 1978).
30. Malecki, Maryann, *Mom & Dad & I Are Having a Baby!* (Seattle: Pennypress, 1979).
31. Mehl, Lewis, C. Brendsel, & G. Peterson, "Children at Birth: Effects and Implications," *J. Sex & Marital Therapy*, 3 (Winter 1977), no. 4.

Chapter 12 • Mindscapes

1. Baldwin (n. 1, ch. 11).
2. Baldwin, Rahima, "The Neurophysiology of Letting Go," *Special Delivery Newsletter*, 3 (Spring 1980), no. 2.
3. Bing, Elisabeth, & Libby Colman, *Having a Baby after 30* (New York: Bantam, 1980).
4. Bing & Colman (n. 4, ch. 11).
5. Colman, Arthur D., & Libby Colman, *Pregnancy: The Psychological Experience* (New York: Seabury, 1973).
6. Courter, Gay, *The Midwife* (Houghton-Mifflin, 1981).
7. Crandon, A. J., "Maternal Anxiety and Obstetric Complications," *J. Psychosomatic Research*, 23 (1979):109–11.
8. Davis, Elizabeth, "Energy Cycles in Pregnancy and Childbirth," *Yoga J.*, 32 (May-June 1980)
9. Deutsch (n. 7, ch. 4).
10. Dworken, Andrea, *Pornography: Men Possessing Women* (New York: G.P. Putnam's Sons, Perigree Books, 1981), pp. 217–18.
11. Erickson, Marilyn T., "The Relationship between Psychological Variables and Specific Complications of Pregnancy, Labor, and Delivery," *J. Psychosomatic Research*, 20 (1976): 207–10.
12. Francis, Babette, "Successful Lactation and Women's Sexuality," La Leche League reprint no. 148 (Franklin Park, Ill.: La Leche League, 1978).
13. Fraiberg, Selma, "How a Baby Learns To Love," La Leche League reprint no. 122 (Franklin Park, Ill.: La Leche League, 1979).
14. Gallagher, S.J., *Love Is a Couple* (New York: William Sadlier, 1976).
15. Gallagher, S. J., *Parents Are Lovers* (New York: William Sadlier, 1972).
16. Gaskin, Ina May, "Ask the Midwives," *Practicing Midwife*, 1 (Fall 1981), no. 14.
17. Gaskin (n. 13, ch. 2).
18. Gass, Robbie, "I Honor You." *Trust in Love* (Ashby, Mass.: Spring Hill Music, 1981).
19. Gunther, Bernard, *Sense Relaxation: Below Your Mind* (Toronto & London: Macmillan, Collier, 1968).
20. Hammer, Signe, *Daughters and Mothers, Mothers and Daughters* (New York: New York Times Book Co., 1975).

21. Harrison, Michelle, "Birth as the First Experience of Mothering," in *21st Century Obstetrics Now!* (n. 50, ch. 2).
22. Hazell, Lester, "Spiritual and Ethical Aspects of Birth: Who Bears the Ultimate Responsibility?" in *21st Century Obstetrics Now!* (n. 50, ch. 2), vol. 1.
23. Hazell (n. 17, ch. 2).
24. Jones, Terry, *Also of Men Born! The Importance of the Pregnant Male* (Milwaukee: ICEA, 1980).
25. Lear, Martha Weinman, *Heartsounds* (New York: Simon & Schuster, 1980).
26. MacDonald, Paula & Dick MacDonald, *Loving Free* (New York: Ballantine, 1973).
27. MacKay, Susan, ed. "Maternal Stress and Pregnancy Outcome," *ICEA Review*, 4 (April 1980), No. 1.
28. Mehl, Lewis, "The Importance of Belief in the Childbirth Process," paper presented at the Annual NAPSAC Conference, Nashville, Tenn., July 1979.
29. Mehl, L., G. H. Peterson, & C. Brendsel, "Psychophysiological Aspects of Birth: Childbirth as Psychotherapy," paper presented at the American Psychiatry Association 1977.
30. Mehl, Lewis, *Mind and Matter: Foundations for Holistic Health* (Berkeley, Cal.: Mindbody Press, 1981).
31. Michaelson, Peter, "Befriending Our Bodies," *Simple Times*, 2 (Winter 1982), no. 1.
32. Montague (n. 31, ch. 2).
33. Newton, Niles, "The Effect of Fear and Disturbances on Labor," in *21st Century Obstetrics Now!* (n. 50, ch. 2), vol. 1.
34. Newton, Niles, *Maternal Emotions* (New York: Paul B. Hoeber, Harper & Bros., 1955).
35. Newton, R.W., et al., "Psychosocial Stress in Pregnancy and Its Relation to the Onset of Premature Labor," *British Med. J.*, 2 (Aug. 1979):411–13.
36. Panuthos, C., *Positive Birthing* (S. Hadley, Mass.: J. F. Bergin, in press.)
37. Peterson, G., et al., "Effects of Childbirth upon Women's Self-Esteem," paper presented at the 13th annual meeting of the American Psychological Association, Toronto, 5 May 1976.
38. Peterson, G., & L. Mehl, "Some Determinants of Maternal Attachment," *Am. J. Psychiatry*, 135 (Oct. 1978), no. 10.
39. Peterson, et al., "The Role of Some Birth-Related Variables in Father Attachment," *Am. J. Orthopsychiatry*, 49 (Apr. 1979), no. 2.
40. Peterson (n. 37, ch. 2).
41. Ray, Sondra, *The Only Diet There Is* (Millbrae, Cal.: Celestial Arts, 1981).
42. Romalis, Coleman (n. 21, ch. 11).
43. Romalis, Shelly (n. 21, ch. 11).
44. Schwartz, Leni, *The World of the Unborn* (New York: Richard Marek, 1980).
45. Simonton, C. O., et al., *Getting Well Again* (New York: Bantam, 1978).
46. Stevens, Richard, "Psychological Strategies of Pain Management in Prepared Childbirth," *Birth & Family J.*, 3 (1977), no. 4.
47. Uddenberg, N., et al., "Reproductive Conflicts: Mental Symptoms during Pregnancy and Time in Labor," *J. Psychosomatic Research*, 20 (1976): 575–81.
48. Wessel, Helen, *Under the Apple Tree* (Fresno, Cal.: Bookmates, 1981).

49. Wood, Robert, *How Do You Feel? A Guide to Your Emotions* (Englewood Cliffs, N.J.: Prentice-Hall, 1974).

Chapter 13 • Planning Your Birth

1. Arms (n. 2, ch. 2).
2. Barry, Cathleen, "The Cutting Edge: A Look at Male Motivation and Gynecology," in *The Women's Health Movement*, ed. Sheryl Ruzek (New York: Praeger, 1972).
3. Bean (n. 2, ch. 6).
4. Bean, Constance, *Methods of Childbirth* (New York: Dolphin, 1974).
5. Beck, Neils, & David Hall, "Natural Childbirth: A Review and Analysis," *Ob. Gyn.*, 52 (Sept. 1978):371.
6. Codman, Ernest, *New England J. Med.* (13 Feb. 1941).
7. Corbin, David, "High Risk Sex," *New Age*, 5 (Apr. 1980), no. 10.
8. Corea (n. 9, ch. 2).
9. Corea (n. 9, ch. 8).
10. Drummond, Hugh, "Playing Doctor: The Trick Is Impersonating God," *Mother Jones* (July 1980).
11. Ehrenreich, Barbara, & Deirdre English, *Witches, Midwives, and Nurses: A History of Woman Healers* (New York: Feminist Press, 1973).
12. Elkins (n. 3, ch. 8).
13. Ettner, F., "Hospital Obstetrics: Do the Benefits Outweigh the Risks?" in *21st Century Obstetrics Now!* (n. 50, ch. 2), vol. 1.
14. Gawain (n. 8, ch. 11).
15. Goodman (n. 9, ch. 11).
16. Gordon, R.E., & K. Gordon, "Some Social-Psychiatric Aspects of Pregnancy and Childbearing," *J. Med. Soc. New Jersey*, (1954):569–72.
17. Harrison (n. 15, ch. 2).
18. Hartman, Rhondda, "How a Childbirth Educator Brings about Change," in *Compulsory Hospitalization* (n. 48, ch. 2), vol. 3.
19. Hesselden, Gatha, "Dealing with Hospitals: A Patient's Perspective," *Medical Self-Care* (Summer 1980).
20. Jordan, Brigette, "Studying Childbirth: The Experience and Methods of a Woman Anthropologist," in Shelly Romalis (n. 21, ch. 11).
21. Kitzinger, Sheila, *Education and Counselling for Childbirth* (London: Cassell & Collier Macmillan, 1977).
22. Kitzinger, Sheila, paper on episiotomy presented in Boston, October 1981.
23. Korte, D., & R. Scaer, "A Survey of Maternal Preferences: What Mothers Want— Not What They Have," in *Compulsory Hospitalization* (n. 48, ch. 2), vol. 3.
24. LeBaron, Charles, *Gentle Vengeance: An Account of the First Year at Harvard Medical School* (New York: Richard Marek, 1981).
25. Makepeace, Emily, "This Is to You, Dr. Ratceller," *Syracuse Advocate*, 3 (1982), no. 2.
26. Marieskind (n. 57, ch. 8).

27. Mazzarella, Pat, "Survey: Why Patients Switch Doctors," *Medical Dimensions* (Dec. 1975).
28. Mehl, L., et al., "Child at Birth: Effects and Implications," *J. Sex & Marital Therapy*, 3 (Winter 1977), no. 4.
29. Melzack, R., et al., "Labor Is Still Painful after Prepared Childbirth Training," *Canadian Med. Assn. J.*, 125 (15 Aug. 1982):357.
30. Mendelsohn, Robert S., *Confessions of a Medical Heretic* (Chicago: Contemporary Books, 1979).
31. Mendelsohn, R., "How To Survive Medical Training without Being Dehumanized," in *21st Century Obstetrics Now!* (n. 50, ch. 2).
32. Mendelsohn (n. 74, ch. 5).
33. Moran, Marilyn, *Birth and the Dialogue of Love* (Leawood, Kan.: New Nativity Press, 1981).
34. *New Nativity Newsletter*, P.O. Box 6223, Leawood, Kan. 66206.
35. *Our Bodies, Ourselves*, Boston Women's Health Book Collective (New York: Simon & Schuster, 1971).
36. Peterson (n. 37, ch. 2).
37. Ratner, Herbert, "History of the Dehumanization of American Obstetrics," in *21st Century Obstetrics Now!* (n. 50, ch. 2).
38. Rich, Adrienne, "The Theft of Childbirth," in Dreifus (n. 14, ch. 8).
39. Romalis, Coleman (n. 21, ch. 11).
40. Romalis, Shelly, "Natural Childbirth and the Reluctant Physician," in Shelly Romalis (n. 21, ch. 11).
41. Rothman, Barbara Katz, "Awake and Aware: On False Consciousness," in Shelly Romalis (n. 21, ch. 11).
42. Scully, Diana, *Men Who Control Women's Health: The Miseducation of Obstetricians and Gynecologists* (Boston: Houghton Mifflin, 1980).
43. Shearer, Elizabeth, "Labor Support," *Childbirth Educator* (Fall 1981).
44. Weiss, Kay, "What Medical Students Learn about Women," in Dreifus (n. 14, ch. 8).
45. Wertz, Dorothy, *Living In: A History of Childbirth in America* (New York: Random House, 1975).
46. Young, Diony, *Changing Childbirth: Family Birth in the Hospital* (Rochester, N.Y.: Childbirth Graphics, Ltd., 1900).
47. Young & Mahan (n. 55, ch. 2).

BREECH

48. Bird, C., & T. McElin, "A 6 Year Perspective Study of Term Breech Deliveries Utilizing the Zatuchni-Andros Prognostic Scoring Index," *Am. J. Ob. Gyn.*, 121 (15 Feb. 1975):552.
49. Ettner (n. 13, this chapter).
50. Gaskin (n. 13, ch. 2).
51. Johnson, E., "Breech Presentation at Term," *Am. J. Ob. Gyn.*, 106 (1970):865.
52. Long, Phyllis, "More Comments on the Delivery of the Breech Baby," *Practicing Midwife*, 2 (Fall 1981), no. 14.

53. Nyles, Margaret, *Textbook for Midwives* (New York: Churchill Livingstone, 1975).
54. Pritchard & MacDonald (n. 41, ch. 2).
55. Ranney, B., "The Gentle Art of External Cephalic Version," *Am. J. Ob. Gyn.*, 116 (193):239.
56. Semchyshyn, S., "Letter to Editor," *Am. J. Ob. Gyn.*, 139 (1 Mar. 1981), no. 5.
57. Souza, Desa, "Postural Exercise Turns Fetus in Breech Position," *Ob. Gyn. News*, 12 (1 Jan. 1977), no. 1.
58. Ylikorkals, O., and A. Hartikainen-Sorri, "Value of External Version in Fetal Malpresentation in Combination with Use of Ultrasound," *Acta Ob. Gyn. Scand.*, 56 (1977):63.

HERPES

59. Gaskin (n. 13, ch. 2).
60. Gunn, Terri, & Mary Stenzel-Poore, *Herpes Handbook* (Portland, Ore.: Venereal Disease Action Council, 1981).
61. Frye, Ann, *National Midwives Assn. Newsletter* (Feb.-Mar. 1979).
62. "Herpes," a bibliography available through the Council for Cesarean Awareness, 5520 S.W. 92nd Ave., Miami, Fla. 33165.
63. Kellerhouse K., & C. Esparza, "Herpes Simplex II," *Mothering* (Winter 1981).
64. Kilbrick, Sidney, "Herpes Simplex Infection at Term," *J. Am. Med. Assn.* 243 (11 Jan. 1980).
65. Marieskind (n. 57, ch. 8).
66. Mitchell, Tom, *You Are Not Alone with Herpes* (Novelty, O.: Skylight, 1980).
67. Richards, Lynn Browne, "Herpes and Cesarean Delivery" (unpublished manuscript, 1981).

Chapter 14 • In Case a Cesarean Is Necessary

1. Cane, Aleta, & Beth Shearer, *Frankly Speaking: A Pamphlet for Cesarean Couples*, 2d ed. (Framingham, Mass.: C/SEC, 1978).
2. Cohen, Nancy, "Minimizing Emotional Sequellae of Cesarean Childbirth," *Birth & Family J.*, 4 (1977), no. 3.
3. C/SEC, *Survey of Hospital Policies & Services for Obstetrical Care* (Framingham, Mass.: C/SEC, 1978).
4. C/SEC, Inc., "Options for Cesarean Childbirth," *C/SEC News*, 5 (1979), no. 2.
5. Enkin, Murray W., "Having a Section Is Having a Baby," *Birth & Family J.*, 4 (1977), no. 3.
6. Hausknecht, Richard, & Joan Heilman, *Having a Cesarean Baby* (New York: Dutton, 1978).
7. Leboyer, Frederick, *Loving Hands* (New York: Knopf, 1976).
8. Marieskind (n. 57, ch. 8).
9. McClellan & Cabianca, "Effects of Early Mother-Infant Contact following Cesarean Birth," *Ob. Gyn.*, 56 (July 1980), no. 1.

10. Meyer, Linda, *Cesarean (R)Evolution*, rev. ed. (Edmonds, Wash.: Chas. Franklin Press. 1981).
11. Montague (n. 31, ch. 2).
12. National Institutes of Health, *Cesarean Childbirth: Final Report of the Consensus Development Conference* (Bethesda, Md.: NIH Office of Research and Reporting, 1981).
13. Shearer, Beth, "NIH Consensus Development Task Force on Cesarean Childbirth: The Process and the Result," *Birth & Family J.*, 8 (1981); no. 1.
14. Schneider, Vimala, *Infant Massage: A Handbook for Loving Parents* (New York: Bantam, 1982).
15. Shulman, Norma, *Labor and Delivery after Cesarean Birth: A Survey of Contemporary Opinion* (Framingham, Mass.: C/SEC, 1978).
16. Worzer, Linda, "Rights of the Cesarean Infant," *C/SEC News*, 5 (1979), no. 1.
17. Young (n. 53, ch. 2).
18. Young & Mahan (n. 55, ch. 2).

❧ About the Contributors

Jini Duffy Fairley, who contributed the material in Chapter 14, cofounded the organization C/SEC, Inc. She has spoken at childbirth conferences all over the United States and Canada. Ms. Fairley has been a La Leche League leader since 1974 and cofounded the first La Leche League group in France. From 1977 to 1980 she served as area coordinator of leaders for La Leche League for eleven European countries. Jini's first child was born by cesarean section, her second child was born vaginally in a hospital in France, and her third child was born at home. Jini, her husband, Michael, and their children, Kevin, Jessica, and Brian, reside in Massachusetts.

Andrew Osborne, who assisted with the section on Informed Consent, in Chapter 8, is a Boston attorney.

Jami Osborne, who assisted with the research, is a VBAC childbirth educator in Boston.

Claudia Panuthos, who assisted substantially in the preparation of Chapter 4, is a licensed independent clinical social worker and founder and director of The People Place, a nonprofit, nontraditional family counseling center. She has been a psychotherapist, consultant, and social service administrator for the past fourteen years. She has authored several articles and books, including *The Emotional Ups and Downs of Childbirth*, *Enlightened Parenthood*, and *Ended Beginnings: Grieving and Healing Pregnancy and Childbearing Loss*. Claudia has lectured throughout the United States and Canada on the emotional aspects of the birthing process. Her training includes transactional analysis and gestalt, bioenergetics, psychodrama, neurolinguistics programing, rebirthings, and other body-mind therapies. Another of her books, *Positive Birthing*, (Boston, Mass.: People Place Press, in press), was written out of her desire to communicate emotional aspects of pregnancy and birth. Claudia is the founder and director of *Offspring*, a national childbirth-education training center and community-based model for counseling and positive birthing.

Catherine Bemis Romeo, who assisted with the research and with the sections on Ultrasound, in Chapter 8, and Siblings at the Birth, in Chapter 11, is a certified childbirth educator and staff therapist at *Offspring*.

᣶ *Index*

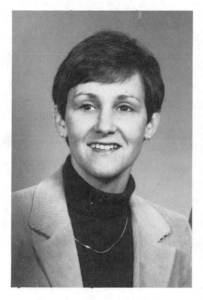 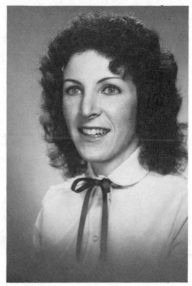

NANCY WAINER COHEN   LOIS J. ESTNER

Nancy Wainer Cohen co-founded C/SEC, INC., the first and now the largest cesarean organization in the country, in 1973, and is a consultant and advisor to the Cesarean Prevention Movement. She is the leading authority on VBAC and has counseled thousands of women on the subject since 1972. Her many articles have dealt with VBAC, cesarean prevention, and positive birthing. Her personal birthing history includes a cesarean delivery for her first child, a vaginal birth in the hospital for her second child, and a vaginal birth at home for her third.

Lois J. Estner, formerly an English teacher, is a VBAC mother, La Leche League leader, and counselor on the topics of breastfeeding, childbirth, and cesarean prevention.

Typography and design by Jeanne Ray Juster
Edited by Jenna Schulman
Set in VIP Electra by Trade Composition Inc., Chicopee, Massachusetts
Printed and bound by Malloy Lithographing, Inc., Ann Arbor, Michigan

---

Paperback cover design by Patricia Greene
Cover photos (left) Suzanne Arms, (right) Edward T. Bissell